W9-DDA-304

Eve Kushner

Experiencing Abortion

A Weaving of Women's Words

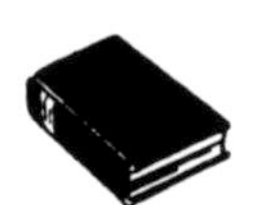

Pre-publication
REVIEWS,
COMMENTARIES,
EVALUATIONS . . .

"Eve Kushner has methodically given a voice to many women for whom abortion has been an invisible experience. Her book is rich in sorting out and describing the complexities of this experience. It reminds us that an abortion is not just a biological severing of a fetus from a woman's womb, but it is also a psychological experience deep with personal meanings. At a conscious or unconscious level it may represent the severing of a potential mother-infant relationship."

Sandra Gómez, PhD, MFCC
Psychotherapist in private practice,
Fremont, CA

"In many respects, the most important debate on abortion is not taking place on television or even in the heated battles of our country's legislative chambers. This is the debate that takes place every day in the minds and hearts of thousands of women who face the dilemma of an unintended pregnancy. *Experiencing Abortion: A Weaving of Women's Words* puts us in touch with women who have had abortions. We hear what they think and feel about their decision and how they have made sense of their experience. Beautifully written and very insightful, Eve Cushner's book is an excellent and sorely needed resource. I will recommend it to both my clients and my colleagues."

Kim Kluger-Bell, MA
Psychotherapist in private practice,
Berkeley, CA

More pre-publication
REVIEWS, COMMENTARIES, EVALUATIONS . . .

"Eve Kushner compassionately and insightfully orchestrates a rich chorus of women's voices in a groundbreaking experiential study of abortion. She takes us beyond political and ethical judgments into the raw realities of this complex life event. Diverse women describe the unexpected emotional impacts of abortion on their lives. They tell us how they worked with these issues and what they learned, in the process, about themselves, loved ones, and society. Kushner shows us the healing and empowering that can come from women facing their experience, understanding it, and sharing it with others. This is a wonderful resource book for women experiencing abortion, for the people who love them, and for the professionals and paraprofessionals working with them."

Carol S. Becker, PhD
Professor of Human Development, California State University, Hayward; Licensed Psychologist, private practice in psychotherapy, Oakland, CA

"Even as a very experienced psychotherapist, I gained many new insights about abortion from Kushner's wise, compassionate, and comprehensive book. Although she speaks directly to women, *Experiencing Abortion* will have immense value for educators and clergy, as well as health clinicians and policy makers."

Audrey T. McCollum, MSW
Psychotherapist in private practice, Etna, NH; Author, *The Chronically Ill Child: A Guide for Parents and Professionals*

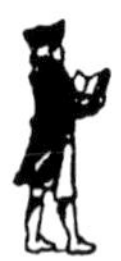

The Harrington Park Press
An Imprint of The Haworth Press, Inc.

NOTES FOR PROFESSIONAL LIBRARIANS AND LIBRARY USERS

This is an original book title published by Harrington Park Press, an imprint of The Haworth Press, Inc. Unless otherwise noted in specific chapters with attribution, materials in this bock have not been previously published elsewhere in any format or language.

CONSERVATION AND PRESERVATION NOTES

All books published by The Haworth Press, Inc. and its imprints are printed on certified ph neutral, acid free book grade paper. This paper meets the minimum requirements of American National Standard for Information Sciences–Permanence of Paper for Printed Material, ANSI Z39.48-1984.

Experiencing Abortion
A Weaving of Women's Words

HAWORTH Innovations in Feminist Studies
Esther Rothblum, PhD and Ellen Cole, PhD
Senior Co-Editors

New, Recent, and Forthcoming Titles:

When Husbands Come Out of the Closet by Jean Schaar Gochros

Prisoners of Ritual: An Odyssey into Female Genital Circumcision in Africa by Hanny Lightfoot-Klein

Foundations for a Feminist Restructuring of the Academic Disciplines edited by Michele Paludi and Gertrude A. Steuernagel

Hippocrates' Handmaidens: Women Married to Physicians by Esther Nitzberg

Waiting: A Diary of Loss and Hope in Pregnancy by Ellen Judith Reich

God's Country: A Case Against Theocracy by Sandy Rapp

Women and Aging: Celebrating Ourselves by Ruth Raymond Thone

Women's Conflicts About Eating and Sexuality: The Relationship Between Food and Sex by Rosalyn M. Meadow and Lillie Weiss

A Woman's Odyssey into Africa: Tracks Across a Life by Hanny Lightfoot-Klein

Anorexia Nervosa and Recovery: A Hunger for Meaning by Karen Way

Women Murdered by the Men They Loved by Constance A. Bean

Reproductive Hazards in the Workplace: Mending Jobs, Managing Pregnancies by Regina Kenen

Our Choices: Women's Personal Decisions About Abortion by Sumi Hoshiko

Tending Inner Gardens: The Healing Art of Feminist Psychotherapy by Lesley Irene Shore

The Way of the Woman Writer by Janet Lynn Roseman

Racism in the Lives of Women: Testimony, Theory, and Guides to Anti-Racist Practice by Jeanne Adleman and Gloria Enguídanos

Advocating for Self: Women's Decisions Concerning Contraception by Peggy Matteson

Feminist Visions of Gender Similarities and Differences by Meredith M. Kimball

Experiencing Abortion: A Weaving of Women's Words by Eve Kushner

Experiencing Abortion
A Weaving of Women's Words

Eve Kushner

Harrington Park Press
An Imprint of The Haworth Press, Inc.
New York • London

Published by

Harrington Park Press, an imprint of The Haworth Press, Inc., 10 Alice Street, Binghamton, NY 13904-1580.

Cover designed by Donna M. Brooks.

Library of Congress Cataloging-in-Publication Data

Kushner, Eve
Experiencing abortion: a weaving of women's words / Eve Kushner.
p. cm.
Includes index.
ISBN 1-56023-902-6 (alk. paper)
1. Abortion–Psychological aspects–Case studies. I. Title.
HQ767.K87 1997
363.4′6–dc20

96-44691
CIP

For Haroon and Crosby

ABOUT THE AUTHOR

Eve Kushner is the President and Founder of Spruced Up Manuscripts, a one-person editing and writing company. Ms. Kushner freelance edits for several book publishers, including Jossey-Bass Publishers; Franklin, Beedle and Associates; and the University of California Press. A writer of personal essays and stories, she has published letters to the editors of several papers, primarily on reproductive issues. In January 1996, *The New York Times* published a letter she wrote about egg donations and, in May 1995, *The San Francisco Chronicle* published her letter on psychological reasons for unplanned pregnancies. Her own unplanned pregnancy opened her eyes to the vast range of issues surrounding unplanned pregnancies and abortion. This led her to undertake five years of research on the topic and interview 115 women who have had abortions.

CONTENTS

Foreword

The voices in this book are familiar, though I have not met these particular women. Their words echo those of the hundreds of women who have come through my door, grappling with an unplanned pregnancy and abortion. For thirteen years, at a Planned Parenthood clinic and in my private psychotherapy practice, I have helped women through all stages of this often difficult experience: the decision making, the surgery, and the period after an abortion. I have seen a wide range of reactions, from relief and fairly calm acceptance, to sadness and confusion, to guilt and suicidal depression. Over the years, I have become increasingly aware of abortion's complexity and the inadequacy of simple formulations.

As I read *Experiencing Abortion*, I was struck by the accuracy with which Eve has captured this complexity. On page after page, I wrote exclamation points in margins as I read words that I have heard women say time and time again. I added more exclamation points and wrote "Yes!" many times as I read Eve's sensitive comments, interpretations, and weaving together of these women's stories. She says about abortion what I have been saying for years, and she has expressed these thoughts in an extremely helpful, accessible way.

Experiencing Abortion is a welcome addition to the scarce literature about the ways in which women cope with abortion. Over the years, I have looked for just such a book to recommend to my clients and colleagues. Many other books that address the emotional impact of abortion offer individual women's stories. While some of my clients have found these books useful, others have found such stories too far removed from their own experiences and could not always identify with these accounts. *Experiencing Abortion* looks closely at each aspect of the abortion experience, offering a map that can help a reader manage overwhelming feelings. At the same time, the book includes a wide variety of examples of how different women have experienced abortion. A reader is likely to find someone with whom she can identify, to see her feelings as valid, and to feel less alone. In this way, *Experiencing Abortion* captures both the uniqueness of each woman's experience and the commonality of our collective experience of abortion.

Another strength of *Experiencing Abortion* is its specific focus on the aftereffects of abortion. Often, women feel the full emotional impact of an abortion only after the procedure. And yet, the period following abortion has been the least addressed by those who offer abortion services and counseling. Many clinics and doctor's offices provide decision-making counseling, as well as counseling on the day of an abortion. Almost none offer postabortion counseling. Much literature available to women and to those who counsel them addresses the decision-making process and how to prepare for an abortion, with little attention to the impact this decision may continue to have on a woman's life. *Experiencing Abortion* focuses on this neglected area and highlights its importance.

I believe it is for political reasons that those of us who support a woman's right to choose have been reluctant to acknowledge that emotional turmoil can both accompany and follow an abortion. In the face of the ongoing controversy over abortion and the real threat of losing the right to choose, it may seem like a luxury to address women's feelings about their abortions. And yet, in reality, many women's experiences take place within the gray area between the two polarized views about abortion. Therapists, health workers, and the women's community can best support women who choose abortion by remaining sensitive to this reality. If we are truly to understand women's experiences of abortion, Eve's insights–and the insights of all the women in this book–urgently need to be heard.

Experiencing Abortion has a nonjudgmental tone. It is at times hard to refrain from judging women who have abortions when we do not consider the complexity of their circumstances. I remember a woman I counseled at Planned Parenthood. She had three abortions in two years, but chose to keep using the rhythm method. I recall feeling puzzled by her insistence on an obviously ineffective method. A year later, she came to my private office for psychotherapy; she wanted help in leaving her battering husband. It was he who had forbidden her to use any other form of birth control. Her situation brought home to me the importance of knowing the full context in which women make reproductive choices. *Experiencing Abortion* reminds us all to remain compassionate in our response to abortion.

Kathy Anolick, MS, MFCC

Preface

The psychiatrists left me alone in the examining room. I sat on the corner of a bench, my knees hugged to my chest. There was nothing to focus on but a big mirror that stretched across one side of the room. Why was there a mirror when I looked so wretched? I had been crying hard. That's how I had ended up in the emergency room. As I thought about everything that had brought me to this place, I became upset again. The doctors returned eventually, asking, "How are you feeling?" "Better," I said. "I cried a little while you were out." "We know," they said. The mirror was two-way. The whole time, I was under observation.

When I first arrived in the emergency room, three men trooped in to interview me. They said they were interns and needed to observe me as a team. I kicked two of them out, explaining that I couldn't talk to men since the abortion and that I couldn't share intimate details with three at once. I figured as long as I was a psychiatric case, I could act as irrationally as I wanted. Two complied and left. Ten minutes later, they returned, saying the sound wasn't good. Would I mind repeating everything I had just said? I looked up near the ceiling to see a black camera pointed in my direction. Grudgingly, I allowed the men to stay and the exam continued. "Please recite the six most recent presidents backward." "Spell your name backward." "Do you have any suicidal tendencies?" I said I kept visualizing slashing my wrist, but that I would never act on it. They weren't so sure and contemplated keeping me overnight. Occasionally, all three men left the room for long periods. They returned and resumed the questioning, much of it repetitive. "Do you feel guilty about the abortion?" I began to explain why I didn't, but they cut me off. "Answer the question. Yes or no. Do you feel guilty about the abortion?"

It dawned on me then how little they understood. These doctors seemed to be relying on clichés they had heard about abortion's effects. It was as if they had never heard a real woman say how she felt about her abortion. Perhaps if I explained my feelings, they would see how wrong their preconceptions were. I spilled out my story bit by bit. They gave their best shot at empathizing. "Well, I think that just sucks, what you've been through," said one, his voice dripping with condescension. I shot him a warning glance and the leader of the three interns told him to knock it off. My best attempts to express myself were reaching deaf ears.

Then again, maybe my feelings were just too strange and complex for anyone to understand. I didn't have any context for them myself. I had coasted through the days before the abortion feeling little pain and, in fact, much happiness and joy. I delighted in certain aspects of my pregnancy and felt very much in love with my boyfriend, Haroon. He had been my companion from the start of this strange journey through pregnancy. It had, in fact, been the defining experience of our short relationship. We were housemates in a condominium close to Dartmouth College, where I was finishing up my senior year, and he was a graduate student. We fell in love quickly, and I moved into his room. Though we always used birth control, I conceived one of the first four times we had sex. It was a month into our relationship and suddenly we were living together and I was pregnant.

The abortion proceeded without many problems, although I ended up in another emergency room that night, vomiting violently for no apparent reason. Emotionally, I felt fine. My clinic had told me to expect mild depression over the next ten days as my hormones changed, but that night and all that week I felt nothing. Of course, I was quite busy, moving to a new apartment, preparing for a month-long publishing program in Denver, and spending time with Haroon before going to the program. As each day passed and proved to be depression-free, I felt relieved. I would be spared the predicted pain.

As soon as I settled into my seat on the plane for Denver, everything changed. I stared at Haroon as he waved to me from the airport, and I felt like we had been ripped apart. He had been through the whole abortion experience with me and now I was flying halfway across the country to a place where no one knew my secrets. I was shocked at the waves of emotion passing through me. I thought I had felt so little because I was clear about wanting an abortion. I now realized that the emotions had been there all along, only I hadn't let them come forward. How could I go to Denver feeling like this? Students come to the program not only to learn about publishing but also to land jobs in fancy publishing houses. I had just graduated summa cum laude from an Ivy League school and didn't feel I could apply for a janitorial job.

In Denver, I had nothing to say to anybody and withdrew into my own private hell. In the bathroom between lectures, I could hear young women laughing by the sinks while I, alone in my stall, changed the bulky, stained pads that I wore as my uterus discharged blood. These women seemed so childish, preoccupied with drinking and meeting men. All I wanted was a meaningful conversation, preferably about what I had been through.

I tried to tell a pregnant woman once, thinking she would understand. We were in the gym, showering after a swim, and I kept staring at her enormous belly. I had never seen a woman naked when she was six months along. As she smoothed moisturizer onto her abdomen, I mentioned that I had been pregnant last month, but that I had lost the pregnancy. She didn't really respond. We talked instead about the changes she was expecting and it hit me that the fruit of her pregnancy was yet to come. Pregnancy wasn't what we had in common; it was only a vehicle that took us to different destinations.

Whom could I talk to, then, about my experience? I wanted to know if I were going crazy, if I would always feel so fragile and volatile, flailing around in the storm of my emotions. One moment I felt furious–at life's unfairness, at doctors, or at anybody who rubbed me the wrong way. The next minute, I was overcome by loss. At the same time, I didn't feel entitled to grieve and didn't understand why I should want to, since I didn't regret my choice. All I knew was that my world had turned upside down and that I couldn't get back to the way I used to feel.

One day I snapped. It started in the bathroom. After the abortion, I had bled for three weeks. A few days after it stopped, I got my period. That day, we were assigned a 500-page novel to read by the following week. Then we got back a homework assignment. Mine had a bad grade and a rude comment. I had thought schoolwork was the one thing I could still do well. The next day, the directors held a meeting to air our gripes about this assignment. I worked up the courage to say something, but was interrupted by a student with frizzy hair. She told me I better get used to the way employers are going to treat me and that this was the real world and did I expect to be pampered all my life?

I said nothing in self-defense, feeling my face get hotter and hotter. When she finished, I ran to the bathroom and let out gasps and splutters and tears. I knew this was an inappropriate place for an outburst, but once I started, I couldn't stop. Finally, seeing myself in such bad shape, I decided to stop hiding in the bathroom like a criminal.

When the meeting ended, I asked the directors if I could speak to them. They made room for me between them on the couch. I launched into my story and began to sob. I didn't care that I was drawing so much attention to myself. I was uncorking my secret and someone was listening. The directors felt I needed a therapist. But it was six at night. Who was available? They decided that the only recourse was the emergency room, where I could see a psychiatrist. I consented, but was scared. Had my life come to this?

* * *

About thirty million abortions have been performed since the procedure became legal in 1973, and countless more occurred before then. Yet somehow, we usually can't find each other when we go through this experience. A taboo on abortion prevents us from discussing it on a personal level. There seems to be no socially acceptable way to come forward and share our stories, to reassure each other that whatever we feel is normal.

I have written *Experiencing Abortion* to help remedy that situation. In this book, women who have gone through abortions reach out to those for whom the experience is new. In a place free of ideological pressure, women say what's really on their minds.

This book is primarily for women who have had abortions. The reader who wants answers quickly can turn right to a pertinent chapter, reading the others in any order. Those who are thinking about ending a pregnancy can also read it to understand the feelings that follow abortion; they might find the Epilogue the most helpful in making their decision or preparing for an abortion. This book should help anyone who wants to know more about how it feels to go through an abortion. Women's lovers, friends, family, clinic workers, and counselors will gain insights into what women feel and need after their abortions.

Experiencing Abortion should help the reader make sense of her own experience. Each chapter tackles a different emotional issue that can arise after an abortion. Within each chapter I tell several stories, each showing a new angle on the chapter's topic. I weave explanations into the stories. The combination of the stories and my text helps the reader gain insights into her experience on both emotional and analytical levels. She can identify with at least some of these women, which will make her feel less alone and perhaps more compassionate with herself. She will also begin to see why she feels and acts as she does.

Those who read this book in search of absolutes ("Abortion makes all women feel the following way. . . .") will not find such definitive statements. It is much more valuable to look at the experience from the inside, with all the specificity and thus the universality that an individual voice can lend to such a discussion, than to examine it from a distance, making general statements that are so vague as to be meaningless. Readers may wonder why I have let women make all the points, rather than interviewing therapists and quoting from books. While I did have a therapist (Kathy Anolick) read the book and help me understand the material better, I feel that the women who have abortions are the real experts on the subject. Those who stand outside the experience, armed with theories, don't know how it feels, any more than the psychiatrists I met in the emergency room.

Experiencing Abortion benefits from a diversity of collected experiences. The 115 women who helped create it range in age from 17 to 75, though many are in their twenties, as is typical nationally for women who have abortions. They come from several races and religions, as well as different education levels and economic statuses. Even the format of their submissions varies; some wrote down their feelings, while others let me tape their responses in a free-form interview. (In all cases, their names have been changed, as have the names of the people they mentioned.) Despite these differences, the cocreators of this book are of like mind on one issue: they want to help other women who might be in the same position they were in just months or even years ago. Almost all of them mention how isolated they felt when they had abortions.

Why is there such widespread isolation? Many times, the people around us simply can't provide what we need after an abortion. They may send flowers, help us make a decision, and accompany us to the procedure. But they cannot always be there, and we may feel uncomfortable asking that of them. The topic may seem so heavy that we worry about burdening our listeners. Even if they can bear the weight of the topic, they may fail to understand our feelings, especially the less straightforward ones.

Take my friend Jane. We had grown close in college, though she was on the debate team and wanted to turn everything into an argument. When I explained my abortion feelings to her, she was in law school, where her passion for logic and rationality had increased. Jane puzzled over why I was depressed after my abortion. I've always supported abortion rights; was I no longer pro-choice? The abortion should have cured my problem–the pregnancy. Plus, I could always have a kid later. Why was I still upset? I appreciated Jane's caring, but all her love couldn't penetrate the barrier I felt between us. What I have described is a rosy picture compared to the support we might receive in other situations. We may be unable to tell people about our abortions, fearing their disapproval, feeling ashamed, or simply thinking the experience too personal to share.

Because we cannot always find support from those we love, we will turn to a book where there is a common understanding. This book is where I belonged that summer in Denver; I needed to meet the women who now fill its pages. Had I known them then, I would have had a sense of community, a sense that others felt as I did. One of the women I interviewed feels similarly. She wants to discuss her abortions, but can never find someone to converse on the level she needs. As a consequence, she says, "I feel like I had to pay some emotional costs, because there's no map on this stuff." This book should help chart that unknown territory.

Acknowledgments

I owe a tremendous amount to the women who contributed their stories to this book. They shared their most private experiences, though most knew nothing about me, and although some had no guarantee that this book would be published. Women came forward despite fears about confidentiality and despite some pain and difficulty in dredging up memories. All the women in this book spent a great deal of energy answering a long, detailed list of questions. Their support for this project made me believe in it all the more. I apologize for being unable to include every astute and moving comment.

Thanks to those who found contributors among friends, sisters, and daughters. I appreciate that people raised this potentially touchy issue with the women in their lives.

In 1991, the Dartmouth General Fellowship Committee awarded me a grant, which was tremendously encouraging. My deepest gratitude goes to them, as well as to Judith White and Sarah Carlson, who helped with my grant proposal.

I owe Kathy Anolick more than I can say. From the beginning, Kathy threw herself behind this project. She pored over every chapter, giving her input on the most microscopic levels. She put considerable time and energy into finding prepublication reviewers for the book. I feel incredibly fortunate that we were in sync as we worked, and that we got to know each other so well in the process. Most of all, I am proud to have Kathy's foreword as the first piece of text in this book.

Many thanks to the following people for refining my approach to the topic: Betsy Black, Josh Horwitz, Tony Horwitz, Audrey McCollum, and Howard Yoon. I am indebted to Dr. Sheldon Kushner, who provided medical feedback. Thanks also to the following people: Carla Freccero, Deborah King, Anne Brooks, Heather Earle, Mary Turco, Robin Finnegan, Lyn Stack, Elizabeth Cotton, Gail Ross, Jan Bouc, Catherine Jones, and Victoria Kelly.

I am grateful to my family (Annetta and Jack Kushner and Reyna Pratt), friends (especially Theresa Wildt), and clients for their support and encouragement through the ups and downs. A special thanks goes to the teachers who made me a better writer: David Wykes, Phil Bosakowski, Tom Yankus, and Charlie Holmes.

I appreciate that The Haworth Press was brave enough to take on a book like this. In particular, I want to thank Ellen Cole and Esther Rothblum, the editors who acquired my manuscript, and Susan Trzeciak Gibson, the production editor who answered all my questions and did a terrific copyediting job.

Many thanks to the following people, who volunteered their time as prepublication reviewers: Carol Becker, Sandra Gómez, Kim Kluger-Bell, and Audrey McCollum.

More than anyone, my husband, Haroon Chaudhri, deserves thanks and gratitude. When Haroon first suggested that I write this book, I thought it was ludicrous, but he helped me see how it could be a reality. Haroon spent hours with me photocopying medical tomes in musty libraries, drove with me to other states to find books, waited in cafes while I interviewed people, and helped me through stuck places. He read every chapter and proposal several times over, and helped me greatly with his big-picture approach. I cannot imagine having written this book without his support.

PART I: RESPONDING TO THE CHANGES

Chapter 1

Moving Through Moodiness

Toni is a 23-year-old African American with an easy smile. She makes frequent eye contact as she rattles off all the feelings she has about her abortions. Only gradually does a dissonance emerge between her animated gestures and her words. As she discusses the three abortions she has had in the last two years–the most recent pregnancy ending four months ago–it turns out she is downright depressed. Toni conceals her unhappiness, hoping that if she focuses on the positive, her bothersome emotions will disappear.

"I don't think I've dealt with all the emotions I have," Toni observes. She explains that when she recalls her abortion experiences, "I'll get deep feelings of sadness and confusion." The feelings, she adds, are "related to being pregnant and having an abortion."

Sometimes an event jogs her feelings. She notes, "I'll be reading a magazine. It's usually related to birth. I'll think of how I could have had children, but I didn't. Then that jars other things." One night she came home to find her roommates watching an HBO special about abortion experiences. Her roommates felt moved by the story, but Toni became distraught. "I sat there bawling," she recalls. Afterward, the feelings lingered. The HBO special and the article may have been designed to elicit emotion, but Toni can become upset by the mere sight of pregnant women; usually, she feels guilt and envy at those times. Even reading an ad to contribute a story for this book "shook up all these emotions."

The intensity and frequency of Toni's feelings bother her. She says that after her third abortion, she felt especially frustrated, "because I couldn't control these feelings. I had these rushes of sadness and anger with myself. It was so many emotions all at once, except for positive ones." To this pile-up of feelings, she adds self-blame for being so emotional. Toni explains, "I felt angry at myself, because I couldn't get over it."

Toni has no road map for her emotional journey. Her preconceptions about what abortion entails have fallen by the wayside. She used to think abortion was "a woman's choice" and "not any big thing," she recalls. "Or all these things that were so vague and distant from the whole situation." Now that she has experienced abortion herself, she still feels uncertain about what an abortion should involve emotionally. She says, "I didn't know anybody that had ever had an abortion. It was never talked about, so you don't know what to expect when it's happening. You want to find someone and say, 'Is this supposed to happen?' When that person's not there, it makes it more difficult." As willing as people are to debate the politics and morality of abortion, few can discuss it on the personal level. Lacking this guidance, Toni laments, "It's almost two years since my first abortion, and I still have feelings about it—sometimes very vivid feelings. When do they die? When do they just become like, 'Oh, well, I had an abortion and I don't think about it'?"

Her friends cannot advise her in this arena because they have not had abortions. Some have tried to support her feelings. "I felt really sad and depressed," says Toni, "and people said, 'That makes sense.'" But they couldn't offer much more help, and sometimes offered much less. Toni muses, "Women who haven't shared this experience . . . it's almost like talking to a wall." Either "you don't get any response," or "their responses are so vague."

To deal with her emotions, Toni has told herself, "Okay, I'm not going to think about the things that make me feel sad." To occupy her mind, she has begun going to the gym, to work, and to the library, where she studies late. She also attends school full-time and has held down two jobs. "I just do everything outside of my house," Toni comments, explaining that at home, she might relax. She adds, "Then my mind drifts. Those are the times when those feelings sneak back up on me."

Toni is so afraid of relaxing that she cannot let herself sleep. She says, "I've been an insomniac for two years, since my first abortion." Toni explains, "Since my abortion, I can't sleep in my mind." Just as sleep patterns change under stress, so do eating habits. Toni observes, "In two years, I've put on fifty pounds, because depression resulted in my overeating." Eating is an easy way of avoiding troubles and finding temporary happiness.

The only time Toni doesn't divert herself from her troubles is at night. She once went to clubs, but after her first pregnancy ended, she worried that people would look at her, know that she'd had an abortion, and judge her. Toni recalls, "I felt really exposed." Now seeing this vulnerability as "just paranoia," she comments, "I realize I'm being silly, because no one can know what you've gone through by looking at you." Toni's feeling of transparency speaks volumes about how much the abortions have dominated her mental life–and how much she tries to resist her feelings so she can carry on with her life.

Toni has employed another defense again pain: forgetting. Despite her "very detail-oriented" memory, which can retrieve names, dates, and faces in an instant, she recalls almost nothing of her third abortion, which she calls the most traumatic, partly because it came only four months after her second abortion. "I remember going for my abortion," Toni recalls, "but I don't remember what day or what it was like." Toni has great insight into this repression: "If I can't remember it, then I can't reflect on it and I can't be sad."

Despite all her ways of avoiding feelings, they manage to surface. As she says of her emotional state after the second abortion, "I chose not to deal with it. But then it was dealing with me." When the emotions sweep over her, she only half-acknowledges them. She says, "Last semester, I'd be walking home from school and I'd start crying. I knew why. But I didn't want to get too deep with it." She fears "feeling those feelings."

At times, she has found crying beneficial. She notes, "I felt like it relieved some of my pressures." She feels awkward about crying in front of her friends and boyfriend, though, fearing they will find her "too dramatic," and also not wanting to "drill the subject into the ground." Plus, crying has not proven entirely therapeutic. "For me," she says, "crying didn't lessen my pain. It hasn't made my memory of this whole situation any easier."

Toni does not know if she deserves relief. She wonders, "Am I supposed to think about this as a reminder, 'Don't let it happen again'?" This comment has a self-punitive tone; she seems to think pain will keep her in line. "I don't know if this is something that I'm supposed to carry with me," she says, as if her emotional burden is a rock to drag behind her in an infernal torture. Despite this inclination to punish herself, Toni knows that she needs to find peace. Thus, she focuses on getting over the experience.

She tried therapy, but didn't feel she could level with the therapist. "It was hard for me to tell someone who didn't know me that I had an abortion, because I didn't want them to judge me," she explains. After her second abortion, Toni told the therapist she'd had one, but didn't mention both. Toni thought, "If she thinks I'm horrible for having one, she must think I'm really horrible for having two." In fact, the therapist didn't respond much at all, except to say that she could tell Toni was holding back something. Even after Toni revealed her secret, therapy wasn't very productive, because, as she says, "I still didn't want to deal with it completely." Toni explains, "I felt I was sitting here talking to this woman who'd never had an abortion–because that was something that we talked about–who probably couldn't understand. So I closed the chapter on it. Then I started to search for people who had had the same experience to bounce emotions off of them."

That is now her main strategy. She explains, "I'm doing that to validate my own emotions because at one point, I really thought I was losing my mind." Toni has sought a postabortion support group, but because abortion has a stigma around it, such groups are rare and she cannot find one. She still sees that as her only answer, saying, "I'm searching so hard so that I can hurry up and get this part of my life over with. I keep thinking that if I join a group in which I can talk about these feelings and not think that there's anything wrong with me, I can proceed to the next part and just push it back into my memory. Right now, no matter how far I try to push it back, something always brings it to the foreground."

Postabortion groups have helped many women; Toni is certainly on the right track. But she also may have to experience her emotions fully, rather than hoping to "get this part of my life over with." One of her reasons for joining such a group is to avoid her emotions. She says that after meeting people who have had abortions, she hopes to "focus on their feelings and emotions, as opposed to dealing with mine."

Until Toni feels able to look at her own experience more closely, she probably won't find relief. It is understandable that she ducks the emotions that assault her; they are not fun to feel. Avoiding them has not helped her, however. It seems that, paradoxically, one must let oneself feel the pain in order to see it come to an end. In this chapter, we will meet women who respond to this challenge in different ways, as well as some who have felt no pain at all. We first encounter Nora, who has shared much of Toni's moodiness.

Nora: "I'm Disturbed at the Process"

Nora, a big-boned 22 year old with a shock of blond hair, refuses to believe anything she is told, particularly the Catholic dogma her father taught her. She laughs, "My dad was so embracing of things with such blind faith that it made me reject all of it immediately. I couldn't see why we couldn't have premarital sex or why I didn't have an orgy with my cousins." When Nora had an unplanned pregnancy eight months ago, her scorn for Catholicism played into her decision. She recalls, "All those films I was shown in Catholic school–those were a big part of my having an abortion, because I was rejecting them." Nora found those pro-life ideas "bogus," "wrong," and "based on nothing."

She took more than scorn into account when she decided to end her pregnancy; as she was still an undergraduate and valued her education highly, her choice was automatic. She viewed her upcoming abortion simply as a legal right she could exercise and expected to feel nothing. Instead, in the weeks afterward, pain and confusion rolled through her in waves. She recalls, "When I was really freaking out, I couldn't even formulate my opinion on it. It was just this feeling of horribleness and you can't even put everything together and see what you're really thinking. It's pure emotional rottenness." She adds, "I'd wake up in the middle of the night and I'd be crying. I felt really empty inside."

Like Toni, Nora doubted her sanity. She recalls, "I thought I was going to go nuts at one point" after the abortion. "One night I just started gasping for air. It was really scary. I've been depressed, but I never thought I was going to lose control of my own head." She couldn't pinpoint the disturbance, except for feeling that she stopped a natural process. It further upset her to feel she had succumbed to pro-life ideology. She says firmly, "I sound like a Catholic here, thinking that this child was real and natural and that I ended his life. I'm disturbed at the process." Nora was shocked that her feelings showed up with a pro-life undertone. She recalls thinking, "This is so trite that I'm having this." She explains, "I was disgusted with myself for having the feeling that I killed something. I was really surprised that I would have that kind of conservative attitude." Rejecting Catholicism but still feeling terrible after her abortion presented a conflict. Nora says, "I felt bad for feeling grief, because I thought I was succumbing to that garbage."

Nora also struggled against her moods because she didn't want to scare off her live-in boyfriend. When she awoke "crying and freaking out," he would ask, "It's the abortion, right?" She hesitated to agree, because she thought the truth would "freak him out." They had only been together four months when the pregnancy came along, and Nora has worried about ruining their relationship. She says, "I get really nervous when I feel sad in front of Adam, because I think that he is going to think I'm just this big, wet mop and that I'm constantly getting depressed." Nora especially did not want to alienate him when she felt so needy and fragile. If he paid her too little attention, she says it "would set something off. I would feel like, 'God, I went through all this because of your penis. Be nice to me.'" Not wanting to rock the boat, she never told him this directly. Besides, he hadn't done anything cruel. "His attention would just be on something else," she says. "But I was much more sensitive to his not paying attention to me. I wanted him to do a lot of mothering."

Now, she says the feelings are "not bothering me every day," and adds, "I guess I worked it out." The storm of feelings moved through her and dissipated in a few weeks, maybe because she succumbed to it whenever it hit, even in the middle of the night.

Olivia: "There Is a Rather Big Hormonal Shift"

Because Nora's strong reaction occurred in the weeks after her abortion, her feelings were probably linked to the hormonal shifts a body goes through when pregnancy ends. The drop in hormone levels may have colored her moods with a painful and frightening intensity. Some people attribute postabortion feelings entirely to this hormonal shift. Olivia, a 46-year-old African American who had an abortion in 1969, understands her own postabortion response this way. "I really believe that there is a rather big hormonal shift," she notes, adding that it lasts "forty-eight hours. Maybe seventy-two." In the first two or three days after her abortion, Olivia felt "isolated, alone, hollow." Likening this response to a postpartum reaction, she refers to "a feeling of loss. A feeling of depression. As a licensed social worker, I wouldn't call it clinical depression, but a loss and a sadness."

Olivia, a self-described "oppression blaster," brings to this discussion a firm rootedness in abortion rights ideology. Arrested for civil rights protests sixteen times in her early teenage years, she is well versed in the slogans any successful activism requires. Thus, she refers to Operation Rescue as Operation Oppress You, and interprets many of her feelings in a social context, rather than a personal one. She says that after her abortion, she felt "bad and ugly and dirty because I came from a society and culture that said, 'That was the wrong decision.'" Not wanting to imply that such feelings are intrinsic to abortion, she hastily adds, "That would have been so if society said that dyeing or cutting your hair were some such-and-such a thing." When abortion "became legal and therefore more socially acceptable," says Olivia, "a lot of the feelings of shame and guilt went away."

Olivia is absolutely correct in how she interprets the feelings that can follow abortion. When society shames us for our abortions, it affects how we mourn, discuss, and accept them. In addition, hormones can rule our moods during and after pregnancy, whether the pregnancy lasts only a few months or goes full term.

This does not tell the full story, however. Neither societal censure nor hormones determine the content of our concerns. To attribute most postabortion reactions to those causes is politically useful, but emotionally too simple. Postabortion responses can vary widely, both in intensity and content. Our personal histories and beliefs, the behavior of those around us, and our social and political worlds can all contribute to our reaction.

WHAT TRIGGERS THE FEELINGS

Hormones cannot explain how, long after the procedure, feelings about one's abortion can reappear with the slightest stimulation. Many women are distressed to find themselves bursting into tears when some event reminds them of their abortions. One 23 year old, who had an abortion two years ago, describes how disconcerting it can be for strong feelings to crash in at inopportune times. She says, "For five months, seeing women with babies really upset me. Sometimes I would cry. Crying when you don't want to and you're like, 'Geez, I wish this didn't happen here.'" As she indicates, it can be upsetting to feel calm and to have an event cause emotional turmoil. We now meet Mindy, who has experienced this often, with a range of triggers.

Mindy: "I Thought I Had Gotten Over It, and Then It All Came Back"

"Going into it, I kept my cool the whole time, didn't I?" Mindy, a lanky 22-year-old brunette, who speaks rapidly and emphatically, turns to her boyfriend for confirmation. "Before you got into the clinic, yeah," Kurt responds. Sturdy, square-jawed Kurt has insisted on being present at the interview, but says little, mostly verifying facts and listening quietly. They have dated since high school, except for a five-month breakup after the abortion. Satisfied with his confirmation, Mindy speaks with more confidence. "Before I got to the clinic, I handled myself exceptionally well, considering. I tried to stay calm. I knew that if I let myself get out of hand, I was going to go off the deep end."

She planned to control her emotions the same way after the procedure. That wasn't the case. After the abortion, Mindy suddenly faced something she had thus far been unable to confront–that she had actually been pregnant. She explains, "I still couldn't believe that that whole thing had happened. I don't think it hit me until I walked out of the clinic. It just came at me, all at once. And for the week after that, I was massively depressed."

Mindy's experience is not unusual. Before an abortion, many of us need to shield ourselves from the alarming fact of the pregnancy and from the emotions that threaten our equilibrium. We shift into autopilot, coping quite calmly with practical details. A comforting denial sets in, along the lines of, "I'll deal with the emotional stuff later."

When the procedure ends, the crisis has passed and any emotions we have deferred can come to the surface. That happened to Mindy after her abortion. She asks, "Right after it was done, I was hysterical for how long?" Kurt responds, "At least thirty, forty hours." Mindy nods. "I just couldn't function. I was hysterical, crying, and all that kind of crap."

The emotional storm took her half by surprise. "It was worse than I thought it would be. I didn't really think it would affect me emotionally as much as it did," she muses, calling her response "a nightmare–a very big nightmare." On the other hand, she acknowledges, "I don't handle any crisis well. I'm a very, very emotional and irrational person." Being wired this way made her response "tenfold what it should have been."

The intensity decreased after those first couple of days, except when commercials for home pregnancy tests or Planned Parenthood reminded her of her experience. She also had trouble on the projected due date, when she realized sadly, "Oh geez, I'd be giving birth right now." One weekend near the one-year anniversary of her abortion, she read an article about women's pregnancy choices. "That ruined my weekend," she recalls. "I thought that I had pretty much gotten over it. And then it all came back to me."

Seeing kids and new mothers has also sparked memories and feelings. She pictures herself as the mother, thinking, "Maybe that would be me pushing the stroller." The odd thing about her new desire for kids is that she has never wanted any. But after her pregnancy, she says, "Every time I saw kids, I was like; 'Oh my God, a baby. It's so cute.'" She finds herself staring at infants often. This new interest in babies may stem from unresolved emotions; she might want a child because she feels grief or guilt for her abortion, and may find that her interest in babies will fade when these feelings do.

Eighteen months after her abortion, Mindy gives contradictory accounts of how much the event is still with her. "I think about it all the time," she says, adding, "It doesn't get me as depressed as it used to." After so much time, "I can cope better," she says. Later, she downgrades her estimate from thinking about it "all the time" to "probably once or twice a week. But it's just a passing thought. It's a part of history." Why the contradiction? Mindy may not want to believe that she is still involved with the experience. She comments, "It's been a year and a half. I can't keep dwelling on it." Mindy concludes, "I guess I'm pretty much okay with it. I've had some time to get over it." Time may indeed have softened her memories, but not wanting to dwell is different from truly feeling at peace. If events easily trip Mindy's emotions, they are probably still unresolved.

When Feelings Crash in

Mindy has listed several events that set off her feelings, including looking at new mothers and babies, seeing commercials, reading articles, and living through the due date and anniversary of the abortion. Here are other triggers that women have cited:

Seeing Certain Kids:

> When I was nanny to a girl who looked like me and would have been the same age as if I had a baby, I became very attached and decided to leave the job. (Lana, age 26, who had abortions at ages 22 and 23)

Having Dreams: giving birth to babies or other creatures, killing animals

> The morning after the abortion, I woke up crying. I had dreamed I was carrying a puppy and had to put it to sleep and didn't want to. (Lana, age 26, who had abortions at ages 22 and 23)

Watching Television or Movies: seeing news about pro-life activities, watching dramas about pregnancy decisions or abortions

> I saw that movie *Eating*. And they started talking about abortion. A week before that, I saw that movie *Switch*. The woman had a baby and she's all, "Oh, I could never have an abortion." Normally, it would just pass over my head. But I was like,

"Why is this happening in these movies?" (Becky, age 25, two months after her abortion)

Hearing References to Pregnancy or Abortion:

I kept hearing these stupid interviews on the radio. Occasionally they would mention something about how abortion is so terrible. I got really upset and shut off the radio. I don't even think about it. Then these pro-lifers come along and remind me. When they said the child didn't have any choice, it made me feel guilty. (Dana, age 27, two years after her abortion)

I went to dinner with a bunch of guys. One was wearing a pro-choice shirt that depicted a hanger crossed out. They started laughing and saying things like, "Just get an Exacto knife, rip it out, get a rusty hanger." I know they couldn't have any idea what I had been through, but I left the table and sobbed for an hour. (Geneva, age 18, one year after her abortion)

Having Sex:

It was hard to have sex initially, because intercourse was the same motion as the abortion. The in-and-out thrusting and that horrible suction noise. . . . Feelings have burst in, especially during lovemaking. It's very weird for men to understand. "You're crying about something that happened way back then, right now!?" (Clarissa, age 30, five years after her abortion)

Going to Gynecological Exams:

I feel in control, generally, but it will hit at odd times. At the gynecologist, being with feet in stirrups, I've cried again. When it hits, it hits hard. (Elissa, age 24, five months after her abortion)

Seeing Friends Become Pregnant and Have Abortions or Babies:

After the abortions, I came across old friends who had had babies, and a few times they were as old as the babies unborn

> to me would have been. I was incredibly jealous and hurt, but felt I deserved to feel that way. (Florence, age 25, who had abortions at ages 18 and 21)

Feeling Lonely or Depressed:

> One evening, while feeling particularly lonely, I thought to myself, "If I'd kept the baby, I'd at least have someone to love me." I cried at this thought, but realized that if that was the only reason I could think of for having a child, then it was a damn good thing I'd aborted. (Zara, age 23, six months after her abortion)

USING EMOTIONS OR LOGIC IN THINKING ABOUT AN ABORTION

In making these comments, these women agree that having an abortion can be emotionally challenging. They accept that they cannot always control the feelings that overcome them. Many other women would disagree. They are completely in control of their postabortion emotions. Juliet, a 42-year-old Caucasian, certainly feels that way.

Juliet: "An Extremely Logical Person"

Juliet describes how she decided on abortion six months ago: "Being an extremely logical person, there was no 'real' choice as to whether to 'do it' or not! It was a clean, cut-and-dry decision to make. There was absolutely *no* way I was going to have a child." Her logical attitude continued during the abortion, during which, she says, "My mood was good, as it usually is. It was like my GYN appointments. Just another doctor in my crotch poking around to find something." Afterward, it was the same thing. "It's over the minute it was over," she says, adding, "After it was done, I mean right afterward, I was already thinking ahead to my day tomorrow. Never looked back, never a second thought about it."

Her experience was easy, partly because she is certain about not wanting children. She says, "I'd rather have a root canal than be pregnant," and quotes W. C. Fields: "Children are like elephants—nice to look at, but I don't want to have one." Given her view on the matter, it is understandable that she felt relieved after her abortion. Certainly, many women feel fine afterward, which is perfectly healthy, normal, and desirable.

Juliet, however, may not really be so resolved. While she claims her abortion "was not a 'biggie'" and that "I gave more thought to where I'm going on vacation," she later contradicts this; in referring to the unprotected sex that got her pregnant, she says, "I promised myself it *will never happen again*" (her emphasis). Certainly, many women vow not to put themselves through another abortion procedure, but Juliet's strong conviction seems odd, since she frequently states that her abortion was no big deal emotionally or physically. In addition, Juliet sent her story in anonymously. She might have done this because she saw no need to indicate her name. Or perhaps she feels uncomfortable on some level. Juliet may feel safer believing that she has no emotion about her abortion. She says she feels proud that, "As a Libra, I try to keep all things in balance. And I'm getting quite good at it." She might minimize anything that disturbs this image of herself as perfectly balanced.

She speaks of her experience with remarkable forcefulness, saying, "It was such a minor thing for me to make a decision. I didn't tell anyone; why should I? I called my doctor and made the appointment. No remorse, no afterthoughts. I just did what was necessary for me. It's my body, my call on the 'what to do.'" Many women feel this way. It seems, however, as if Juliet may be protecting herself, that perhaps she has feelings she cannot bear to acknowledge. We will now meet Ada, who also has experienced no negative feelings about her abortion, but who describes her experience in a very different tone.

Ada: The Farm, Zero Population Growth, and Existentialism

"I have sometimes wondered why the abortion I had in 1975 was not devastating and has not had a major impact on my life," says Ada, who is white and 58. "I speculated whether this might be due to massive denial, but I now understand some of the reasons I was able to cope well with the abortion physically, mentally, and spiritually."

Ada's views on abortion derive from her childhood in England and Australia. She notes, "I grew up on a farm seeing copulation, birth, and death as natural, everyday events. I learned that a good farmer does not have animals that cannot be properly fed and so, from an early age, I understood that when lambs and calves were castrated, newborn kittens drowned, or a cow aborted, this was a responsible and 'kind' thing to do." Ada adds, "I knew that when an unmarried girl got pregnant, she was 'in trouble' and had four alternatives." Those were marriage, suicide, adoption, or an illegal abortion. She continues, "I grew up thinking of abortion not as a moral issue, but simply as one of the more risky solutions to the practical problem of unwanted pregnancy."

As Ada became an adult, she took in new ideas about population growth that confirmed these early beliefs. She and her husband Reuben decided "that it was not right to bring more children into an overpopulated world while there were always children waiting for adoption," and "that we should do no more than replace ourselves in the world." In other words, two people should leave behind no more than two children.

Ada and Reuben adopted a child and gave birth to another. Then Ada's IUD failed and confronted them with another pregnancy. Not only would a third child conflict with their belief in rearing just two, but it would be very difficult for them to support three kids. "I do not recall that we had to agonize at all over the decision to abort this pregnancy," says Ada. "The choice was clear." Ada's philosophies further confirmed the decision. She notes, "Having read a good deal of existential philosophy, I believed that a 'right' choice is the choice that is made with due consideration and for which full responsibility is taken."

Ada had an emotionally painless abortion and attributes this to her way of approaching the situation. Her beliefs helped clarify her decision, "eased the experience of abortion," and enabled her "to live comfortably with the consequences" of her choice.

Only recently has she wondered about the child she did not have. She recalls "one occasion, about twenty years after the abortion, when I fantasized about what the aborted child might have been like as an adult, but this was not a painful experience." Rather than resisting her emotional side, Ada has searched for more emotion. "I feel vaguely guilty about the *lack* of difficulty and intensity," she says, adding, "I might accuse myself of being cold and callous if I did not know myself to be a sensitive and caring person."

Emotions Versus Logic: Different Perspectives on the Issue

Ada probes herself for guilt, because she would like to see evidence that she is sensitive and caring. She values her emotional side and welcomes any feelings that arise. Many women share her attitude; they allow themselves to feel whatever feelings they have about their abortions. The following comments reflect this perspective:

> I started to realize that I'm not going to get over this if I can't be with my feelings and just be sad if I have to be sad. But I try to wait till I get home to start crying. (Becky, age 25, two months after her abortion)

> I don't think I'm even close to totally healing, but praying to the baby helps–it's a safe time and I cry whenever I do. A little release, a bit at a time. (Elissa, age 24, five months after her abortion)

Some people feel so strongly that emotions must accompany an abortion experience that they expect every woman to feel pain about her abortion; they feel intolerant of those who have no negative feelings. For instance, one 22 year old who has had an abortion says, "I think you're a cold person if it doesn't hit you. You've got a screw loose if you can do it and have no problem with it at all." Part of such an outlook derives from antichoice views of abortion. Those who oppose abortion insist that guilt is an inevitable reaction and even hope, in a punitive way, that women feel guilty after abortions. This attitude is prevalent in society, even among those who call themselves pro-choice. Women who pick up on it may berate themselves if they have felt no pain. For instance, a year after her abortion, another 22 year old recalls, "I felt awful for not feeling guilty or crying whenever I saw kids. I thought something was wrong with me for not feeling bad."

In contrast to this outlook, some women feel it is important to use logic rather than emotion in the course of an abortion experience.

They think rationality is normal and even essential in this situation. As one 35 year old puts it, ten years after her abortion, "I've blocked a lot of that stuff out. I'm not doing it deliberately, but you have to go on, you have to enjoy your life. What good is it if you're tearing yourself apart?" Valuing logic in an abortion experience can lead some women to devalue and even scorn emotion as shameful and weak. For instance, after three abortions in her twenties, one thirty-eight year old says, "The emotion-laden, theatrical approach to life is sheer stupidity. The rose glasses of sentiment need to be ripped off and the matter examined coolly and objectively." If women sense this attitude in society, they may become intolerant of their own emotions. The following comment, from a 20 year old who ended a pregnancy six weeks ago, reflects how some women blame themselves for feeling emotional about their abortions: "I thought, maybe I'm crazy because I'm the only one who can't see that this is the logical thing to do. Maybe I'm being too emotional. Maybe I should be more rational."

Some people feel it is vital for the heart and mind to work together, both in making the decision and in reacting to an abortion experience. The following comments reflect how some women have sought and achieved harmony when they have had abortions.

> I felt I made a life decision about the emotional and physical well-being not only of myself, but of the child-to-be. It was one of the best decisions I've ever made. It was an emotional decision, of course, but it was based on rationality. (Zelda, age 39, four years after her abortion)

> I went on with my life–neither denying nor focusing on the issue, but dealing with the moment-to-moment feelings as best I could. The only issue is the occasional sadness about the lost potential represented by the lost pregnancy. But usually I am able to balance that by thinking about quality of life for that child. (Lynn, age 40, who had abortions at ages 17 and 33)

This third approach–balancing emotions and logic–seems to make the most sense. It is ideal to work from the head and heart as one proceeds through an abortion experience, especially if logic and emotions agree with each other. If, however, only one part presents itself, that is fine as well. One can no more prod oneself to feel emotions that simply aren't there than one can force oneself to fall in love. What a relief to feel no emotion and to be spared pain! On the other end of the spectrum, if logic is absent, let emotion steer the way. Those emotions have a logic of their own and demand attention as they drive toward resolution. Now we will meet Annika, who struggled to balance logic and emotions.

Annika: "I Pushed the Feelings Aside, Because I Wanted to Function"

"I can be very intellect-oriented, but I'm also a very emotional person," explains Annika, age 31. Her appearance corroborates this description. Her tailored suit speaks of intellect and seriousness; her European accent lends sophistication to her voice. At the same time, her delicate build makes her look vulnerable. As she recalls the unplanned pregnancy she had five years ago, she says, "The really emotional part couldn't deal with it at all. It was the part that just wanted to rejoice in being pregnant."

She had to focus on her rational side and not indulge fantasies of carrying her pregnancy to term, because her relationship with her boyfriend, Phil, had conflicts. She recalls, "We were very much in love. But we had completely different expectations of life. I want children; he didn't want any children. The paradox of this whole situation was that he wanted me to have the child." Phil had gone through an abortion with an ex-girlfriend and did not want to take what he perceived to be another life. Faced with his opposition to her abortion, Annika says, "I felt like I had to be really clear-headed." She tried to "think really rationally" and remind herself, "This doesn't mean he really wants this child."

Annika considered her options, none of which appealed to her. Rather than surveying her choices and joyfully choosing one, Annika wondered, "How am I going to get out of those three options?" She rejected birth and adoption and backed into abortion by default. She notes, "I just halfway decided. It didn't really feel like I was saying, 'What I'm going to do is "a" and it's going to be the best thing.' I never was there. I was completely ambivalent. Even though I felt like a bigger part of me was leaning toward not having" the child, "there was a part that wanted to hold onto it."

Because she felt "so pushed" into being rational to counter Phil's irrationality, she says, "I didn't really allow myself to sit with the feelings. I tried to push them aside, because I wanted to function." Only when she slept did she stop blocking out those feelings; they came forth in dreams. She dreamed once of having a baby and awoke distraught, realizing that she had "repressed" the part of her "that really wanted to hold this child, to cuddle it and love it."

Annika had to wait five weeks in a state of "complete turmoil" until the fetus became large enough for a safe abortion. During this time, Annika felt unsure whether she could terminate a pregnancy that she partly wanted. At the abortion, her ambivalence became intolerable. When her doctor described the procedure he would perform, she began "crying like crazy" and "couldn't even listen to this." Later, she thought back to this moment and wondered, "Why didn't anybody rescue me then? Why didn't anybody say, 'You seem really upset about it. Do you want to think about this some more, or come back when you're feeling better?'" Annika felt so much pain that she could not face up to the decision she had halfway made; she wanted someone else to take responsibility for her choice. Because no one did, she proceeded.

After the doctor numbed her cervix, Annika says, "I just took one look at this vacuum, and started to cry hysterically. I was thinking, 'Oh my God, this poor thing. What am I doing to it?'" Annika recalls, "Even the moment that the procedure happened, I was so torn." During the abortion, "I was crying the whole time. I remember thinking I had to pull myself together as much as I could and that was as much as I could ask myself to do."

When the procedure ended, Annika kept sobbing. Her gynecologist tried to comfort her, and her friend, who had come to the procedure with her, said with concern, "Annika, you have got to let go." She could not. In the following months, Annika's pain continued, and she did not know how to cope with it, so she began to block it out. For the next year, she diverted her attention from her feelings by staying busy. She remembers, "I just tried to move on and keep going with my life. And with what I had wanted for my life. I really got myself head over heels into school and was a straight-A student." Ironically, her studies were all about emotions; she was training to become a therapist. Her self-diagnosis? She muses, "I was severely depressed, definitely. I was in serious trauma."

She knew this because every so often, her feelings would "break out." She recalls, "I'd read something; I'd hear something on the news about abortion." It could be a "poem or some picture of a baby I saw. Anything could trigger it." She would cry about it for hours. One event that unleashed her feelings occurred back in Europe; when her brother's wife conceived happily, Annika felt extreme envy. She explains, "It brought up this thing of 'mine would have been the first grandchild to be born.'" Even now, she occasionally wonders about her potential child, who would have been four soon. She says, "I think about what this life would have been like and what personality it would have had or what it would have looked like. There's a sadness about having taken something that was unique."

WORKING THROUGH THE FEELINGS

It is often tempting to hope such feelings will go away. Sometimes people think that because an abortion is irreversible, their feelings about it cannot change either. For example, six weeks after her abortion, one 20 year old says of her experience, "It's over. The only thing left is the feeling that it should never have happened. But it's resolved, because I can't do anything about it. I'm just hoping that it'll just go away with time." Another woman, age 27, has a similar attitude, even though her experience occurred two years ago. She comments, "I still have some bad feelings, but then I don't want to make myself feel too bad. And I have good feelings, too. I guess I've gotten over it, because I just feel like there's nothing more I can do about it. I have to be done with it. I don't want to sit around moping over something I can't change." These women may find that their emotions linger for a long time. They might feel relief faster if they try to resolve their feelings.

Annika looked closely at hers, and after five years, occasional thoughts about the fetus are all that remain of her previous pain. It literally took a large jolt for Annika to realize how much help she needed. On October 17, 1989, the one-year anniversary of her abortion, a huge earthquake rocked the San Francisco Bay Area, where she lived. She speculates on why that event clued her in to her emotional needs: "People say that some traumatic event brings up" repressed feelings. The anniversary of the abortion also rekindled her emotions. Shaken into a hyperawareness of her life, Annika could no longer deny what she had experienced in the last year. She says, "I knew that periodically I would have those phases of breaking down and just feeling terrible, terrible, terrible. And when I was feeling that way, I had no sense of ever getting out of that. There was a sense of I'm going to die or feel like this for the rest of my life. And I knew I needed help with it."

Annika started both individual and group therapy. Individual therapy, she says, "really helped me out, because I had so much pain around this that I didn't even dare to look at it." She feared that if she examined her pain, "it was going to explode" and she was "going to be left with nothing." Although this fear made it hard to go to therapy, where she spent sessions sobbing, she muses, "It was good for me to do that. I couldn't repress this anymore." In therapy, she looked at her sorrow about the abortion and about being unable to "undo this." It took nearly two years to make peace with her abortion, but it was worth every minute. Annika observes, "I felt in a better place emotionally. I felt better about who I was, too, because that's just not the way I approach life," she says, referring to her former, numb state. Group therapy also helped, enabling her to see that others were "just as deeply affected by it" as she. Annika recalls, "I had felt so isolated with it. I had felt like maybe something is wrong with me that I'm having such a hard time dealing with this."

Now, as her professional life as a therapist begins, Annika has formed her own postabortion group. Because five years have passed since her abortion and she has worked through the issues so thoroughly, she says she feels capable of "hearing all those stories without freaking out about my own stuff." Annika has started the group because she understands so well the value of exploring emotions and seeking resolution. As much as she tried to block out her feelings in the beginning, she eventually realized that they would not disappear on their own. She had to reenter the old pain before she could reach a peaceful state. "When I was in therapy working through the really painful stuff," Annika recalls, "it was absolutely awful and I felt terrible for a long time, but it was necessary to do that." She advises women to seek individual or group therapy, "or to get themselves emotional support otherwise. And really to face the issues around it."

Chapter 2

Coping with Stress and Regaining Control

Until last year, Marilyn, who is 28 and Caucasian, was accustomed to having things go well. Then, she had an unplanned pregnancy, which she ended eleven months ago. Consequently, she and her fiancé broke up. After that, she broke two ribs in a bicycle accident and discovered that she had herpes. Reeling off this list of troubles and the way they made her feel, she says apologetically, "I must sound like Susie Misfortune, but nothing this bad ever happened to me before. For twenty-seven years I had done whatever I wanted! Then I had this year of terrible things."

Marilyn comes across as fairly controlled, though not uptight. She speaks quickly and articulately, connecting personal and political issues with ease and exhibiting a sophisticated vocabulary. A PhD candidate at a top-notch school, Marilyn acknowledges that exercising her intelligence is central to her identity, and does not jibe with motherhood. When she became pregnant and zoomed in on the idea of being a wife and mother, she suddenly froze. Marilyn explains, "I had come to view motherhood as a demeaning job. And I thought, 'You're not going to be doing any writing. You're going to be taking care of a baby and making a home.'" Marilyn adds, "I could not just go and be a Bohemian mom."

Nothing in Marilyn's past had prepared her for this role. On the contrary, she cites "years of conditioning that I had against having a child." When Marilyn was a teenager, her mother began expressing fears that Marilyn would have an accidental pregnancy. Soon, Marilyn thought, "Now, there's the worst thing that can happen to you." She put "a lot of effort into avoiding getting pregnant. Being very sexually active, but not wanting to have that be a consequence.

Spending a lot of money. Going to doctors. Developing a lot of habits, all geared toward not ruining my school trajectory."

Saying, "Pregnancy is a loss of control over your body," she adds, "I always hated my menstrual periods" and "was terrified by the effect that they have on my thinking and behavior and emotions." Marilyn resents "having this uterus that does whatever it wants, doesn't consult me, and is supposed to dictate this whole life cycle. Which it has for a long time for many people. And I did not want to be part of that."

Marilyn resisted joining the ranks, the women throughout history who have not had any say over their reproduction. She could not simply yield this control. Her Italian fiancé, Stefano, had a very different attitude about pregnancy, however. Explaining that many Italians see having children as "a natural thing to do" and expect women just to "go with it," she comments, "That's not completely crazy. Perhaps my middle-class, achievement-oriented condition killed a certain possibility that was in my life."

Wanting a high degree of control over her affairs, Marilyn was distressed not only by the seeming unmanageability of pregnancy, but also by the terrible timing. She conceived in Italy, where she studied and Stefano lived, but did not discover the pregnancy until they were traveling in the United States, surrounded by Marilyn's family. She describes the atmosphere: "There's my mother, father, sister, and grandma. They have this whoopee, fun vacation. And I've got to accompany them around everywhere." Marilyn considered concealing her condition from the family while she and Stefano decided what to do. She knew, however, that it would be simplest to be up-front and therefore explained the situation to them. "I told my mom first," Marilyn says, and her mom spread the word. Marilyn recalls, "She told my dad. And she's not capable of hiding anything from her mom, so she even told my grandmother. That's not something I would have anticipated." Suddenly, Marilyn had no control over her secret. She says that while "this horrible thing" was happening, her relatives surrounded her like a "Chinese family, where the young couple is home with the extended family. Everybody knows, which makes me feel worse."

Amid this chaos, Marilyn and Stefano tried to think clearly about their options. Birth or abortion. Living in Italy or the United States.

Marilyn's career versus motherhood. Under the best circumstances, Marilyn has a hard time making decisions. In this situation, it was excruciating to make an "irrevocable" choice about the pregnancy. Eventually, they decided on abortion. Shortly afterward, Marilyn and Stefano's romance fell apart. She explains, "It was the abortion that broke us up." Marilyn calls this breakup "the worst thing that ever happened to me," explaining, "I was unprepared for it to end and I reacted in a totally unexpected way. I don't really understand it myself."

After these losses, Marilyn felt "traumatized." She returned to the United States to a doctoral program that no longer felt important. That fall, she made a "careless" left turn on her bicycle and fell, breaking her ribs. Marilyn attributes the accident to more than bad luck. She explains, "I was suicidally depressed and I was not being very careful with my life in the normal way that you would be." Marilyn acknowledges that bike accidents can happen to anyone and notes, "I don't mean to make everything into a huge melodrama. But when bad things are happening to you, they all seem connected. It's like a plan."

Two months later, as Marilyn healed from the accident, she noticed some strange symptoms, which turned out to be herpes. Marilyn theorizes that the herpes outbreak, too, may be connected to the other unhappy events. She says, "The high emotional stress and the abortion followed by the bike accident probably made the latent herpes come out."

This series of problems left Marilyn with a "severely incapacitating" depression, which lasted a long time. She realizes that no one thing made her depressed; rather, the way one trauma followed on the heels of another overwhelmed her. It seems, even eleven months later, as if "the whole thing is still going on." Still, things have begun to improve for Marilyn. She says that eight months after the abortion, "I began to feel like a human being again and capable of having a life." The depression was worst six months after the abortion, when she discovered the herpes; it then started to lift. Marilyn speculates, "Partly it just ran its course. You can only be depressed for so long. I would say that I was suicidally depressed. And that either ends in suicide, or it ends."

Marilyn has touched on some key points that we will cover in this chapter. She describes how each crisis seemed to cause the next and how the concomitance overwhelmed her. She suddenly found herself with a very complicated life, where dealing with one problem meant facing others at the same time.

MANAGING WHAT FEELS UNMANAGEABLE

Marilyn noted that her pregnancy, abortion, and subsequent troubles seemed all the more traumatic because they were the worst things she had ever faced. This feeling may have been enhanced because her mother had set pregnancy up as the one crisis that could disrupt Marilyn's life. A pregnancy and abortion may not seem stressful for women who feel they have gone through more taxing experiences. For instance, one 44 year old who has had three abortions since her twenties notes, "It was like getting four molars pulled. I consider that a bigger deal, because you can't eat for like four weeks." Similarly, a 49 year old cites other difficulties that greatly outweigh the abortion she had at 28. She says, "I have had much worse problems in my life: a disabled child, financial hardship, health problems. Compared to the real, living issues in my life, the abortion was a blip on the screen."

Many other women do find it stressful to go through pregnancies and abortions. Pregnancies rarely come into stress-free lives; instead, they land on top of schedules already bursting at the seams and present a large problem to be solved in a very short time. Making a decision and arranging an abortion can add to the stress. There are usually quite a lot of tasks to accomplish. We have at least one pregnancy test, if not several; make a decision; locate an accessible, affordable abortion facility; find money, or speak to an insurance company about coverage; and schedule as many as three visits to the facility. Meanwhile, we may feel nauseous, dizzy, and exhausted. On top of this, we have to keep up with our daily duties and may have important and challenging talks about the pregnancy with a lover, friends, and family.

At the abortion facility, we may find more stressful situations. Dealing with the paperwork, insurance regulations, and short-tempered receptionists has made more than one woman burst into tears. Adding to that, we may encounter protesters outside the abortion facility, have communication problems with the personnel, or discover unexpected facts about our bodies at the procedure. We may also feel quite a lot of stress if the procedure does not go well. On rare occasions, we may have an incomplete abortion or develop an infection, dragging the experience out for weeks. Abortion is a medically simple and frequently performed procedure; it is unusual to develop problems. If complications do develop, though, they can create extra stress. Because medical aspects are one part of the experience we cannot control, it can be frustrating to have problems in that area.

The abortion promises to relieve much of the stress of the pregnancy, and for many women it does. As one 23 year old comments six months after her second abortion, "Both of my experiences were stressful up to the abortion only. After the abortion, life was (and is) great–it's like I've been given a new lease on life." For others of us, however, an abortion triggers a barrage of unexpected feelings, making us feel that we have lost control of our emotions. In fact, the stress can make us moodier than usual, adding to the confusion.

One 19 year old who had an abortion a year and a half ago describes how stress affected her: "While I was pregnant and for the first few weeks after the abortion, I felt extremely overwhelmed. Everything I did seemed more difficult than it had to be." As she indicates, stress can make even small tasks feel unmanageable. We may find it difficult to stand back from challenges and figure out a course of action. In this state of panic, we might also find that we are scatterbrained. That was the case for a 21 year old who had an abortion two years ago. "I was so disorganized," she recalls. "I lost a Romantic poetry notebook that had amazing notes in it for my class." She was frustrated because she "couldn't systematically get things done and move forward." Under stress, we may find that we have more to cope with, but that our emotional resources have been depleted. We might feel too burdened to handle the tasks we face.

In a stressful situation, we may feel tough or numb, coping robotically with the challenges thrust before us. One 25 year old who had an abortion a year ago recalls her mental state during pregnancy: "Numb. Lack of mood. Not nervous or anything. Autopilot. . . . I coped by living, trying to organize my life, and by telling myself that it simply wasn't the time." Another woman, a 17 year old who also had an abortion a year ago, comments: "I was very calm when I called for my pregnancy test results. Actually, I could be described as an automaton. I already knew, as if it had been programmed. I just said 'Okay. Thank you.' After I hung up, I closed my eyes for a brief moment, letting it really sink in. I can't say I was surprised. I react very calmly in stressful, hectic situations. On the surface, of course. My mind was racing." As both of these speakers indicate, this numbness can help us get through a difficult time, rather than falling to pieces under the stress. The numbness usually wears off when we are no longer stunned by the turn of events.

WHEN OTHER PROBLEMS BECOME ENTANGLED

Often, an unplanned pregnancy falls into our lives because we are already under severe stress. We may have been stretched too thin to attend to matters of contraception, perhaps forgetting a pill one morning amid a host of other concerns. We may even welcome pregnancy as a stabilizing force in a time of chaos; consciously or unconsciously, we may try to conceive. Pregnancy may seem like an appealing way to escape career turmoil or to bring happiness into a troubled romance. We might fantasize about how a baby could solve our problems, until a positive pregnancy test comes, making us suddenly realize how carrying to term won't work at all. For reasons such as these, we may find that our pregnancy comes at the worst possible time, when we already have more in our lives than we can handle.

Meredith: "First I Try to Kill Myself, and Then I'm Pregnant"

Twenty-one-year-old Meredith, who is white, certainly conceived during a hectic time. She was 19 or 20 when she had her third unplanned pregnancy. Her life had never been stable. Her past included a mother who left her in infancy, sexual abuse at the hands of the grandfather who raised her, a six-month marriage at 18 to a man in his forties, and abortions at 17 and 18. A dyslexic, Meredith had dropped out of high school and had worked in cocktail lounges. When she conceived for the third time, she had no job and was living with her boyfriend, Mario, who was nearly 50.

She describes the situation: "By this point, I was so fucked up I was seeing a shrink. He was giving me antidepressants and calming pills. If you just looked at my life, the main damn reason I was depressed was 'cause I wasn't working. I didn't have a place in life or any kind of competence. I was totally dependent on Mario. I lived by the fucking television set. No wonder I was depressed. I didn't need a fucking psychiatrist to tell me that. Of course, I would have preferred to take some drugs or have this guy tell me what to do, because that was much simpler." She speaks bitterly about the psychiatrist: "The guy got a lot of money. Two hundred dollars an hour. Talk about decadence and Prozac and Tranxene and Thorazine and Xanax." As Meredith thinks of the pills she took, her mind moves quickly to the alcohol she consumed at that time. She says, "We bought lots of wine and enjoyed that very much. I especially liked drinking by myself."

Meredith's depression and substance use did not help her relationship with Mario. She gives him a lot of credit for sticking by her, explaining, "He really was fantastic. He wasn't necessarily helpful, but I think that he loved me enough to be there even when I was really off the wall. And I was very off the wall." She acknowledges, "It was miserable to be around me. I was always depressed. I think I just took the entire backlog of my life and dumped it on Mario." He began to avoid her, staying out late drinking. In her solitude, Meredith used cocaine, which she calls "this great thing that enabled me to drink more." When they were together, they fought. She recalls, "We really couldn't stand the sight of each other. We couldn't go through a day without wanting to kill each other. And I was lying to myself. He was sick of me lying to myself and he was lying to himself."

One day, they had a big fight in which "some hurtful things were said. But I think he meant them," Meredith observes. She realized the relationship might end and comments, "I couldn't bear the thought of his leaving me, 'cause I couldn't function without him." Meredith attempted suicide. She recalls, "The funny thing is, I tried to kill myself with a bottle of Prozac." She wrote Mario an elaborate goodbye letter with instructions on what to do with the cat. Meredith continues, "Much to my surprise, I woke up the next day. If you take more than like fifty capsules, there's a safety release in the medicine that dissolves in your stomach so you can't do that. You may get very sick, but you can't die."

That same week, Meredith discovered she was pregnant and realized that she had been for a while. She describes her astonishment: "I didn't plan to get pregnant. It wasn't even a thought in my head." Suddenly, things made sense. Meredith laments, "If only I'd known I was" pregnant. "That was probably part of the reason I was so depressed. Every time I've been pregnant and every time I get my period, I am a typical PMS candidate. I'm very emotional and high-strung in general. When my hormones do things, I go crazy."

Despite her shock, she was thrilled; a baby represented new hope in this time of misery. Meredith recalls, "I was very excited. It was like I had forgotten what I had just done to myself–trying to kill myself. My focus shifted. I bought all these baby books." Mario, however, was less enthusiastic. Meredith understands how he felt. She says, "It's just a hell of a lot to hit Mario with. First I try to kill myself, and then I'm pregnant."

Realizing that the fetus could be damaged, especially because of the Prozac overdose, she and Mario consulted a genetic counselor. They wanted "to make sense of this thing" and to allay their worries with professional advice. Meredith spits out, "What a fucking joke of a job they have. Two hundred and fifty dollars and all they could tell me was, 'We don't know very much about Prozac, but there's a possibility that the child could be retarded.'" Meredith rolls her eyes, saying, "Then again, it could have been totally healthy." Meredith laments, "I needed that false hope, you know?"

Reluctantly, she decided to have an abortion. She recalls how hard this was for her: "I did not want to give the baby up. I felt terrible that I had to do that. I was getting the anesthetic and the doctor was about to inject it into me. I said, 'I'm sorry,' and I started crying. I just felt like, I wish I could reason my way out of this one."

It was hard for her to take the pregnancy and abortion on top of the suicide attempt. Adding to the odd timing, Meredith had visited an abortion clinic that week. Her friend had ended a pregnancy and needed support. Meredith explained the procedure and accompanied her to the clinic, thinking, "Ha, my days with that are over!"

Even now, Meredith finds the coincidences too bizarre to believe. She says, "This is all in a week. One, two, three."

The synchronicity is strange and the events are unusual. But there is nothing uncommon about the fact that a complicated story lies behind Meredith's conception and her decision to end the pregnancy. Many of us bring complex histories into a pregnancy. Our other problems and the challenges in our abortion experiences can easily become entangled, each making the others harder. When we look back on a pregnancy or abortion, several parts of our lives will probably come into the picture at the same time.

Ricki: "It Feels Stressful, Because I'm Trying to Catch Up Now"

As we cope with an unplanned pregnancy and abortion, one problem can cause another, much as a snowball becomes larger as it rolls downhill. We have seen how this may have been the case for Marilyn; the pregnancy and abortion caused her to call off her engagement, which made her depressed, which might have contributed to her bike accident. All this stress then made her herpes active. In her case, the links are speculative. We now meet Ricki, in whose case the cause-and-effect relationship is quite obvious.

Ricki, a 20-year-old African American, had an abortion six weeks ago. She remains very much involved with it, because her pregnancy caused problems she is still trying to solve. Her pregnancy occurred at the end of a semester and her grades suffered as a result. Ricki failed a class because she "blew off the final." In another class, she "was running an A," but again says, "I blew off the final and I got a B in it." Ricki wonders, "How did I get a B in this class? It was such an easy class. I'm attributing it to that," she says, referring to stress, "because I can't see any other reason I messed up."

Ricki is trying to have the failed class deleted from her record. Not wanting to use the abortion as her excuse, she will tell school officials, "I was having allergy-related problems. That's the reason I didn't do well." This is not a lie. Stress from the pregnancy and from school made Ricki's asthma acute. She says, "I even went to the hospital a few times last semester. I'm trying to use that excuse, instead of the abortion. It's probably a combination, but I'm not going to tell them that part," she says, alluding to the abortion.

If Ricki's excuse doesn't work, she will have to repeat the class she failed, which would bring traces of the fall semester's problems into spring. She already feels the effects of her previous problems on her current life, explaining that she has "added stress" this semester, "because I want to try to make up my mistakes from last semester." Ricki seems quite driven about this. She says forcefully, "I need to catch up, I need to study, I need to get all A's this semester because of last semester. So, I'm shifting focus."

In addition to this pressure, Ricki has found it stressful to hide the abortion from her family members, who would disapprove. In answer to her mother's questions about why Ricki was hospitalized with asthma, Ricki said, "Stress from school." She also attributed it to arguments with her boyfriend, Wayne. Ricki was pregnant over Christmas vacation and spent time at her parents' house, trying not to let them see how sick she felt. She managed to conceal her pregnancy, but not without some ironic moments. Suspecting that she hadn't done well on her finals, Ricki shared her concerns with her mom. She expected her mother to be angry. Instead, Ricki's mom said consolingly, "I'm not mad at you. We're proud of you. You're in school. At least you didn't drop out of school and get pregnant." Ricki said, "Oh, yeah, at least I didn't do that."

The strange thing about her mother's words was that her family doesn't usually mention this topic. Her mother may have raised the issue because, as Ricki says, "Before I knew I was pregnant, I kept talking about being serious with Wayne. And being married." Her family responded, "We don't want you to get married, because you might end up getting pregnant. Then you'll drop out of school." Ricki says with exasperation, "I started that conversation with them before I got pregnant. But they won't let that go." Ricki's reaction to such discussions? She comments, "You feel hot under the collar because you know you're pregnant." Certainly, such talks didn't help lower her stress level.

TRYING TO CONTROL LIFE'S VAGARIES

When Ricki conceived after a rare instance of not using protection, she learned what we all learn with unplanned pregnancies—some parts of life are beyond our control. Contraception is within our command, certainly, but we cannot dictate when we will or will not conceive. For some of us, this can be very frustrating, especially if we have large needs to control our lives. Ricki has that need. She says, "I'm the kind of person who sits down one night and plans out what I want to do for five years. Maybe I'm a control freak. I try to control every variable. I'm going to get married this time. I'm going to go to this school."

Insistent on mapping out her future and refusing to believe that unforeseen events can occur, Ricki was stunned to conceive against her will. She says, "It goes against the sense that I have lots of control. It's a stupid mistake and I'm not supposed to act stupid. I'm supposed to make intelligent decisions and be able to control almost all variables in my life." She has had trouble accepting that her life went off course with the pregnancy. Ricki explains that when she discovered the conception, her reaction was, "This is not part of the plan." She adds, "I was baffled. I'm supposed to go to school, graduate in four years, get married, go to law school, he goes to med school. I had it all planned out."

If, like Ricki, we discover that our plans do not hold, we may need to accept that we cannot always call the shots. This can make us feel vulnerable. It may seem that if unplanned pregnancy can happen to us, anything can. One 25 year old who had an abortion eight weeks ago has this point of view now. She says, "It's really made me feel like I'm not invulnerable. I went through that in high school when two of my friends died in a car accident and one of my friends got cancer." She notes that back then, all of this trauma "wasn't happening to me," so she still felt somewhat protected. When she conceived, however, she says it "really made me feel like anything could happen to me." Now, she fears rape, among other things, and comments, "Coming back late at night, I run through the parking lot now. I never did that before. I would just walk. Even if it were two o'clock in the morning and I was by myself. I always felt like, it can't happen to me." After an unplanned pregnancy, we may be more aware that no protective bubble deflects tragedy from our lives. Sensing our vulnerability can make us more cautious in a sensible way, or it can make us feel overly concerned about controlling our environments.

A need to control may come from our histories. Survivors of sexual abuse, in particular, may confront this issue. Cassie, age 25, has recently had memories of incest. This information helps her understand why she has always needed to have her affairs in perfect order. She says, "I'm finding out that incest survivors tend to be controlled. I hated moving into an apartment once where a friend had already been living. I felt like I was living in somebody else's house. Her stuff was all over the place. I wanted my stuff to be there. Right now, I control the stupidest things at home. When my husband sleeps, he trashes the bed. And I want him to make it. And if he forgets to make it on occasion, that should be an, 'Oh well, I'll just make it.' But it's not. For me, it blows up into this total, 'He's defying me. I want this bed made.' I'm finding that I have to be very much in control of things. And I'm afraid to let go of the control."

When Cassie had abortions at 22 and 24, she had trouble adjusting to aspects of her experiences in which she lacked control. She recalls of the pregnancies, "I was so angry that this happened to me. I did not choose this to happen. I did not want this at all. I was very upset about that." After each abortion, she felt depressed for a while and says, "The emotions bothered me, because I was not in control of those." Trying to avoid pregnancy after her abortions has been vital. She says, "I want to be able to have a little button, a little switch that I can turn on and off in myself so I will not get pregnant." Before her second abortion, Cassie consulted doctors about tubal ligation, because, as she says, "I never wanted children and I never wanted to go through pregnancy or abortion again." The doctors refused to tie her tubes, due to her youth. Lacking the control she needs, Cassie says, "It angers me that I don't have more control. I get angry at the government and other groups that aren't working harder to give me more control."

Cassie feels strongly about this issue, and she did not even conceive because of a birth control failure. Those of us who have been through method failures and abortions may have an even more acute need for reproductive control. In an effort to avoid pregnancy, we may find ourselves using three methods at a time, paying close attention to when we are most likely to conceive, and feeling anxious if periods are late. Sometimes, these efforts turn from caution into compulsiveness. Because another unplanned pregnancy may seem completely unacceptable, we may become rigid about contraception or sex.

After an abortion, we may also find ourselves being more controlled about other aspects of our lives, such as how much we eat or exercise. If the hormones of pregnancy made us gain weight, we may direct lots of attention to this matter. Twenty-eight-year-old Talia, who had an abortion four months ago, says, "I am having trouble controlling my weight right now, a problem I really have not had. I have a huge belly and I can't stand it. I am walking every day and eating less, but it's so hard!" Because our uteri can seem so hard to master, it may seem appealing to clamp down on the things we can control.

The more out of control we feel, the more we try to dictate the way things should proceed. After an abortion, we might begin to impose order on our futures–the most uncontrollable thing we face. Talia has felt compulsive not only about her weight, but also about her life. She says, "Lately I am obsessed with having order in my life, a plan. The abortion has made me think about my future, whereas before I lived mainly day to day." A pregnancy or abortion can make us evaluate our lives and see whether they match our ideals. Because so many of us end pregnancies to protect our future plans, we may be much more conscious of our life choices after an abortion.

Some of us think that having an abortion is a powerful way to assert control in our lives. We see unplanned pregnancy as usurping our power and feel that by ending the pregnancy, we can steer our lives in a chosen direction. One 40-year-old Asian American named Lynn had abortions at 17 and 33. Lynn says that the abortions have confirmed "my ability to choose the direction of my life." They allowed to her to control her affairs and to feel, "I can influence my life. I am not subject purely to 'fate' or the authority of others." Lynn's choices gave her not only a "feeling of control," but also "confidence" in her decision making. This control and confidence have "remained for the most part intact" in all the years that have passed since her abortions.

We have met several women for whom control is vital; nearly all are either women of color or incest survivors. Women in these two groups may never have received encouragement to take control of their lives. Even many white women who were not molested have learned, in effect, that passivity is more feminine. For women raised with the sense that their lives were not theirs to lead, unplanned pregnancy may have served to reinforce this feeling. It is all the more exciting, then, when previously passive women discover that they can indeed call the shots in their own lives, that they can decide what they want and carry out these wishes. In this sense, an abortion can serve as a way to exercise their voice, a way to assert, "This is who I am, and this is what I do not want." We now meet an incest survivor who began to say these things after she conceived.

Bernice: "It Was the First Time I've Taken Complete Control of My Life"

As 41-year-old Bernice recalls her Midwestern Catholic girlhood in a family of nine children, the years disappear and the tears of anger and grief return in a flash. Her mother, a pro-life leader in the community, forced Bernice's 14-year-old sister to carry a pregnancy to term and give the child up for adoption. Bernice's father and uncle molested probably every girl in the family; the silence surrounding incest is still too strong to break after all these years, so Bernice does not know how many of her sisters were affected.

She knows how the sexual abuse affected her, though. Bernice says, "The way my sex life has been throughout my life had to do with being a victim of incest. Having sex wasn't that big a deal for me, even being brought up a good, little Catholic girl." She laughs hard at these last words, adding, "It's all such bullshit. They tell you this stuff in church, and then your father crawls into bed with you at night. And nobody talks about it."

Bernice slept with several people in her teens, figuring that since she lost her virginity so young, she must be a bad girl, and what did it matter anyway? She never used birth control. She had little information; plus, using contraception would have meant taking charge of her life, which was alien to her. She recalls, "I was just completely out of control. Everybody else had control over my life–my friends, my family, my boyfriends, whoever." She did whatever anyone else wanted her to do. At age 18, she became pregnant, and a strong conviction arose within her–she would not let her mother force her to carry to term. Bernice would do anything in her power to end this unwanted pregnancy.

It was 1972 and New York was the only place for Midwestern women to obtain an abortion. After her friends made arrangements, Bernice flew to New York and ended the pregnancy. She notes the significance of this event: "It was the first time that I've taken complete control of my life and made it go the way I wanted it to go. Made things happen because I wanted my life to go in a specific direction. Nobody else had any say over what happened. It made me realize that there were things I could do to control my life."

Bernice was stunned at the power she had assumed for the first time. She explains, "I always felt I had no control as far as the incest was concerned. But once I got pregnant, I could do something about that. I could say no. And it would be no. And it was no. I could say no to this. I could never say no to the other. I could try to say no, but it would never do any good." As Bernice speaks, her words become repetitious, as if she is recreating the way she kept realizing that she could take charge. She was surprised not only that she could assume this control, but also that it was possible to change her behavior at all. She explains, "Instead of letting people talk me into doing things their way or instead of letting things slide and going, 'Oh, whatever happens, happens,' which is what I did a lot with my life, it was new and strange that I just all of a sudden sat up and said, 'No, wait, this is not something I want. This is not going to happen.'" When Bernice conceived again at age 20, she felt the same way–determined to control her destiny by ending the pregnancy.

It would be nice if the abortions changed Bernice's passivity forever, but that is too simplistic. She did not become permanently empowered. Instead, she reacted decisively when emergencies arose. Bernice says, "They were isolated incidents," adding, "In my twenties, I was mostly not in control, even when I thought I was." Bernice says she still does not "have as much control over myself, my environment, my emotional life as I would like." Incest leaves a long legacy, and Bernice's struggle with control continues.

The abortions, however, stand out as turning points when she began to be the way she wants to be. Bernice asserts that the abortions helped her recapture "a part of me that existed when I was very young, but then when my father started to abuse me, it got buried. Having to make these decisions," saying "'This is what I need to do,' and going through with it" all "made me stronger. It made me feel more confident in myself and made me see the person that I actually was"–a person "who had just gotten smothered over the years."

An unplanned pregnancy can wrest control from us and an abortion can seem overwhelming, especially if it is not straightforward emotionally or physically. When these events make us feel that our lives are unmanageable, stress levels can be high, indeed. But Bernice's story shows how abortion can also act in the opposite way, countering the stress of pregnancy and enabling us to decree what kind of life we would like to lead.

Chapter 3

The Empowering Force of Anger

As Wanda, who is 23 and Caucasian, speaks of the man who impregnated her and left, her anger seems as fresh as when he slighted her. She drifts into the present tense, saying, "I am nineteen years old. You are thirty. You have no concept about how to treat people." Then Wanda snaps back into her current reality and says, "I truly hated him."

Wanda still hates him, and for good reason—he reneged on their arrangement. When Wanda conceived, they had only dated a few months. Wanda decided on abortion, and she and Stuart agreed to begin dating again after the procedure. She explains, "We didn't know each other very well and this was a hard thing to deal with. When it was over, we could just start the relationship over." She figured he'd still be there for her.

Instead, Stuart pulled out of the relationship gradually. First, he waffled about financing the abortion. Wanda recalls, "He was going to pay for the whole thing, and then he gave me a sob story about how bad his finances were. I was like, 'Please don't pay for all of it. I'll pay for half.' Here I am waiting tables. He's a stockbroker." Stuart promised to visit Wanda after the procedure, but only came once; he arrived four hours late, staying for ten minutes. He returned none of Wanda's calls. She later learned that while she'd had the abortion, he had played golf at a country club next to the clinic.

Having had no contact with him since that time, Wanda says, "There's absolutely no sense of closure." Part of her wants to call Stuart and let him have it. But another part of her thinks, "Why would I even want to talk to this man?" She feels that "he wouldn't care one way or another." Wanda may be right, but his response may not be as important as she thinks. Even if he reacted badly or met her anger with complete silence, she might feel better letting him know how he hurt her. That way, she might not feel so powerless. Wanda has considered taking action, but in a combative way; she has fantasized about revenge and karma. Besides these vindictive thoughts, she harbors a lot of blame. She says, "I really have to put a lot of it on him because I think it could have been easier."

Wanda's first abortion experience was not easy, and she holds not only Stuart responsible, but also the clinic. Wanda's abortion occurred at fifteen weeks. The procedure lasted two days. The clinic staff inserted laminaria in her cervix so that it would dilate overnight, and sent her home without preparing her for the terrible cramps she would feel. That evening, in great pain, Wanda called a hospital; the staff said she was having contractions. Wanda cannot believe the clinic didn't warn her of this.

The clinic's staff members were impersonal. Their attitude was almost, "Here's another one. Get her over with." Wanda says, "It was like a cattle haul. They brought us all in at the same time." Wanda does not feel that the clinic considered patients' needs. Those in the waiting room could hear noises from the operating room. Wanda observes, "They didn't have the room soundproofed. You could hear the machine. So it was like waiting to be branded." Once Wanda arrived in the operating room, the clinic staff did an ultrasound and told her, "The baby's perfectly healthy." Wanda thought sarcastically, "Thank you. That's just what I needed to know." Wanda saw the ultrasound picture of her fifteen-week fetus, which disturbed her. After the procedure, as Wanda awoke from the anesthesia, she anxiously asked a nurse, "Am I all right?" The nurse responded, "You're fine," and pouted, "You pulled my hair." Wanda recalls thinking, "I've got bigger fish to fry at the moment." She adds, "Even in my state I was like, 'A little sympathy would be nice.'"

Sympathy is not what Wanda received when she drove up to the clinic for her follow-up exam. Picketers crowded around her car carrying pictures of babies' heads impaled on scalpels and yelling, "Don't kill your baby!" Unable to face the mob, Wanda drove away and called the clinic to cancel her appointment. They provided an escort for her. Still, a protester shoved a disturbing piece of literature into Wanda's hand.

As Wanda walked into the clinic, she stared at the protesters and wondered, "You don't think I felt anything about this? You think I did this like ordering a cheeseburger in a restaurant? You want me to feel bad? Fine, I feel bad." Wanda may feel badly, but she stands by her decision all the way. She describes the grim financial realities motherhood would have brought: "When you're nineteen years old, you're looking at welfare. For you and someone else! Right-to-life, yeah. What about quality of life?" Wanda has felt a great deal of pain about her abortion and continues to resent that pro-life people dare to accuse her of callousness. "I don't know if they think we're running in there, 'I'm going to have an abortion! I can't wait!'" she says with mock glee. Wanda felt no such joy as she ended her pregnancy or as she coped with insensitivity from Stuart, clinic staff members, and picketers.

Wanda has listed three groups women often resent after abortions: their partners (or men in general), medical staff members, and those who attack abortion rights. Women may also feel angry at family and friends, at themselves, and at the situation in which they have found themselves. We will see how women have handled this anger. First, though, we explore reasons for this rage, beginning with anger about gender inequities.

ANGER ABOUT THE RELATIONS BETWEEN MEN AND WOMEN

Women who have had eye-opening experiences with men may question why gender relations are the way they are. Why do men have so much freedom in the sexual arena? Why are women saddled with responsibility for birth control and pregnancy? Odessa, a Jewish woman in her mid-thirties, has asked such questions.

Odessa: "I Altered My Body So Men Could Do Whatever They Wanted"

Sixteen years ago, Odessa was date raped and impregnated. She told the man that she was pregnant and planned to have an abortion.

He reassured her that it wouldn't hurt, saying "it was just like going to the dentist and having teeth pulled." It turned out to be quite painful, and the doctors did nothing to assuage her discomfort. Noting that they were male, Odessa recalls, "The doctors were very insensitive. I had to talk them into giving me Valium in a time of great stress. I had to be present and talk them into it. They finally gave me the Valium, but they were patronizing and said there wasn't going to be pain, which wasn't true. The Valium helped a lot. It wasn't a big deal. They were acting like I was a drug addict." The procedure turned out to be incomplete and she had to have it repeated; again, Odessa went through hell trying to obtain painkillers from the clinicians.

These experiences reinforced attitudes Odessa already had about "how women are treated" in Western medicine. The rape and the difficulty with the doctors also bolstered her beliefs about how men and women relate to each other in general. Odessa says, "The experience confirmed some of the ways I felt about the patriarchy. It changed how I was going to deal with men. It strengthened my feminism." Odessa is not specific about these changes. It may be significant, however, that she later came out as a lesbian.

Odessa feels infuriated by the unequal efforts women and men make in avoiding pregnancy. This anger comes out of her own experience. Noting that she always used birth control faithfully, she sees it as ludicrous that she had to deal with a pregnancy, especially one conceived through rape. After the rape, Odessa slept with men for several years and "really resented that women have to do all the work around contraception." She thought, "What if I never have a child? All those years of using birth control!" She didn't want to have her tubes tied, figuring, "Why should I have to get my tubes tied so men can have carefree sex with me?" Odessa comments, "I felt like I always had to be taking responsibility and altering my body so men could do whatever they wanted."

She says she feels further enraged because, "There is birth control for men, but in my experience, most men do not actively involve themselves in using it." Odessa thinks men shirk this responsibility because they cannot relate to the need to prevent pregnancy. Lacking any sense of partnership with them in this arena, she feels alienated from men.

"Men Can Walk Away from Sex; Women Are Slaves to Their Bodies"

Odessa is not alone. Many women feel enraged at the men who have impregnated and abandoned them, leaving women to deal with birth control, pregnancy, and abortion, as if men have nothing to do with reproduction. Some men have even denied that they could impregnate women. One 27 year old who has had abortions at ages 24 and 26 encountered this with her second conception. She notes, "This person I was dating lied to me and told me he was sterile. I will never again believe a man." Even when men acknowledge their part in causing pregnancy, we may resent them for leaving behind their sperm, a substance that can wreak havoc in our lives. Because men are not the ones who conceive, they seem to have much more sexual freedom. Some women find this infuriating, as the next two comments show.

> [Right after her abortion] I'm waddling home from the hospital and this guy goes, "Hey babe, hey babe." I was like "Oh my God! It's because of you fuckers that I'm like feeling like shit." I was totally hating penises. The guy is able to walk away free and honk horns at women, while women have to get abortions. (Nora, age 22, eight months after her abortion)
>
> The difficult part is realizing that men can walk away from sex without worrying about consequences, whereas women are slaves to their bodies. (Georgia, age 46, who had abortions at ages 23 and 27)

Even the men who know about the pregnancies that they partly caused may not support us through births and childrearing or abortions. Women who cope with such serious matters by themselves may feel very alone–and quite angry.

ANGER AT CLINIC STAFF

Our anger at men may derive from the way male clinic staff members have treated us during our abortion experience. If a man is part of our medical staff, he is often the doctor and may have power over both the female staff members and the women who seek abortions. If he is at all insensitive, it may reinforce any anger we already feel toward men.

Sometimes, the gender of the clinic workers has nothing to do with anger we may harbor toward them. Like Wanda, we may feel that female staff members were rude, abrupt, insensitive, or impersonal. While we are at an abortion facility, we are quite vulnerable, and clinic workers' kindness or coldness may be magnified in our eyes. Here are some ways in which women have resented the way they were treated during abortions.

If Counseling Seems Insensitive or Pushy:

> While I was on the table, they were trying to pressure me into using the pill. I was just like, "Talk to me about it later." I thought that was pretty awful. Like, "Now, now, little dumb animal, should we put birth control in your feed?" (Marilyn, age 28, 11 months after her abortion)

If Staff Members Speak Down to Us or Act Judgmental of Our Choice:

> The doctor was an asshole. While I was on the table, I asked him a question. I was so nervous that I couldn't even hear his answer. He said, "Hello! Are you listening?" in a very rude tone. I'll never forget or forgive that jerk as long as I live. (Evelyn, age 18, ten days after her abortion)

If Staff Members Treat Us with a Lack of Respect:

> [At her first abortion] I was treated well by everyone, except one male doctor. He rammed three of his fingers into my vagina and was very cold. When I screamed "ouch," he shook his head and said I had to go under. I felt worthless. (Florence, age 25, who had abortions at ages 18 and 21)

> [At her second abortion] I remember the crew of doctors and nurses laughing and goofing off. This was serious to me. I was deeply offended and felt abandoned. I felt pain and screamed loud. The doctors told me to shut up or they would stop the

procedure, because I would scare the other patients. (Florence, age 25, who had abortions at ages 18 and 21)

Peggy: "I'm Mad at the Whole Hospital"

Peggy, a 26-year-old African American, shares this rage at the clinic staff members who performed her second abortion six weeks ago. She feels that the communication was terrible and that she was misled. When Peggy called her HMO, they said that the nurse would explain the procedure at the first appointment and that Peggy would return another time to have the procedure done. Instead, when Peggy arrived, the nurse said that they would insert laminaria to dilate her cervix and that the actual abortion would happen the next day. Peggy recalls, "I'm sitting there feeling trapped in a way. We had already talked about having the abortion, so I might as well have it."

Peggy felt torn, because she did not really want the abortion. She says, "In my heart, I felt like I wanted the baby." Her boyfriend, Charles, had urged her to end the pregnancy, however, because he already had two kids and wanted no more children. As Peggy spoke to the nurse and contemplated having the laminaria inserted, she became distraught. The nurse asked, "You sure you want this?" Peggy recalls, "I kept thinking about him, that he wants me to go through this and he'll be pleased, and just get it over with." The nurse asked repeatedly whether Peggy was sure about the abortion, and told her, "You don't want to go through this in a state of turmoil." Still, Peggy feels that the nurse could have done more, saying, "You need to talk to the counselor first." The nurse did not offer this option and Peggy finally consented to have the procedure. She recalls, "I lay down on the bed. At that point I started crying." As they inserted the seaweed laminaria, the nurse held Peggy's hand. Peggy says of this gesture, "I think it was only because I started crying. I don't think she would have if I didn't."

That night, Charles was furious that Peggy had begun to end the pregnancy without telling him. She considered calling off the abortion, but had grave concerns; they had told her that if they took the seaweed out, there would be a 50-50 chance that she would lose the pregnancy. Peggy decided to continue with the abortion, figuring, "I've been this far and the seaweed's in there." She returned to the

HMO the next day even less enthusiastic than before about ending the pregnancy. A nurse approached her and said, "I'm going to clean you inside and outside with Betadine." Peggy says, "She took this stick with cotton on one end dipped in Betadine and it's freezing cold. She just shoves it in there and it hurt so bad. I felt like I was being raped. It was the worst feeling in my life. It wasn't her body she was cleaning. It didn't hurt her. It hurt the hell out of me!"

When the procedure ended, the doctor told Peggy, "It's over. You did so well." Peggy says, "I was so pissed. I was mad at him and all the nurses, the whole hospital." In the next weeks, Peggy wanted a follow-up exam, but was told this was unnecessary. Outraged, Peggy notes, "If I felt that I wanted a checkup after this procedure, it shouldn't be a problem." Peggy is absolutely right; a post-op exam is advisable and is usually mandatory in an abortion facility. She resents her HMO's lack of concern, saying, "It doesn't matter to them."

Peggy's experience seems mixed. The staff members were somewhat caring and partially insensitive. They should have been clear with her that the laminaria would be inserted during the first appointment and should have examined her two weeks later. Peggy may be angry, however, for reasons other than those she stated. She appears to be mad at Charles and at herself for ending the pregnancy. The clinic workers may be an easy target for all that anger–it could be that she holds them responsible for the decision, displacing her anger onto them. It is perhaps easier to be mad at the "whole hospital" than at Charles or herself.

ANGER AT THE ANTIABORTION MOVEMENT AND CATHOLICISM

Some women are angry after a clinic visit, but not at the staff. Instead, many women resent those who picket abortion facilities and hurl abuse. We may harbor great anger toward those who judge our choice and infringe on our rights. The following comments show this rage.

Anger at Those Who Oppose Abortion:

> I'm a black woman. If I have the child, you better be ready to take care of that child, because it's going to go into foster

care–a system that doesn't want it. Most pro-life people aren't willing to do that. If half the people in the pro-life movement adopted children, there would be no unadoptable children. Until all the children are adopted, I think no one has any right to say anything. (Sabine, age 23, two years after her abortion)

Anger at Catholicism for Its Stance on Abortion:

> Long before my first abortion, the Catholic church lost its grip on my mind. I feel sorry, though, for the woman who is still trapped by the Vatican patriarchy, is poor as dirt, already has six kids she can't feed, and her church says, "A gift from God!" A hell of a gift: no food, no inoculations, no clothes, and guaranteed fifteen-plus years of dependency. (Gabriella, age 38, who had abortions at ages 22, 24, and 26)

We may feel enraged that many in the antiabortion movement have no concept of our individual situations and have the gall to impose narrow-minded, unrealistic views on us.

Bernice: "A Completely Unrealistic Attitude"

Bernice, age 41, bears much of the resentment these women express, both out of her political convictions and her personal experience. Bernice becomes enraged when anything threatens reproductive rights. Her personal history is less mainstream. Bernice was one of nine children. Her mother, the local pro-life leader, forced her 14 year old, Bernice's sister, to carry a pregnancy to term and to give the child up for adoption. Bernice's mother had thirteen pregnancies. She only began using birth control when her doctor said she would die if she had another child. First, she consulted her priests about the matter.

Given the Catholic atmosphere in which Bernice grew up, she blames the church "for screwing up my attitude so much that I just got stupid." By "stupid" behavior, Bernice means using no birth control, which allowed her to conceive at ages 18 and 20–pregnancies she ended. After putting herself down, she catches the error in her logic and says sarcastically, "I'm stupid, right? Not the men or anyone else I was with." She flipflops two more times on the matter, saying, "I just feel like it was something that I could have known better. But then how could I have known better if no one taught me?"

As a teenager, Bernice had little information about sexual decisions. Bernice mainly holds the church responsible for not dispensing information and for denying that teenagers will have sex. Bernice comments, "All they ever told you was, 'Don't do it.'" They provided "nothing about birth control, nothing about abortion, nothing about anything else. Just don't have sex." Bernice finds this "a completely unrealistic attitude," arguing that teenagers throughout history have had sex. Bernice thinks it is despicable that the church tries to shame young women into abstinence and finds this approach unhelpful to young minds. She says if teens attempt to make an informed decision about sex by asking, "Why shouldn't I have sex?", the church simply responds, "Because it's not right. Because good girls don't do that." The church issues condemnation without exploring the issue further. Lacking useful guidelines, Bernice conceived twice and ended up having two abortions–certainly not the outcome the church had in mind when it withheld information.

ANGER AT A GENERAL LACK OF SUPPORT

Unlike Bernice, who bristles at the church's unhelpfulness, 25-year-old Becky resents that her loved ones have been unhelpful since her abortion two months ago. She is stunned that her friends and family have taken no interest in her emotional needs and don't seem to care that she is in pain. Becky keeps waiting for someone to notice that she is unhappy and to respond in a loving way, but no one has provided this support.

Becky met with such apathy from the beginning of her crisis. When she told people she was going to have an abortion, no one challenged her. Becky was ambivalent about her choice, and wanted some resistance so she could articulate her reasons out loud. She sought such opposition from several people. Becky found a therapist and told her, "I'm pregnant and I'm going to have an abortion next week." The therapist never questioned this decision. Nor did her HMO, which offered no abortion counseling, treating abortion "like a procedure." Becky's boyfriend felt that abortion was the best solution and told her, "I can't financially and I'm not ready emotionally to be a father." It angers her that he favored abortion, perhaps because he based this decision on his needs, not hers.

Her family also leaned toward abortion for her because it met their needs. Becky's father is a clergyman, and Becky thinks her parents would have been embarrassed for their unmarried daughter to come to services with a swelling abdomen. She muses, "Were they really thinking of me, or themselves?" Becky believes they saw her abortion as a way to wrap the problem in a "neat little package" so no one else would know. Making matters worse, Becky's mom asked her to tell her 17-year-old sister about the pregnancy so that it wouldn't happen to her. Becky laments, "I felt like I was being used."

Since the abortion, the people in Becky's life have continued to draw a blank about how to respond to her emotionally. She fumes, "Because there weren't any big physical problems, no one was really understanding." She needed their help. Becky explains, "I was freaked out. Nothing has ever happened this big in my life before. All these feelings were coming at me and I didn't know how to cope." She wanted to hear, "I know this is hard for you now. And everything's going to be okay." Instead, people said, "You'll get over it." Becky comments, "No one really validated how hard it was for me." People's inadequate responses made Becky feel isolated. She explains, "I was feeling really alone, because I had all this anger at everyone. I felt like everyone let me down."

Becky understands, though, that there may be a difference between how people acted and how they felt. She muses, "No one made a big deal, but I wonder what everyone was thinking. I'm sure my parents were more affected by it than they let on." She realizes that although people seemed distant, they were probably trying to hide their discomfort. Becky has tried to see it from their point of view. She says, "I thought about how I've reacted to people when someone close to them has died. It's hard, because you can't really say anything that will make them feel better. I guess that's how people were with me."

Becky realizes that "people can only give a certain amount," that they have withheld support out of their own limitations, not because they want to cause her pain. Perhaps the people in Becky's life are not as aware of the emotional drama going on within her as she thinks. Whatever the reasons for their silence, Becky is enraged to find that she can go through the biggest crisis of her life without much apparent concern from others.

ANGER AT THE SITUATION AND AT OURSELVES

During a pregnancy and abortion experience, we may resent the situation in which we find ourselves. We might feel angry that we are pregnant and that we have to cope with extra stress. If so, we may blame God or the fetus for "causing" the pregnancy. The following comments show such anger about being pregnant.

> After I found out I was pregnant, I punched myself in the abdomen out of anger. Anger not at myself or at Dwight, but at the "child" for being a pain in the ass and forcing me to do things I didn't have the patience or money to do. (Regina, age 25, seven years after her abortion)

> [With her first terminated pregnancy] I definitely felt a lot of anger about my pregnancy. I wasn't mad at anyone, really. Just mad that I had to deal with the hassle of getting an abortion–and mad that being pregnant and waiting to have an abortion were consuming my thoughts and time. I wanted to just go on with my life as usual. I didn't want to have to deal with it. (Nicola, age 25, who had abortions three years ago and two weeks ago)

It can be hard to live with such anger when no person or institution is particularly accountable. This anger, however, may fade when the stress of the situation ends.

What may be harder to handle than anger at the world is rage at ourselves. After discovering an unplanned pregnancy, we may blame ourselves for the partner we chose, for forgoing birth control (or for not using it diligently), and for how we make the decision to have an abortion. After an abortion, we may lambast ourselves for our choice and for feeling the "wrong" amount of emotion. The next comments show how some of us direct rage at ourselves.

> I am so angry at myself for getting pregnant, for messing up the fetus with substances, and for aborting it. I don't think I'll ever forgive myself. (Evelyn, age 18, ten days after her abortion; Evelyn is pro-life)

> Both times, I was mad at myself for not being more careful. I'm surprised at how much blame I placed on myself for getting pregnant, but if I placed blame on the guy, it would feel like I was giving him power. (Nicola, age 25, who had abortions three years ago and two weeks ago)

The second speaker indicates that she feels more in control by blaming herself. Taking the blame may feel right, particularly if we make a habit of criticizing ourselves. Self-blame may also be easier than accepting others' shortcomings. It may not, however, be justified.

Ricki: "I Felt Like a Hypocrite"

We may feel angry at ourselves if we have gone against our own moral code. Twenty-year-old Ricki, who is a Black Muslim, opposes abortion and has been mad at herself since she had an abortion six weeks ago. She had the hardest time the night after the abortion. She recalls, "I woke up in the middle of the night and I felt so bad. I was crying all night. I felt really low, like I was the stupidest person on earth." Ricki says she felt stupid "for everything I did. Stupid for getting pregnant in the first place. Stupid for letting him talk me into having an abortion. I just started hating him," she says, referring to her boyfriend, Wayne. Ricki continues, "I was mad at everything. I felt like I couldn't take the event back." She blames herself for having conceived at all, saying, "I knew what I could have done to stop it and I didn't." She and Wayne usually used contraception, but had no condoms once or twice and went ahead with sex anyway. Ricki also assails herself for being sexually active before marriage, saying, "If I had not had sex in the first place, then it wouldn't have happened." What bothers Ricki most is having had an abortion when she thinks abortion is wrong. She says that at first, "I felt like a hypocrite, because I'm professing that I don't believe in this, but I see myself doing it."

THE DANGERS OF UNRESOLVED ANGER

Ricki finds it hard to live with herself after transgressing her values. Anger at oneself can be difficult to withstand, sometimes leading to depression. When any type of anger persists for a long time, we can become stuck. We may invest a lot of energy into maintaining our anger, thinking it essential to keep saying that we are right and another is wrong. Acknowledging our own role in, say, an abortion, may feel too frightening. We may need to protect ourselves by heaping blame on someone else. Ricki has tried this approach.

Blaming Other People

In her discomfort with breaking her moral code, Ricki began to wonder, "How can I justify this to myself to make myself not feel that way?" Then, she came up with the key: "I started blaming other people: 'I wouldn't have done it if he didn't want me to do it or if my parents supported me.'" Ricki has great insight here into what many of us do unconsciously–when we cannot bear to take responsibility for our actions, we try to blame others.

Ricki mainly blames Wayne for her abortion. Although he also opposes abortion, he focused on practical concerns when Ricki conceived. He pointed out that she would have to drop out of school for lack of money. When Wayne insisted, "You have no choice. You have to do this," Ricki felt "trapped." He quickly treated the decision as a moot issue. She says, "We talked about it for a few minutes and that was it. Every time I tried to bring it up after that, he was like, 'There's nothing we can do about it.'" Ricki splutters, "He made it sound like a math problem, like there's only one answer."

Ricki had an abortion after all, and feels that Wayne forced her to do this. Her anger at him is quite understandable. He neither gave her the space to explore her feelings, nor respected that her wishes might be different from his own. In her anger, she feels like a victim of his strong will. Ricki will probably have to keep blaming him because it is too uncomfortable for her to look at her own role in choosing abortion. Her anger at him–which covers up anger at herself–may last a long time.

Powerlessness

Ricki feels powerless within a relationship in which her feelings have been ignored and with a pregnancy that felt impossible to bring to term. It seems that she began to believe what Wayne told her–that she had no choice. If we feel as powerless as Ricki, we might begin to think of ourselves as victims. In this mindset, we might shrug off all responsibility for our actions. Feeling that someone has wronged us, we may feel entitled to do anything to avenge ourselves. We might not stop at one or two instances of revenge, instead waging a continual war. We may have become the aggressors, but, still feeling powerless, we might be blind to the effect we have on others. All we know is that we were treated unjustly and that nothing can remedy this. There are three dangers here: first, we may harm other people; second, we may overlook our own ability to redress injustice; third, the anger might fester, hardening into bitterness and hurting us more than anyone else.

RESOLVING ANGER

Anger is not always dangerous. It is a necessary response to injustice and attack. A lack of anger would be worrisome, meaning that we didn't care if others hurt us. Some of us may act indifferent because we are afraid to let anger surface, because it might be explosive. We might also worry that anger is unfeminine. It is important to acknowledge our anger, to let those feelings come forward, and to realize that such feelings are not destructive, in and of themselves. The key is what we do with the anger.

It may be helpful to step back from the situation before taking action. We may need to understand our own position a little better. Why are we angry? What need of ours did someone overlook? Once we establish our own stance, we might try to understand what others have brought to the conflict. Did they hurt us out of malice or mere thoughtlessness? Assessing people's motivations can make it seem more manageable to deal with those people. We may decide that they are trying to meet needs of their own through their hurtful actions.

Understanding Men

We might ask why men treat women as they do. For instance, we may try to explain why so many men shirk their contraceptive responsibility. Could it be that some men don't have a strong sense of cause and effect where sex and pregnancy are concerned? It may take the edge off our anger if we consider that men may not be out to get us. Perhaps they simply "don't get it." In many ways, the two genders don't understand each other well, and an area such as birth control that can require cooperation just exacerbates the problem. It can be enlightening to realize that men sometimes feel angry and helpless because women wield so much power over pregnancy; a woman can lie about using birth control and can decide the fate of a pregnancy. It would help the two genders come a little closer if we acknowledge how vulnerable we each are to the other's whims in these matters.

It is also important to realize that many men do support women. Countless men wear condoms, not just out of concern about contracting diseases, but also out of a sense of responsibility. Men frequently give women space to make decisions about pregnancies. Many men accompany women to abortions, holding their hands during the procedures and taking care of them afterward. Men often remain committed to women after abortions, and couples frequently feel closer because they have withstood this crisis together.

Understanding Clinic Workers

A man and woman may hurt each other in an attempt to meet their own needs—needs that may have little to do with the other person. Similarly, when clinic staff members act disrespectfully toward women having abortions, the clinic workers' actions may have little to do with the patients. Melba, a 46-year-old Caucasian doctor, has insight into this issue. She points out that surgery is very demanding. She says, "In order to be attentive, focused, and disciplined, there is an emotional distancing." She adds, "You cannot allow your own emotional vulnerability to get in the way of your own judgment and attention when you're in the midst of a surgical procedure." Melba opines that in medical school, students are invited into different specialties partly based on their personalities.

Melba believes that an ability to be detached is seen as a boon in surgery, so colder people are more likely to become surgeons.

When Melba performed abortions in a feminist clinic from 1977 to 1979, the clinic staff tried to reinforce this distance between doctor and patient. Distrusting doctors, the staff members wanted doctors to function as surgical technicians, rather than connecting with patients. Once, when Melba put a comforting hand on a patient's shoulder, they pulled her arm away. The clinic workers attacked Melba whenever she addressed patients' emotional concerns about abortion. She explains that for the clinic staff, "There was tremendous denial that abortion was not just a physical experience." In having this point of view, the clinic workers were responding to pressures in the political furor over abortion.

Because of the demands of their job, the clinic workers may be cold toward the patient, on occasion. They may be frustrated to see so many unintended pregnancies. They might feel hopeless because some women use birth control erratically, or not at all. Caring for several clients despite stretched financial and emotional resources may cause staff members to feel stressed, and they might take these concerns out on the occasional patient. It can be hard for clinic workers to treat each client as unique. This is no excuse for coldness. But it may help to remember that clinic staff are under great pressure, facing zealots who will shoot them with pleasure and a society that stigmatizes their work. Clinic workers may find it hard to keep giving. It is also important to note that there are many wonderful clinic workers of both genders who have helped thousands of women feel supported.

Accepting People's Limitations

Clearly, many clinic staff members have limits on what they can give us, as do many men. This can be disappointing if we go through an abortion experience depending on their kindness, and meet instead with neglect or even cruelty. We can rage against them, but once the clinic workers and men drop out of our lives, they will not hear our complaints. Instead, our anger will reverberate in our heads, bothering only us. At some point, it may feel better to let go of this anger, to move beyond it, accepting other people's limitations. This is not the same as excusing their behavior. Relinquishing our anger may be more akin to saying that this battle is going nowhere and that there are better ways for us to spend our energy.

One 24 year old has experience with letting go of anger. Since Elissa had an abortion five months ago, her boyfriend has been hot and cold toward her. She has felt enraged and hurt. Now, Elissa tries to set aside her anger and accept him for what he is. She says, "In order not to be bitter and overtaken by anger and sourness, I turned those feelings into compassion. The only way I could sleep at night was to realize that he just wasn't able to give me what I needed. I can't be mad at his inabilities. I must recognize them and pray for him." This approach is not easy. Elissa recalls, "I was torn to pieces. I felt like I was dancing around his feelings and I was the one who went through the hell. But I truly found compassion and it was the only way I could keep going with some sort of peace." Recognizing what he can and cannot provide has given Elissa realistic expectations and has ended her cycles of hope and disappointment.

Taking Action

It may not be satisfying to accept people's limits if we feel we can help them change. We may want to harness the energy behind our anger and use it to right the wrongs. Some of us take anger to a higher level, acting on convictions about how things should be different, feeling powerful in this way, instead of focusing on how we were mistreated.

Brittany, a 22-year-old Caucasian, took action after receiving deplorable treatment at a feminist clinic three years ago. Brittany liked some features of the clinic, but says, "I didn't like the way they were talking to me." They told her, "It's a fetus" and "a tissue," not "a baby," the term Brittany prefers. She found their approach "very forceful." Smacking her hands together, she imitates how the clinic workers implied, "There's nothing wrong with what you're doing." She did not find their method reassuring and says, "There wasn't really an opening for me to have an opinion. It was like, 'This is the way it is.'" She finds their attitude unnecessary, saying, "I think they were used to having to reassure people about it." Perhaps they harbored some ambivalence and wanted to reassure themselves about the procedure. In any case, Brittany did not benefit from their approach.

She has very different ideas about what would ease the experience. She says, "There really needs to be space for people to feel horrible about having an abortion. To cry their eyes out, or to feel like killers," as opposed to being persuaded otherwise. Brittany believes clinic staff shouldn't insist, "It's not a baby," but might say, "This is another person that you care a lot about. This must be hard for you."

Brittany couldn't have an abortion at that facility. For financial reasons, she had to have it at her HMO, which met her emotional needs even less. The clinic workers did not seem interested in talking to her. Brittany says with much frustration, "I did not feel like there was anyone who had given thought to anything beside the procedure."

Enraged about how hard it was to find a facility sensitive to her needs, Brittany volunteered at the first facility, the feminist clinic. She explains, "I thought they really needed some help figuring out how to counsel people where they weren't pushing their views of abortion on people." She went twice to learn how to counsel, before her schedule made this volunteer work impossible. In those two visits, she was appalled at how much the counselors imposed their beliefs on the patients. Brittany notes, "I remember their really feeling strongly that they needed to calm people down when they were crying. One woman didn't want to open her legs for an abortion and they all tried to talk her into opening her legs." Brittany says the clinic workers' attitude toward hesitant women was one of impatience and frustration, along the lines of, "Oh, God, why do these women feel this way?"

Brittany had a second abortion one year later at her HMO. Again, she felt frustrated by how the staff members acted. She explains, "The nurse who said she would stay with me through it left the room for the abortion and didn't come back until it was over." Afterward, she lay in the recovery room and cried about the abortion. The clinic workers tried to comfort her out of her tears, murmuring, "Don't cry now," or "You're all right. It's over." Brittany understands that they uttered these words with good intentions. She comments, however, "I don't think it was that helpful to have people trying to stop me from crying."

Brittany feels unsatisfied with these emotional experiences, but carries neither a sense of hurt nor burning anger. She has tried to fix injustices. Now, she grapples with "how to be most powerful in addressing" abortion issues and how to make "the world at large in regard to abortion more how I want it to be. Figuring out what the steps are." Not every unjust situation can be fixed with simple steps. But Brittany's approach seems more rewarding than fuming in silence or feeling like a victim who cannot influence the world.

Chapter 4

Allowing Ourselves to Grieve the Losses

Since Wanda had an abortion at 19, she has moved across the country and fallen in love with a new partner. Four years have passed, but Wanda occasionally still feels grief about that abortion. As she recalls how the feelings returned one night, her green eyes become round, and she sweeps her straight, red hair behind one ear. She says, "My boyfriend and I were getting ready to go to sleep. And I looked up and said, 'Honey, I'm really upset about this.'" He did not understand, so Wanda insisted, "I miss it. I miss that child. I lost something." Wanda remembers panicking and yelling, "You don't understand. There's something gone!" She adds, "It's like I went into the room, they gave me the anesthetic, and all of a sudden something's gone that I will never, ever get back."

Before her abortion, Wanda did not expect to feel this way. She thought, "People get pregnant and if you want, you can have an abortion. It's no big deal. I wasn't anywhere near prepared for the things that I was going to feel."

Wanda did not have a typical abortion in some ways. Caught in denial, she put off recognizing that she was pregnant and finally had her abortion at fifteen weeks. The second-trimester abortion was difficult physically. After having laminaria inserted to dilate her cervix, she returned home, unaware that the laminaria would stimulate contractions. Wanda discovered that the only way to relieve her pain was to crawl.

After she had the abortion the next day, she went home to bleak circumstances. Her car had broken down and she lived in a town where a car was essential. Her boyfriend had stopped returning her calls, and her brother felt awkward about the abortion, so he did not look in on her much. She recalls, "I was completely by myself. It was pouring rain. I had no food in the house. And after being pregnant for fifteen weeks, I was a mess." Wanda details how she spent her time: "The first day-and-a-half, I was pretty much in bed. It really took a lot out of me. Most of the time, I just sat inside, stared out the window, looked at the rain, and cried. For days." Wanda lights another cigarette and recalls how empty she felt: "I had nothing left but a memory of crawling around on a floor and screaming my head off." She felt not only that she had lost the fetus, but that she had somehow lost a bit of herself. A month after the abortion, she wrote in her journal, "During that ten-minute procedure, I destroyed just the tiniest bit of Wanda. That's kind of hard to get a grip on."

Since that time, Wanda has had another unplanned pregnancy. Eight months ago, her birth control pills failed. She and her boyfriend are in a reasonably secure, loving relationship, so having the baby was a definite possibility. On the other hand, neither of them have finished college and their career prospects seemed pretty dismal. Financially, they were not in the best position. And they still felt quite young. Still, because Wanda's first abortion had caused her so much distress, she gave the second decision ample consideration. She finally decided on abortion again, but spent five days with the fetus, speaking to it, eating food she thought it might enjoy, and saying goodbye.

Wanda describes how she feels now: "This time, I feel like I miss something maybe even a little bit more, because I gave this one more the benefit of the doubt of actually having feelings or thoughts or being involved with my life with Colin. And this one had a lot more identity." Because she tried to imagine the fetus as it would be after birth and how it would affect their lives, this fetus was more developed in her mind than the first.

Thinking it "completely acceptable" to grieve after an abortion, Wanda has mourned for each fetus. She refuses, however, to imagine what the fetus could have become. Wanda says, "I accepted quite a while ago that that's something I'll never know." She notes that when families lose a child, they often assume the kid would have grown up to be a superstar. Wanda cautions, "You don't know that. He could have been a junkie. You can project all you want, but you don't know. So why waste your time and energy creating a life existence and personality for someone who's not there anymore?"

Wanting to put her grief to a better use, Wanda has run a support group for HIV-positive men. She told the members her reason for joining: "I had an abortion and I feel like there's a little part of me missing or that I took a little something away from the world." By running the group, she gave something back. In the group, Wanda came face to face with people's grief and loss, as well as her own. Although her abortion losses caused her great pain, she did not shy away from experiencing those feelings again. Perhaps she joined the support group so that she could restimulate her sense of loss and resolve her feelings about her abortions. Acknowledging that she has not closed the file on those losses, she comments, "I don't know if I look at it as a situation that can ever be totally resolved." Nor does she know if it is possible to feel blasé about her abortions, if there will ever be a day when she can shrug and say, "That's just something I did." The "hurt," she comments, is "an ongoing thing." She believes that her grief may indeed ebb someday. But, she notes, "That's not what I'm looking for." Wanda is more interested in accepting her abortions and feeling the grief they have brought than in dulling her pain.

Wanda's story shows some of the losses one can feel after an abortion and illustrates a good way to act on grief. In this chapter, we will explore loss and grief more fully as they might arise in an abortion experience, and ways of responding to this grief.

LOSSES SUSTAINED IN THE ABORTION EXPERIENCE

After an abortion, some of us feel no loss at all—only gains. We may feel relieved that the abortion has restored freedom and that the challenges of the pregnancy have made us grow. We may also rejoice in seeing an end to nausea, swollen breasts, and a lack of energy.

Others dislike ending pregnancy's physical aspects. Pregnancy can bring pride in fertility and femininity, excitement, a sense of being special, uncontracepted sex, an increase in libido, extra calories each day with impunity, and, if we have never carried to term, a preview of how that might be. We may feel sad to lose these assets.

The most obvious loss sustained in an abortion is that of the fetus. Grief about this loss may take us entirely by surprise. We cannot anticipate how sad we will feel about most losses. An abortion, which can bring complicated feelings anyway, is even less predictable. Grief about a fetus may feel irrational. Why would we feel loss if we chose to have an abortion? Probably because we developed some feelings for the fetus. It is possible to become very attached to a pregnancy, even in a few weeks. The fetus may take on special significance for us. Each of us defines that significance differently. We now meet Clarissa, a 30-year-old Caucasian who had an unusual relationship with her fetus.

Clarissa: "I Could Feel the Second That Spirit Left My Body"

Clarissa describes the abortion she had five years ago: "I swear I could feel the second that spirit left my body. It was as if I were having a tug of war with this soul. Like holding onto the hand of a child and someone is pulling from the other side, its arms being jerked at both ends until in the end it's just gone. All of a sudden no resistance–no pulling. Everything is over. At that moment, I wailed. I never thought I would feel such deep sadness, that it would feel like such a real loss of a person who never existed." Later that day, Clarissa was "a raving, screaming, crying, hysterical, angry, mournful mess."

Part of her pain came from a pact she made with the fetus's spirit when she conceived. She recalls that as she and her boyfriend made love, "I felt like there was a spirit of the child, a soul there, and I had a conversation with it. It was asking if it was okay to come to me. I assured it, it was. That no matter what, I would protect and take care of it."

When she discovered that she was in fact pregnant, Clarissa was going to carry to term. She explains, "I was happy. The positive feelings came from the beauty of conceiving life. It's just an incredible feeling and I see it as a blessing, a gift. Since I cared deeply for the father, it was a good thing until I saw how unmutual it all was." Her boyfriend objected to the pregnancy. He wanted to be a responsible dad and did not feel that he could be at that point. Clarissa considered his needs and those of the child and agreed to have an abortion.

In the two weeks after she made this decision, she says it was "terrible" to carry the pregnancy. She embarked on a new relationship with the fetus, smoking and drinking in front of her boyfriend "in a vindictive manner" so he would see her pain. She comments, "I never envisioned my uterus or the contents. I didn't want to know anything more about it." Clarissa had to block out the fetus, maybe to prevent herself from feeling attached to it, or perhaps because she felt guilty about breaking her promise. Even now, she feels quite guilty and sad about that breach of faith. She says, "I betrayed this soul, whether it was real or not. I betrayed myself, at least." Clarissa adds, "In my spiritual world, that was a very serious betrayal and I regret this very much. I'm a lot more careful about promises in the tangible world." Clarissa felt attached to the fetus and gave it her word, losing in one instant both a potential child and part of her integrity.

"Giving up the Dream"

When a pregnancy ends, we lose any dreams we had for the pregnancy or fetus. Twenty-five-year-old Cassie feels that pain ten months after her second abortion. At first, she and her boyfriend, Todd, decided to keep that pregnancy. They went to Nevada for a quickie wedding and began to dream about the child they would have. She explains how far they got in visualizing the pregnancy: "We bought a disk called 'Songs To Be Born By.' And we had thought about getting a beeper so that he would know if I went into labor. And finding a quiet place to live. I was thinking about baby clothes. Cute little things I could buy."

Then reality set in, involving Cassie's sickness, their money problems, and Todd's depression about his menial job. Suddenly, the pregnancy seemed impossible. Cassie recalls, "There was still that little part of us that wanted to go ahead and do it. But for the most part, we couldn't. And I felt like it was circumstances beyond our control. If we'd had the money, we could have done it." As Cassie speaks about this time in their lives, she cries easily. Her sadness has to do with "giving up the dream." She notes, "If everything had been perfect, I wouldn't have been sick throughout my pregnancy, we would have had money, and we'd have this baby that would just bring love and joy and absolutely no trouble to our lives. I knew that wasn't realistic, but it was cool to think about."

Cassie has lost her dreams about that second pregnancy, but she can still dream of future pregnancies. For others of us, this is not true after an abortion. We may decide to rule out any more unplanned pregnancies and have a tubal ligation; alternatively, our partners might have vasectomies. In such cases, we part with both a particular pregnancy and with our childbearing potential, an often cherished aspect of womanhood.

For Fern, abortion went hand in hand with closing the door on motherhood. At age 32, when Fern found herself unexpectedly pregnant, she made a larger decision than whether to carry this pregnancy to term. With thirteen years' hindsight, she says, "I knew in choosing abortion that I was not only saying 'no' to that pregnancy. I was also saying 'no' to ever being a mother. I had much more grief about that. I wondered, 'What would it be like? Am I going to regret never having the experience?'" She had never imagined herself as a mother, but wanted to explore the possibility.

Fern spent a lot of time speaking with the fetus's spirit and doing visualizations to imagine her life with or without this child. By focusing so much on her feelings about this pregnancy, she found after the abortion that she had already mourned the loss of the fetus. She still had a keener sense of loss about rejecting maternity. Fern had to accept that motherhood is not her chosen path. She has achieved that resolution over time, especially as she has made career choices that would not have meshed well with motherhood. In addition, Fern laughs, "It's helped to hear from several psychics that I've had many lifetimes where I've been a mother and that that's not what this life is about for me."

"Part of Myself Died"

In giving up a possibility, both Fern and Cassie relinquished parts of their dreams or their futures, which were central to their senses of self. Other women feel much more directly that they have lost part of themselves through an abortion. Two years after her abortion, one 22 year old comments, "I feel like I became darker the day of my abortion. Heavier. Some pure light-hearted part of myself died that day." If we have an unplanned pregnancy or abortion when we are young, we might feel that it takes away our youthfulness or our ability to be carefree. One 41 year old, who was molested during her early years, notes surprisingly that at her first abortion at 18, she felt "the loss of girlhood even more than when I first had sex. I think I felt a loss of innocence." If we perceived ourselves as "good girls" before the pregnancy or abortion, we might think that this is no longer true and may feel sad about that. It can be quite painful to feel that we have lost a valued part of ourselves. The more we believe that the pregnancy and abortion go against our sense of self, the harder we will find it to accept these experiences.

To say that part of oneself is lost, however, need not be negative. We may lose naiveté or narrow-mindedness, clearing the way for growth and empathy. One 22 year old expresses positive feelings about how her abortion at 20 changed her sense of self: "I felt loss to a certain extent, but I felt that by denying the birth of another, I could give birth to myself." The experience we gain may become a valued part of who we are.

Still, we may grieve that our life has brought us unexpected pain, that it has deviated from the course we hoped it would take. One 22 year old feels sorrowful about this four years after her pregnancy ended. She says, "I feel sad that I had to have an abortion. I feel sad that I had to get pregnant at a time when I couldn't have a child. I feel sad that I had to choose to give up my child. I feel sad that I was not responsible in my sexual activity." Like this woman, we may feel unhappy that we had to go through unnecessary troubles. A 31 year old feels this way nine years after her abortion. First, she was date raped. Then, she found out she was pregnant and decided on abortion. Her roommate alerted the local antiabortion group. This unfortunate woman recalls, "The most painful part had to do with being harassed by a right-to-life group trying to talk me out of it. They even went to my church to tell the youth minister what I was doing. I never went back to church after that. I feel sad that I was harassed by the right-to-life group–and how they shamed me for my choice." Sometimes, when life has brought us trauma such as this woman describes, it is harder to see the loss as making room for a gain. Maturity, wisdom, and strength can take root, but trust and optimism may have been destroyed.

Simply by conceiving an unplanned pregnancy, we may feel that we have lost security. Life may seem chaotic, unfair, and perhaps unmanageable. If we conceived because birth control failed, we may find it hard to trust contraception in the future. Sex may seem less safe and less fun, which can represent a terrible loss of freedom.

Lost Relationships, Old and New

As we go through an abortion, we may compare it to other instances of loss. Sometimes, the loss of a fetus pales in comparison to losing a person we have seen, known, and loved. A 35 year old explains how the abortion she had ten years ago was a relatively small loss compared with the deaths of her grandmother and dog, and the loss of her husband, who had to be put in a mental hospital. Another woman, age 42, concurs, six months after her abortion: "I only grieve about the deaths of my loved ones (friends and family). This was neither. This was nothing compared to the loss of my loved ones, either from cancer or AIDS. That's a rough experience to go through, watching your loved ones die slowly each day. The abortion was easy."

A loss tends to bring other losses to mind. After an abortion, we may miss people who have left our lives. One 25 year old found this to be true right after the abortion she had ten months ago. She comments, "After the abortion, I started feeling a lot of sadness about my relationship with my father. He sexually and emotionally abused almost every member of my family. I hadn't had contact with him for two years, but I had never felt sad about it before." As we grieve about our abortions, we may find ourselves tending to wounds sustained in old relationships.

Going through an unplanned pregnancy and abortion can also cause us to face ruptures in current relationships. Quite often, an unexpected pregnancy can put pressure on a romance, causing disagreements or a lack of communication. Sometimes a pregnancy can lead a couple to examine their future together and to decide that they are better off apart. Losing a relationship as well as a pregnancy can be terribly painful and complicated.

After an abortion, we can also lose people in another sense. They may not leave our lives, but they may disappoint us, making us realize that the bonds were not as strong as we thought. Friends and family may react to our news in ways we do not expect, which might lead us to reevaluate those relationships. Whether a relationship suffers only in the moment or in the long term, we might grieve the loss involved in this disappointment.

Emerald: "I Needed People to Be There for Me"

Emerald, a 35-year-old Caucasian, has felt this deep disappointment in others since her second abortion, six months ago. Several people disappointed her when she most needed them. She recalls being angry at the health care providers, who [she] felt didn't take my sense of my own body seriously." These clinicians pooh-poohed her accurate feeling that her abortion was incomplete. She also felt "extremely angry" at her friend's response to the abortion. This friend was "acting out issues around her own pregnancies and abortions." Emerald adds, "I have rage and loss over my ex-partner." Emerald and Gaylin had broken up before they conceived, but continued to have sex. After Emerald discovered her pregnancy, she planned to keep the baby and felt extremely excited. Initially supportive, Gaylin then slipped back into substance abuse and became hostile toward Emerald. Hurt and angry, she ended the relationship for good.

Emerald usually supports other people and says, "I am not often in these types of situations where, whammo, suddenly I need you to be there for me." Because her request for help was so rare and so acute, she found it difficult to forgive those who could not come to her assistance. She says, "In the most pragmatic kind of way, I can't afford to keep around people who don't give me support. So I mostly choose to let them go."

Emerald sees that her anger and grief are interlinked. She says, "I always consider anger a sign pointing at sadness and disappointment"; underneath any anger is a great deal of hurt. She has tried to focus on her sadness by exploring why others were unable to help her. She speculates that they were uncomfortable about pregnancy, abortion, and her feelings. She refers to both her friend and the clinic workers as she muses, "If people have any issues about babies or grief or abortions, and then you go through this very messy abortion in which you are grieving a lot because you really wanted the baby, and the abortion turns out to be incomplete and it's not all nice and neat, it can't be put away in a shoebox up on the top shelf of your closet–if all that, then you are going to see their response to these issues in themselves. How do they feel about their grief, their baby/abortion issues? Are they in denial? Do they minimize? Do they act out? Whatever they do around their own shit, they will do around yours." What Emerald means is that other people's odd responses to our abortions may have nothing to do with us, only with their own unresolved feelings about pregnancy or abortion.

Feelings That Can Accompany Grief

Emerald realizes that her anger is a natural response to losing not only the people she loved, but also the fetus. Emerald has experienced grief about the fetus with both of her abortions. She says that after the first abortion at age 25, "I felt some sadness, but now, having had a second abortion, I realize this sadness was extremely slight." During her second abortion, she says, "I had a keen sense of a soul 'floating around' waiting to incarnate and it was pretty much agony to say goodbye." Since the abortion, she has felt such intense grief and sadness that she has trouble believing that she won't "feel sadness forever."

Her grief takes many forms, including jealousy about "people with kids, especially if they are doing better economically." Money is largely what prevents Emerald from having children right now. She copes with this envy by reminding herself how much work it is to be a mother. At other times, Emerald's grief makes her retreat from the world. Initially, she withdrew "as part of the grief process." She says, "I did not go overboard in other involvements." Like Emerald, we may wish to lick our wounds in private, not feeling that we have the strength to socialize.

Emerald has named many of the feelings that can accompany grief, including anger, disappointment, jealousy, and withdrawal. She has not mentioned a few others. As we grieve, we may go in and out of denial, unable to believe on some level that we have indeed lost what we have. After an abortion, we might block out what we have just been through, feeling as if the whole thing never happened.

Sometimes we do not feel the loss of an abortion in emotional terms, but in the way our bodies react. After the procedure, we may feel physically and emotionally empty. Our bodies may go through a grieving process of their own. One 38 year old recalls how this happened to her fourteen years ago: "I was having terrible lower abdominal cramps every day. I remember lying in bed holding my abdomen, crying with pain and sadness. The physician said this reaction was not typical, but some women did have this sort of reaction. He reassured me that in a short time, probably after a complete menstrual cycle, the cramps would subside. And they did. The physical grieving ended." The bodily mourning may not end so quickly. Six months after her second abortion, a 23 year old describes the way her body continues to experience the loss: "Some remnants of a sadness–a clenching of my legs as if in the stirrups, a flop in my stomach, second-long flashes–sometimes invade my body rather than my mind. My mind is the rational one, recognizing an experience to be reasoned with. My body, however, has a memory of its own." This woman may grieve through her body because she does not want sad memories to come into her "rational" mind. She may not feel that it is acceptable to grieve for the pregnancies she ended. If so, she is not alone.

THE CHALLENGES OF ABORTION GRIEF

After an abortion, women often wonder, "Do I have the right to grieve a loss I chose? If I feel sad, does it mean the choice was wrong?" We now meet Meredith, who has felt that she does not have the right to grieve after her abortions.

Meredith: "Your House Is Dirty, You Clean It, and That's the End of It"

Meredith, who is white and 21, has had three abortions since she was 17. Each one brought some pain, but the last was the hardest. She planned to carry the pregnancy to term, but then realized that she probably damaged the fetus by taking drugs and overdosing on Prozac in a suicide attempt. Reluctantly, she had a third abortion.

It was hard for Meredith to lose her dreams about this pregnancy, dreams that sustained her in a time of great depression. She explains that before she decided on abortion, "All these thoughts go through your head. You start buying cribs in your head. You can't wait for the fetus to grow. You can't wait to watch the progress. And then it's all over. Then you've got this stupid maternity shirt and this stack of books, and you're never gonna use them." What did Meredith do with these belongings? She answers resolutely, "Gave them away. Fast as I could. Just put it out of my sight."

Meredith has tried to do the same with her feelings. She sustained another great loss in her last abortion, but tries not to dwell on it. "I lost the hope that Mario and I were getting closer together," she says. Meredith and Mario had had an off-and-on relationship since she was 16. He was thirty years older than Meredith and she depended on him in ways that felt unhealthy to her, which accounted for much of her depression in the first place. The abortion sealed the fate of their crumbling relationship. As it ended, she often imagined having children with Mario. She thought, "If only I were older and I met him when he met his second wife, then I could have had a kid with him." Meredith adds quickly, "But that's a good way to torture yourself," thus whisking away those troublesome thoughts.

In not allowing herself to dwell on these losses, Meredith enforces what she feels to be other people's attitudes about grieving abortion losses. She picked up on these attitudes early, when her parents made her end her first pregnancy. She notes that her parents "didn't want to talk about it at all. They wanted it over. And as far as grief, there was absolutely no need for grief. It was just like cleaning your house. Your house is dirty, you clean it, and that's the end of it." When she had another abortion a year later, she could not grieve because, she says, "I was too busy running." Her personal life had become quite complicated, and she found it easier to avoid thinking about her problems. Meredith continues, "And the third time, I just felt again that I couldn't grieve. I was grieving to some extent internally, but I didn't give it too much time or thought, because it just didn't seem like I would be allowed to."

Most of this constraint on grief came from her interaction with other people, from their "limited amount of understanding" of her experience. Meredith also sensed that if she communicated her feelings to Mario, her grief would "put a barrier" between the two of them. She adds, "I thought it would certainly hurt the relationship. On an intellectual level a person can understand you are going through a certain experience, but emotionally, they're at a loss." The rest of the prohibition on grief came from within. Meredith considers grieving "a waste of time" and says, "It just didn't fit into my getting on with my life." Grief seems not only inefficient to her, but also quite frightening. She muses, "If I allowed myself to think about the possibilities, I'd go crazy. I think that's part of the grief and I'm not sure I would allow that." When she refers to "the possibilities," she means those of the fetus and those of her relationship with Mario.

Claiming the Right to Grieve After an Abortion

Meredith's circumstances are unusual, but many of us share her hesitance to grieve, partly because society does not tolerate any type of grief for long. Forty-four-year-old Beth, who has had five pregnancy losses, knows this well. She had an abortion at age 27. After that, she tried to carry to term, but had a miscarriage and two stillbirths. At age 40, she conceived again by accident and could not face the pain of another stillbirth. With mixed feelings, she had an abortion. She recalls, "I had this enormous sense of grief afterward. I've learned later that grief is normal; grief is okay. It's human. It's appropriate. But when you're going through it, you think you're the only one who's ever been there. And you think either that something is terribly wrong with you, or you're crazy. Society has such terrible constraints around all that. Even when it's a legitimated, public grief that people know about, our society has a very short time span for grief. You're supposed to be stoic, you're supposed to get over it, and you're supposed to be okay in a week or a month."

We may feel that society allows even less time for grieving the loss of a fetus that many assume we did not value and that most people never knew about. Because of the secrecy surrounding abortion and most people's desire to push this uncomfortable subject into the closet, we pick up messages that we should forget about an abortion immediately after the procedure. People often treat an abortion as a practical solution to a problem, not recognizing the depth of grief we may feel. Beth addresses this attitude when she says, "It didn't happen, so how are you supposed to have feelings about it afterward? If you can't tell people that this was part of your experience, how can you process those feelings?"

Even if we do tell others about our abortions, we may not receive the support or understanding we need. Because others have never known the fetus, they cannot even respond out of their own feelings of loss, unlike if a neighborhood dog dies. When 28-year-old Yvette was pregnant three months ago, she shared her news with her jailed father and a guy who sat next to her at work. Her father devoted only one sentence of his next letter to the topic. Yvette's co-worker "acted like it was nothing." He said, "Oh, too bad. But you're going to get it taken care of, right?" Yvette says, "I expected for the two weeks before the abortion, and for some time after, that he would be really considerate. Instead, he wasn't at all. He acted as if nothing was going on." Yvette says with exasperation, "Obviously, he was uncomfortable with it. Either that, or he just didn't think it was a big deal." She adds, "It struck me through the whole thing that people are very unsympathetic about it. Even if you're not close to someone, certainly you can have some feeling for what they're going through. People give more attention to someone who's going through a divorce or got their apartment ripped off than I got." As Yvette found, many people cannot handle abortion on a personal level. The issue is too charged. The people Yvette told may also lack empathy and might react this way with any issue.

It can be very painful to grieve without others' knowledge or support. One 22 year old has grieved in isolation about her abortions. She had one five years ago, another just three months ago, and says, "My abortions have caused me so much anguish. It's the biggest letdown in the world. Going through this big, awful ordeal and coming out with nothing to show for it. It's such a disappointment. There's no describing the loss. It's a death you mourn alone, not even able to talk about it."

Forty-five-year-old Nadine shares this loneliness. She performed an herbal abortion at age 27 with the support of a wise woman who prayed while Nadine ended the pregnancy. Before the abortion, Nadine told a friend about her plans, but her friend scoffed that an herbal abortion would never work. With a sad voice, Nadine recalls how she felt: "I realized how lonely, how really lonely. . . . 'Cause all I had was this woman who most people call a witch. I just didn't have support. And that makes me very sad." The loneliness stays with her after all these years. The lack of support affected how she grieved that abortion. She says that back then, "I really didn't know about grief. Talking about it was not acceptable, so I just went on and lived my life. My biggest sadness is just that I can't talk about it in the culture, let alone grieve in an open way."

Nadine has a solution. She says, "I think it would be most appropriate to grieve together," to have a "ritual. The whole thing is such a lonely business that I believe in a lot of networking and women coming together around this issue. It should be a communal grieving. I don't think abortion is such a big deal. It's just another procedure in life. But the fact that it's denied and not put in its proper perspective is the pain."

Thirty-one-year-old Annika agrees that a ritual is crucial. She sees the problem as lying in the abortion procedure itself. Annika calls the procedure she underwent five years ago "extremely cold and mechanical." She points out that while a person's death occasions a funeral and memorial services, "There was nothing of that for this life. This whole procedure and how it was dealt with medically seemed so cold and so removed from an actual death." She adds, "I think I would have liked to have the remains and bury them." If Annika had been able to do this, she says, "It would have felt like I had acknowledged to a greater extent the significance of this. This wasn't just something inconvenient that I had to get rid of and that was thrown in the garbage. I didn't want to look at it that way." The way in which clinic workers whisk away the fetus comes very close to how society treats abortion on an emotional level—the common feeling is that it should be out of sight and out of mind.

The prohibition on abortion grief partly results from the controversy surrounding abortion. The antichoice side points to postabortion grief as a sign of wrongdoing. Twenty-five-year-old Mariel, who had an abortion ten months ago, explains how this aspect affected her. She says, "I thought you should just feel relieved that it's over. I felt confused by grief, loss, and sadness. I associated those feelings with pro-life people who say that you'll feel those things because you made the wrong decision." She says of these emotions, "I feel that those are a normal part of many women's experiences. They are not evidence that they shouldn't have had abortions." Mariel would like to have understood this from the start and notes, "I wish someone had told me that it's okay to feel sad and it didn't mean that I made the wrong choice or that I wasn't really pro-choice."

Twenty-five-year-old Cassie felt similar pressures after her abortions at ages 22 and 24. "I felt like if in any way I was unhappy, then I was just fueling the antichoice fires," she notes, adding, "I wasn't letting myself mourn. I was under the impression that if I did, I was denying that this was a good choice for me." Cassie resolved this issue by grieving for some kittens that died right after her first abortion. She cries as she recalls laying one of them to rest: "I took the cat outside and I dug a hole and I buried it. And I got on a nice outfit and I put on some music and I had a little funeral." As sad as it must have been for Cassie to witness those cats' deaths, her tears may also be for the fetus she lost. It may have been easier for her to mourn a proxy, a visible, soft, lovable kitten. Indeed, using a proxy for the fetus and performing a ritual can help in resolving grief.

Several Western women feel encouraged that the Japanese have a ritual for grieving abortion losses. People erect shrines to the aborted, miscarried, and stillborn. Represented by a statue, the lost offspring receives a form and a name, creating an identity. Participants are purified, usually with smoke from incense, and make offerings to the figurine, allowing them to care for and connect with the fetus's spirit ("Beliefs," Peter Steinfels, *The New York Times*, August 15, 1992, A7). While Westerners often interpret this as a positive way to respond to abortion, author Helen Hardacre argues otherwise in *Marketing the Menacing Fetus in Japan*. In her view, the Japanese ritual stems from a misogynistic attempt to scare women, who hear that the spirits of the fetus will attack them and that they will suffer spiritual and physical consequences unless they donate a costly statue and pay priests a hefty sum to perform rites. Created in the 1960s, the ritual has no Buddhist basis.

For women seeking a ritual in the United States, a Zen center in the San Francisco area conducts memorial ceremonies for women who have had abortions or miscarriages. Kimberley Snow's book, *Keys to the Open Gate: A Women's Spirituality Sourcebook*, describes this ceremony and other possible rituals. It is noteworthy that one can find abortion rituals only of New Age or Eastern origins, not in mainstream America, which would rather ignore death in general and abortion experiences in particular.

Aside from the fact that we do not commonly ritualize abortion in this society, we may also have trouble grieving if we believe abortion is bad. We might see crying as a luxury in which we do not deserve to indulge, especially if we feel we have been selfish in having an abortion. Because we played an active role in bringing about the loss, we may not feel justified in mourning. We might even want to deny ourselves relief from our pain. After her abortion at age 18, one woman thought this way. Seven years later, she notes, "I felt I had to punish myself by grieving intensely, or else I wouldn't be forgiven by myself or God." Grief is neither a punishment nor a luxury. Instead, it is a tool to help us heal after a loss. The idea is to acknowledge and release pain over what we have lost. Then, we can resolve our feelings and move on in our lives.

RESOLVING GRIEF

What does it take to work through the feelings of grief? Is it just a matter of crying until there are no more tears left, or is something more involved? We now meet Brittany, who has grieved in different ways after each of her abortions.

Brittany: "You Are Irreplaceable; I Will Never Forget You"

Four years ago, Brittany, who is white and 22, had a daughter, Courtney. She very much wanted another child, but when she and Courtney's father, Dean, accidentally conceived again a year later, Brittany did not want to impinge on Courtney's infancy with another baby. With much sadness, Brittany had an abortion for Courtney's sake.

After the procedure, Brittany held on tightly to her feelings about the fetus, not wanting to "completely lose touch with that baby." Like Brittany, we may feel that we have to cling to our memory of the pregnancy so that it does not slip into oblivion. We may feel that as long as the fetus is alive in our minds, it still exists in some form. As the sole guardian of its memory, we may think we have betrayed the fetus if we stop grieving its loss. Brittany's way of staying connected to the fetus, one she thought of as a boy, was to name him and write him the following letter:

> Dear Morgan,
>
> I think of you so often, and wish you could be here, loving and learning with us. I miss you so much! I don't know if there is a way for you to return to me. But I hope in my heart of deep hearts that you do. I love you so much. If you cannot return some day, I want to give you this message: You are irreplaceable. I will never forget you. I will always wonder about you and all of your talents and interests. You have always been completely lovable and I will always love you. I know that your specialness is reflected in every special person that I know. When I see newborns, I wish that we could have met. The thought of *you* is wonderful! Please know that I want the best for you and I'm sorry that things aren't together well right now. December 1 is a day that is your day, my love. I am so sorry for the reason. Please be well. I love you,
>
> Mama
>
> P.S. I will do the best that I can for you *always*!

It can help to act on grief, as Brittany did; writing a letter probably made her feel less powerless in the face of loss. Naming the fetus like this is also a good idea; if grief feels overwhelming, it may help to realize that the loss is very specific. Brittany planned further actions; she consoled herself by saying, "I know that I'm going to have another child and that helps me. I want to be pregnant again." She intended to fill the void with a new baby.

Brittany did, in fact, conceive again a year later. She felt great excitement about the pregnancy and planned to carry it to term. Dean expressed doubts about having another child, though. He already had his hands full parenting Courtney and felt unhappy in his job. Dean wanted to develop his career, not have a second child dependent on them. To top it all off, Dean and Brittany were not even romantically involved when Brittany conceived; they had simply had sex one afternoon when she picked up Courtney from his house.

Dean and Brittany struggled over the pregnancy decision, but Brittany finally decided to have an abortion. She held out hopes that she, Dean, and Courtney could be a family again, and figured that carrying this pregnancy to term would alienate Dean forever. She sacrificed this pregnancy for the sake of a romance that didn't quite exist. After the abortion, Brittany felt "lost." She had no set relationship with Dean and no pregnancy.

As Brittany grappled with feelings of loss after her second abortion, she rejected the way she once consoled herself by hoping to conceive again soon. She recalls how after the first abortion, she needed "something to think about to serve as a comfort." She remembers saying to someone, "Maybe the spirit of this one will return in another baby," and observes, "It was this way of holding onto something where I wouldn't have to grieve it."

With her second abortion, Brittany did not take comfort in that idea. Someone in her peer counseling program said to her, "Try telling me that you're never going to have any more children." Brittany recalls, "I told him that I was never going to have any more children. And cried and cried and cried and cried. Certainly, that's not a decision that I've decided that I'm going to proceed with. But it was good for me to consider, so that I was able to grieve." She realizes that this exercise was essential, because it made her keep saying goodbye to the fetus. She says she is glad that the counselor "wasn't comforting me and letting me hold onto this comfort. He was actually ripping it away and saying, 'What is it going to feel like when you have to face what has happened?'" Brittany thinks it is unwise to "use the future as a comfort for something that's already happened." She does not want to base her decision to have more children on unresolved grief about her abortions. Brittany knows she cannot have children simply as replacements for ended pregnancies, or as ways to let the souls of past fetuses come forward. She says that when the counselor forced her to face this, "I realized that a lot of the spiritual beliefs that I was holding onto were because I had feelings that I hadn't gotten out yet about particular experiences. The more I've gotten to do that, the more I haven't needed those things."

Brittany raises an excellent point. It may be easier–but more dangerous–to accept losses by thinking of how we can replace them. After an abortion, it is natural to think of a new pregnancy as a great substitute. We may even regard the abortion as a sacrifice to our future parenthood. A 26 year old holds this point of view two years after her abortion. She says, "I can justify the abortion as a necessary sacrifice to be a better, well-adjusted parent in the future. I hope I can follow through." She advises other women, "Your sacrifice now will help your future." There are merits in regarding abortion as a sacrifice to all sorts of future development, but this may prevent us from grappling with the loss that we confront now. Plus, it puts a lot of pressure on us to achieve certain things in the future, things that simply may not be in the cards.

There is no need to look so far into the future for a gain–the growth many of us acquire during an abortion experience may serve this need. Brittany says her first abortion helped her mature. In fact, she calls her second experience easier, explaining, "I've grown a lot out of my experience with the first one." She adds, "I have been able to resolve some of my feelings about abortion and loss. And was further along on that continuum." As Brittany surveys her pregnancy losses, she now sees not only something forfeited, but also recognizes what she can keep forever–knowledge, experience, and growth.

Chapter 5

Relief: Now and Later

Josie, who is 26 and white, has changed her life radically in two years. She recalls that back then, "I was in a really out of control period. I was avoiding life issues by partying and hanging around with a crowd that kept me below my potential." She dated Lloyd, who was more committed to another woman. Josie says, "Although I didn't realize it, our relationship was really immature and based on liquor, sex, and decadent fun."

Josie sees these problems as having started quite a while ago. She says, "I grew up sheltered, went straight into college after high school, and was having a difficult time taking care of myself and dealing with the real world." She certainly wanted to take on the world when she graduated from college. Josie explains, "My double major had taught me to expect" a "high-paying corporate job." She adds, "When I didn't immediately get that job, my self-esteem plummeted, and I floundered for over a year until I became pregnant." The pregnancy served as a wake-up call. Josie muses, "Suddenly finding myself penniless, jobless, resourceless, spouseless, and pregnant was the shock I needed to finally force myself to get my life together. Being pregnant made me realize the severity of my situation and gave me the impetus to do something about it."

She thought about her options for a day or so, then decided on abortion quite easily. "Abortion really was my only alternative," she says, both because of the tattered state of her life, and because she had partied so much before realizing she was pregnant.

Prior to the abortion, Josie was consumed with fear. She recalls, "I wanted to know if it would hurt, if I would die on the operating table, what I could do to facilitate an easier procedure." It turns out Josie had nothing to worry about. Sounding like a representative for the abortion facility, Josie says with obvious sincerity, "It had a real hospital feel that was really comforting. I had excellent care and I highly recommend" that facility. She wanted general anesthesia, but had some concerns. She discussed this with the doctors and decided on a heavy sedative and a local anesthetic. To calm her fears about the procedure, Josie says she "made every nurse I came in contact with explain every detail to me, until I felt like I knew enough about it that I could perform an abortion myself."

The result of all this careful discussion? Josie rejoices, "It worked out great. The actual procedure was so quick and painless that I hardly realized that it had begun. I expected the machine to produce a loud, clanging sound instead of the quiet hum." Many women do find the machine noisy; Josie's heavy sedative may have reduced the sound to a murmur in her ears. Looking back, she comments, "I was pleasantly surprised that the procedure turned out not to be as big a deal and not as intense as I anticipated." Josie adds, "I wish someone had put it in the proper perspective for me. I recently told a friend that getting my cavity filled was more invasive, more stressful, and more painful than my abortion. Women aren't half as scared of the dentist as they are of Planned Parenthood."

Emotionally, the procedure went well. Josie recalls that the nurse "kept talking to me about college and asking me questions to keep me pleasantly distracted. She caressed my head during the procedure. That simple act of kindness was so comforting. I wept a little bit, not from pain, but because this nurse treated me with such tenderness." It can be upsetting to have only a nurse as a source of emotional support at the procedure, but Josie didn't see it that way. She says that Lloyd, who was supposed to arrive at the facility as Josie checked in, "wound up showing up just as I was released. It was just as well," she concludes, explaining, "I was proud of myself for taking care of everything alone."

Josie used the facility's medical technology to reassure herself about the morality of her choice. She asked to see fetal pictures that corresponded to the length of her pregnancy. Josie adds, "I studied my own ultrasound and actually looked at the aborted tissue, just to make sure I wouldn't see any teeny feet or limbs or head. It was comforting for me to know that I was aborting a lima-bean-sized lump of tissue, rather than a fully formed infant." Josie was pregnant for four weeks before her abortion. Doctors will not perform abortions as soon as four weeks, because they might not be able to locate a tiny embryo during the procedure. Josie knew this and says, "I lied about the dates of my period, so the doctors would think that I was further along." Although it can be dangerous for doctors to have incorrect information, this strategy helped Josie feel better about having an abortion. Josie took this relief about the morality of her choice a step further. A nonpracticing Jew, she comments, "Because the abortion itself was so smooth and relatively painless, I took it as a sign from God that I had made the right decision."

She had solved her immediate problem—the pregnancy—and could have returned to the life she knew before she conceived. Instead, Josie recognized an opportunity to give her life a makeover. She says, "I concentrated on getting into a stable, monogamous relationship, I quit running around and sleeping around, and I worked really hard to get into a job where I feel valued and enjoy my work." Josie says that after five months, "I was employed in an advertising agency, had a new studio apartment, and I was out of the old circle of friends." As Josie looks back, she concludes, "That unplanned pregnancy was about the best thing that could have happened to me at the time."

Josie felt relief at many stages of her abortion experience. As her fears about the procedure diminished, she felt at ease. After learning about fetal development, she felt reassured that she had made the right choice. Later, Josie saw how the unplanned pregnancy helped her on a large scale. In this chapter, we will look at how other women have felt relief, both immediately after the surgery and as their lives have progressed.

WHEN IMMEDIATE FEARS DISSIPATE

Most of us approach the abortion procedure with great anxiety, as we would any operation. If we are to be awake during an abortion, we may worry about how much pain there will be and how we will feel as the fetus leaves our body. In a clinic or hospital situation, there can be hours of waiting prior to the procedure, time in which we sit, think, and worry. When the actual procedure arrives, every detail counts. How the clinic workers treat us is of paramount importance. Simone, who had her abortion in a hospital, explains how significant the medical staff's behavior was during her experience.

Depending on the Kindness of Clinic Workers

Thirty-nine-year-old Simone, who is white, brought great ambivalence into the abortion she had a year ago. She knew she wanted to have a child in the future, but felt stretched thin by the demands of raising her 17 month old and coping with a full-time career in transition. Her husband Vic also faced turbulence in his career when Simone conceived. They felt torn between their desire for a second child and the feeling that the whole family would enter a dark, hopeless period if Simone carried the pregnancy to term. They decided on abortion, but Simone could not embrace the decision wholeheartedly. The anxiety about her choice melded with fears about how physically painful and invasive the procedure would be. She came to the hospital "absolutely terrified."

Simone was quite relieved to find the procedure less invasive than she had feared. Before the procedure, however, the clinicians put her fears to rest. She recalls, "The nurse practitioner explained everything." The counselor was "positive about the decision," which helped. Then Simone and Vic met the doctor and inquired about her attitude toward abortion. The doctor responded, "I feel like what I'm doing is really important," and they felt pleased that she did not treat the procedure "like it was some back-alley thing."

Simone notes, "I expected much more ambivalence on the part of the professionals." She had thought that they would feel as uncertain about her decision as she did. Plus, as she explains, "I went into it thinking that there is a taboo about it and you get stigmatized. In the midst of this vulnerable period, you get treated with contempt and disdain." Simone's mother had this experience when she ended a pregnancy in the 1970s. She was a middle-aged woman who shouldn't have been having kids, but the nurses regarded her "with disdain." Simone's friend, who had an abortion in the deep South, was also "treated with contempt by the very people who were doing the procedure." Simone had feared that. To convey how vulnerable women at an abortion facility are, she adds, "You're at the mercy of doctors and nurses." Referring to this potentially bad treatment at the hands of the staff, Simone comments, "I was amazed and pleased to find that that wasn't the case. The experience was so positive. It didn't leave me with a sense that I had done something awful." Instead, the staff members valued their work, which felt affirming.

Like Simone, we may be so vulnerable before an abortion that if the clinic workers are kind, we feel immense gratitude. Josie has mentioned that she wept at the nurse's caress. A 22 year old who received good treatment five years ago feels similarly thankful. She says, "I feel incredible love for the way they treated me. I feel like they saved my life and I can never repay them fully."

Paige: "I Was Very Thankful My Boyfriend Was There to Support Me"

Twenty-two-year-old Paige, a Palestinian American, shares this gratitude for the support she received. In her case, it came from her boyfriend. Paige dreaded having an abortion alone. When her boyfriend came with her to the procedure, she felt thankful and relieved. Her abortion experience had begun so badly that she did not expect this positive outcome.

When Paige discovered she was pregnant four years ago, she initially received almost no emotional help from the only people who knew–her cousin, friends, and boyfriend. She notes, "My boyfriend was there sometimes, but he also seemed emotionally absent. In fact, he wanted to break up with me a week before I was going to have the procedure." Paige knew they had a bad relationship, one based on sex. Still, she needed his support and reassurance. He decided that he would come with her to the procedure, but that afterward, he did not want to be together anymore. Paige consented to this arrangement, probably because she was so vulnerable at the time. She recalls that during her pregnancy, "I was lonely and many times depressed. I cried a lot." Her boyfriend actually proved supportive, warm, and kind during this period.

On the day of Paige's abortion, people were supposed to picket the clinic. "Thank God this did not happen," says Paige. Once inside the clinic, she felt quite anxious. She recalls, "I just wanted to get the thing over with. I anticipated pain and discomfort. I felt ashamed. I did not want anyone to see me." She worried that people pitied her. It turned out, though, that, as she says, "The people at Planned Parenthood were very kind and helpful. They tried their best to make me feel comfortable and were very discreet."

Their support was nice, but her boyfriend's was vital. She says, "He was with me the whole time. He tried to cheer me up. In the procedure room, I could tell he was nervous, too. But he held my hand. I looked at his face most of the time. It was incredibly helpful. To go through the procedure by myself would have been ten times worse."

Paige and her boyfriend broke up after the abortion, as planned, and even that event afforded her some relief, because their alliance had been so uneasy. She says, "We were very different. If I had not gotten pregnant, we would have broken up a long time ago." She adds that she felt glad to end the relationship because "I was still very resentful of him for the way he had wanted to break up with me before the procedure." Now, four years later, she has let go of this anger. She explains, "I understand what we were both going through at the time and don't blame him. I know he did what he could for the person he was. I am thankful that he was able to support me in the way that he did."

Relief About the Level of Anesthesia

Like Paige, 22-year-old Brittany had certain emotional needs to meet when she went through abortions at ages 19 and 20. Seeing an anesthetic as a type of emotional "numbing," she chose to have no anesthetic with each procedure. She cried at both procedures, which felt like an important release. The physical pain of the procedure helped her tears flow. She feels "really happy" about how having no anesthesia affected her emotional experience, so much so that she wrote the clinic a note about this positive aspect. To her, it was a relief to control this part of her experience and to let out her sadness.

Brittany's point of view is rare. Many of us feel the need for some respite from the pain. The following examples show how other women have tried to meet their emotional and physical needs by choosing to have more anesthesia than they might have had.

Local Anesthesia with a Tranquilizer

Twenty-eight-year-old Marilyn, who went through an emotional maelstrom before her abortion eleven months ago, told the clinic workers, "Whatever you can give me here, give me, because I'm emotionally exhausted. I've had enough carrying on. I'm sure I will experience this deeply, both before and after, but I don't want any physical pain and I don't want to feel any worse." Her request proved beneficial. She took a Valium and says of the physical pain, "It wasn't as bad as some of the menstrual problems that I've had. There was one moment where I felt like, 'My God, I can't stand it anymore.' Then it stopped. It was actually very fast."

General Anesthesia

At 22, Cassie remained awake during an abortion. At the time, she had chlamydia, but did not know it. Because this disease scarred her reproductive organs, she felt "a tremendous amount of pain" during the procedure. When she had her second abortion at age 24, Cassie chose to be asleep, which turned out to be a great decision. A year later, Cassie explains, "I hate pain and I'm very uncomfortable when I go to a gynecologist. Not having to be awake through the exam and the abortion helped a lot." Cassie has recently remembered that she was sexually abused during her childhood. This could explain her discomfort about gynecological exams; they can feel invasive, much like sexual abuse. An abortion procedure could trigger the same feelings for her. For these reasons, general anesthesia was the right choice for Cassie.

Medically, being asleep for a first-trimester abortion is often unnecessary and is riskier than having a local anesthetic, so clinic workers may discourage general anesthesia. Emotionally, however, there are several reasons that being tranquilized like Marilyn or being unconscious like Cassie may ease the whole experience of abortion.

Donna: "I Wept a Little–Relief and Sadness; It's Over"

The stress we feel before an abortion can yield to tremendous relief afterward. Donna, who is white and 42, did not expect to feel her load lighten in this way when she had an abortion two years ago. The counselors in the preabortion interview told her, "A lot of women feel great afterward." She responded, "I won't feel great." But, she says, "My first sensation was relief. I wept a little, alone—relief and sadness. It's over."

Donna brought a lot of emotional anxiety into the procedure, initially unsure about her choice. She had three boys, and felt drawn to the thought of meeting the child that "might have been my girl." But Donna and her husband felt overwhelmed by the demands of raising 2-year-old twins and a 5 year old. They decided to end the pregnancy.

Abortion was not new to Donna; she had had one at age 22. But that was nearly two decades ago. As Donna approached this current abortion, she feared the physical pain and coped by making herself stay calm. She wrote in her journal the next day, "I did very well. I was a model patient. I didn't jump or squirm. I took care of myself, a mature woman doing what was necessary. They appreciated that. I hadn't wanted to put this burden on myself, insist to myself that I had to *behave well*—but when the time came, that was what I needed to do, for me to get through it as easily as I could."

Her composure may have helped, but what was even more vital was that, as she says, the procedure "hurt less than I thought it might. It was far less frightening and demanding and painful than childbirth. It was most like being at the dentist." After the procedure, when Donna fell on the juice and cookies in the recovery room, a new analogy occurred to her. It's like giving blood, she thought in her "suddenly cheery relief." Driving home from the procedure alone, she felt "close to elated. No cramps, no blood. Just fine." She did end up feeling some "emotional discomfort" two days later. Overall, though, her fears proved unnecessary, and all the energy that fueled that anxiety dissolved into relief.

"My Insides Were Free, No Longer Choked up"

After an abortion, we may feel relieved that not only our emotional difficulties, but also our physical problems have ended. If the pregnancy has felt like an illness, we may rejoice that we feel so much better after the procedure. Here are some ways women have experienced this relief about the physical changes that follow an abortion procedure.

When Pregnancy Symptoms Disappear

Thirty-two-year-old Oriana has had abortions at 18, 19, 25, and 30. She says that afterward, "A lot of times, the primary feeling is one of relief. It's such a relief not to feel nauseous and not to feel that sense of invasion and that something is going to be interrupting your life." Oriana describes how she feels when the first trimester of pregnancy ends, either because of abortion or because she is carrying the pregnancy to term: "I feel like I am a real person again. God, I don't have to sleep twenty-four hours a day. And the thought of food doesn't make me want to gag. Just getting my life back, having more energy. My first three months are usually so strongly screwed up that I just turn into a lump and zombie."

When We Begin Bleeding

We may feel relieved when we begin to bleed as the uterus heals. Twenty-three-year-old Darian rejoiced six months ago when she saw blood after her procedure. She recalls, "I was so happy to see it. It meant that it was over–my insides were free, no longer choked up with this situation. I loved the sight of that blood." We may also feel relieved if the bleeding is lighter than we anticipated.

When We Get Our Period Again

Darian says, "I was ecstatic at the sight of my first normal period (I was so afraid it would never come, that they missed something and I was still pregnant . . . horrors)." Veronica, age 21, had an abortion a year ago and agrees that her first period was a source of joy. She recalls, "I felt really relieved the first time I had my period again. I never thought I would be glad to have my period! It just made it like, okay, things are really back to normal."

Any of these bodily changes may serve as milestones, places where we breathe a sigh of relief that the pregnancy and abortion are finally over.

RELIEF ABOUT BEING CHILD-FREE

As the urgency of ending the pregnancy ceases, we may feel less concerned about the physical aspects and more involved in the emotional part of the experience. At several points, we may reassess our decision. For example, 22-year-old Nora looks back on her abortion eight months later and feels more glad than ever not to have a child. During her pregnancy, she felt a mothering instinct come over her. Knowing that having a child would be impossible, she bought a puppy. She immediately associated the puppy with the fetus, calling the dog a "symbol of what I would have had." Unlike a child, a dog is "something I can deal with," says Nora. "It's not a child that I have to cope with for years and educate." As months passed and the projected due date grew closer, Nora only felt more at ease about her decision to have the abortion. She says, "I was thinking about it over Christmas: 'Shit, I'd be really pregnant now.' I definitely was thinking in January, 'God, I'd have a ten-day-old kid right now.' I'm glad I don't." Nora occasionally runs into a young woman who gave birth around the time Nora had her abortion. Nora says, "When I look at her, I'm pretty happy that I had the abortion, because I didn't want to be in her position." Nora feels relieved about the ongoing freedom of having no children.

Zelda, who is 39, white, and child-free, has felt that liberty for a long time. Becoming pregnant four years ago briefly threatened her freedom. She had an abortion and immediately had a tremendous sense of relief, both about ending the physical burdens of pregnancy and about calling the shots in her own life. Zelda says, "I felt empowered, like I had followed through with an extremely significant decision in my life. After the abortion, I went on a picnic and went swimming. I was training for a triathlon, so the pregnancy really put a damper on my training activities." She says that when she dove in, "It felt great to be back. I let myself float and closed my eyes and experienced having my body back, having my life back. Having a kid and being a single parent were definitely not what I wanted."

Zelda mentions single parenthood because she had a poor relationship with her partner. Finding herself pregnant by a man with whom she had no future filled her with anxiety. Zelda notes, "I came from a single parent home and I would *never* impose that life on another." Making matters worse, Zelda hated the physical state of pregnancy. She says, "I just wanted 'it' out. I was ill almost from the start." She had great trouble yielding to her body's changes and recalls "not liking my body very much, because it was feeling out of control, like something was taking over and I could no longer feel the way I wanted."

She says the only good part about conceiving was "a little positive feeling about, 'Yeah, I can create life.'" Although this feeling was "little" for Zelda, the way a positive pregnancy test confirms our fertility may be the first thing we feel relieved about in the course of an abortion experience. As one 30 year old says of her unplanned pregnancy six years ago, "The only positive feelings were the fact that I could get pregnant. I've done a lot of drugs and feared sterility." Since Zelda did not fear infertility or want children in the future, she felt no overwhelming happiness to find out she could conceive.

Zelda's negative feelings about her pregnancy afforded great relief about her abortion. Four years later, this relief leaves little room for doubt about her choice. Zelda notes, "Sometimes I think about how old the child would have been and have a tinge of remorse. But then I think about how I would not be pursuing things I wanted to pursue." She adds, "I thought I might feel more regret about it, but didn't and still don't to this day."

"I'm glad I didn't put any of society's guilt on me," Zelda observes, referring to the way many of us take in messages that abortion is wrong, even if we are pro-choice. Our guilt can interfere with feeling relief. We may even feel guilty for being relieved, because it might seem callous. Zelda did not have this problem. She says, "It felt great to really know I had made the right decision. I'm glad I allowed myself to acknowledge that and be okay about accepting my guiltlessness." Zelda continues, "I never had a problem with 'Did I do the right thing?' I always felt I did." She explains how her spiritual views of abortion helped her remain guilt-free: "I believed that an unwanted child should not be brought into the world and that the spirit doesn't enter the body until the child is born healthy and viable. That helped me not to feel guilty about having an abortion. I don't believe that having an abortion was a 'sin.' I was considering the life of the child. I was making a selfless decision, because I would want the best life possible for a child and knew I would not be able to provide that." Being able to avoid guilt and believe so strongly in her decision came as a relief to someone who thought she "was supposed to feel more guilty."

Rather than taking in pro-life criticisms of her decision, Zelda was more attuned to pro-choice voices after her abortion. She says, "I was extremely grateful to the women who have fought so hard to give us this right. I realized even more how having abortion available to us is a freedom and a right that many women don't have." Zelda's gratitude to abortion rights activists is a type of relief; when she faced an unwanted pregnancy, those women's efforts provided the help she needed. Now, Zelda wants to assist other women by offering the following advice: "Don't feel guilty. Believe in yourself and your ability and right to make a decision that will affect your life in a positive way."

WHEN UNFORESEEN CIRCUMSTANCES CONFIRM OUR CHOICES

In the years after an abortion, our lives may change so that we look back on our decisions and feel relieved once again. Events that we could never have predicted can cast a new light on our choices. These later circumstances may include problems that crop up, personal growth that could not have happened with a baby, or giving birth when the time is right.

Lynn: Later Troubles and Successes

Lynn is a 40-year-old Asian American whose problems and achievements confirm that her two abortions were good decisions. Lynn explains that having an abortion at age 17 "enabled me to continue my education, avoid family and community censure, and not be forced either to raise a child while a child, or marry while too young for the responsibilities." Lynn went on to marry and to carry two planned pregnancies to term at ages 24 and 26. Unfortunately, she divorced some years later.

At 33, while building a solid career, she accidentally conceived again. She decided to end the pregnancy, a choice she calls "easier" than the first abortion decision, "only in that I was sure that had I not had the first one, my life would have been very different, I suspect in negative ways. The reasons I was having the second abortion were much the same, so I was confident that it was the right choice." Just as the first abortion allowed her to develop herself, the second let her keep pursuing a career. Lynn considered her finances as she made this decision, and felt pleased that the abortion allowed her to stay afloat; she says, "A third child would have plunged me almost irretrievably into poverty."

As time has passed, Lynn has faced financial and emotional challenges in raising her two children alone. Their life feels to Lynn "like the upper end of poverty." On "very rare occasions," when Lynn wonders what her life would be like with two more kids, she reminds herself that "trying to provide for the two boys is already a constant financial and emotional struggle" and that having four "would have been disastrous for us all." Lynn summarizes the situation in the following way: "Now that my boys are sixteen and fourteen and we struggle to respect each other and keep communication alive, I am even more certain that the two abortions I had were the best decisions for my life."

"Knowing What I Know Now, We Really Did Make the Right Choice"

Lynn feels that two more children would have brought her greater challenges than she could have handled. Abortion allowed her to avoid these problems and minimize the ones she currently faces. Sometimes, trouble unrelated to children can fall into our lives after an abortion, and we may be glad that we did not involve a child in the melee.

Randi, who is 35 and Caucasian, feels this way about the abortion she had a decade ago. When she was 25 and her husband Carl was 27, they conceived accidentally. She says that back then, "Neither one of us was ready to be parents." Although they wanted children, she notes that a baby "just wasn't right at this time in our lives." There were also financial constraints. In addition, Randi faced a tenure decision.

Emotionally, the decision was a bit difficult. Randi says that during the two days in which she knew she was pregnant, "I remember crying. I remember saying, 'I want this baby.' I remember romanticizing about the idea and forgetting about the work. Saying, 'Oh, I'll get tenure in the final year.' I can still feel myself gradually letting the romantic fantasies go away and knowing that someday I still was going to be able to do this."

After Randi had an abortion, she felt relieved and confirmed in her choice. She comments, "I don't have any regrets at all. It was absolutely the right decision. There's not a question in my mind." She says of Carl, "He never questioned it."

She then makes a key point: "In hindsight, it was even more right." Carl "has a mental illness, which didn't surface until a year and a half after the abortion." He "flipped out" one day and ended up in a mental hospital. The relationship eventually fell apart. Six years later, they divorced. Randi later had a baby on her own. Ten years after the abortion, Randi can say, "If anything, his illness, which then precipitated the divorce, made me even more sure that terminating the pregnancy was the right thing to do."

Forty-two-year-old Carrie, who is white, has a similar story, although the breakdown that casts a positive light on her abortion was her own. When she conceived at 35, she and Olin had dated for just five months and were unsure of their future together. Deciding on abortion was difficult because Carrie wanted kids very much and was midway through her thirties. She and Olin agreed, however, that a child was too much pressure to put on such a new romance. She had an abortion and the relationship ended up thriving. Within a few months, they married. Seventeen months after the abortion, they had a child. The next period, however, proved rocky. Carrie was an addict and both of her parents were alcoholics. She had not yet dealt with those issues, and they demanded urgent resolution "about a year after Duncan was born." Carrie entered a twelve-step program.

Seven years have passed since Carrie's abortion. She and Olin have had another child and their marriage is solid. While she had the abortion because she was unsure about the relationship's strength, and although the romance has lasted, Carrie does not regret her decision. She explains, "The rightness of the situation was pretty obvious." Carrie muses about how different her life would have been if she had carried that first pregnancy to term: "Seeing that I went into a twelve-step program within the first year of my child's life, I don't think we would have survived as a family." She considers that idea for a moment and adds, "If we did, it would have been even more wrenching. I would have hit bottom more quickly and I'm not so sure that the relationship would have survived." Carrie nods and then says, "Knowing what I know now, we really did make the right choice."

Simone: "Yes, This Is the Right Time to Have a Child"

Carrie waited to have a child until her relationship with Olin could better accommodate a third person. Unlike Carrie, 39-year-old Simone already had one child when she conceived again. Her 17 month old and the turbulence of her and her husband's careers made their lives much too complicated to allow for a new child. Tragically, they very much wanted a second child and planned on trying to conceive soon—just not that soon. They worried about the psychological damage they might inflict on the whole family if they could not devote enough loving time to each child. With heavy hearts, they ended that pregnancy. Earlier in this chapter, we saw how Simone went into the hospital "absolutely terrified," and how the clinic workers' attitudes afforded her much relief.

Seven months after the abortion, at the time the second child would have been born, she and Vic conceived again happily; Simone is now halfway through this pregnancy. Her family has settled into a more manageable routine. Simone says contentedly, "I have the real sense of what it feels like to be pregnant with Vic when it is the right time, when it is a good time, when I have the time, when I can concentrate on it." Now, she says, "I'm not psychologically worn out and still reeling from the impact of the pregnancy," or from her career transition "and all that pressure that went along with it." She adds, "I know that I can set my work schedule up so that I have the time to spend with this child." This last pregnancy has let her know that, "Yes, this is the right time to have a child." Feeling so good about her current pregnancy, Simone feels more resolved about the abortion. She comments, "Even though it's still painful, and even though I wish I never had to make that decision, I still look back on it and say it was the right decision for us at that time."

PART II: WORKING TOWARD ACCEPTANCE

Chapter 6

Lifting the Veil of Denial

Yvette is a 28 year old of Scandinavian beauty. Speaking openly and passionately about her abortion, she becomes so worked up that rings of perspiration spread from her armpits down her grey dress. The dress flares out at the waist, revealing a plump abdomen. Yvette begins to talk about how she has gained twenty-two pounds since she discovered her pregnancy, which she ended three months ago. The conversation turns to the movie *Eating*, which has a scene about abortion and focuses on weight issues. Yvette saw the film two weeks ago, but draws a blank on the scene in which two women discuss their abortions. "At what part were they talking about their abortions?" she laughs, realizing that she should be able to recall this. When she hears a summary of the scene, she responds excitedly, "Oh right! Look how quickly I repressed that! Now I remember. The French woman and the other woman." She pauses to reflect. "It made me sad, but I can't remember what they said now." Yvette listens to an abridged version of the conversation. "God," she says with amazement, "I really am a little bit in denial." She laughs in disbelief at how much she has forgotten. Then Yvette digs a little deeper. "I do remember I was sort of sad when they were talking and she was crying." Was Yvette sad because it reminded her of her own experience? She muses, "It's quite possible that I was, and what I'm doing is I'm trying not to think about it. I'm busy repressing it a lot. Which is good and bad."

Yvette calls this denial "amazing for somebody who's been in therapy for so long." She has spent years looking at her family troubles and her past, which includes being an addict from ages 15 to 21, dropping out of high school, and having an abortion at age 16. In therapy, she doesn't usually avoid things for long. She lets go of old feelings by discussing them. "I haven't with this," she says, explaining, "I don't want to indulge it. I don't want to have too much feeling about it." She figures she probably will look at her feelings "once more time has passed."

Just as Yvette fears her emotions now, she felt apprehensive before her abortion. She says she hoped it "would be like when I was sixteen," when she had an abortion and treated it "like it never happened." She says, "I don't think that I really ever experienced it like this one." That may be because she was on drugs at the time. "I was an addict then," Yvette points out, "so you can't think of me as a thinking, normal human being." Her earlier abortion did not prepare her for this recent one. She says, "I didn't expect to feel this much at all." She does not want to be numb, and sees denying feelings as very unhealthy. But she hoped that with this latest abortion, it would be easy to go on, where "once it was over, it was over." She muses, "I certainly didn't expect this range of stuff to come up."

The breadth and depth of her emotions have frightened her, especially right after the procedure. She recalls, "The day after my abortion, I dealt with it a lot. I allowed myself to grieve it. My therapy session was two days later. I talked about it a little bit." That session was difficult for her. She recalls sharing her macabre thoughts about the clinic workers who performed her abortion. Yvette says she had images of them as "satanic types" in a horror movie, who smiled "as they had me drugged" and "as they ripped my baby" away. These images made Yvette feel "terrible, because they really were wonderful and very supportive." In describing these thoughts to the therapist, Yvette says, "I started really crying and I didn't want to." She explains, "I felt like maybe I would cry for days and I just wouldn't stop." Yvette held back in the moment, but says, "I cried that whole next day." The pain scared her. She notes, "After that, I just wanted to put it behind me." Yvette has not cried again about her abortion experience.

Her feelings then surfaced in another way. She recalls, "For about two weeks afterward, I was anxious. I kept imagining that I had an infection." She called the medical staff, who assured Yvette that she would have severe cramps and pain if she truly had an infection. Yvette explains why she imagined an infection when there was none: "The real reason I was that anxious was I was repressing all these feelings from the abortion."

It has taken Yvette a while to remember how she reacted to her abortion. At first, she says she was only affected for one day. Then she shares other memories. Yvette muses, "As I was talking to you, I contradicted myself a couple of times and forgot to mention stuff." Why? She explains, "I've been trying not to think about" the abortion.

She jumped at the chance to speak about her feelings in an interview, but Yvette feels nervous about stirring up feelings that have been frozen for nearly three months. She says, "After today, I don't know what will happen." Yvette finds herself pulled in two directions. She is tempted to stay numb, to hide in a comforting denial. Another part of her, the part that has led her out of addiction and into therapy, knows that she should look at her feelings more closely and resolve any conflicts.

Many of us share her struggle, using denial at several stages in our experiences with pregnancy and abortion. Denial certainly serves a good purpose as it spares us from facing what we are not yet ready to face. It cushions big blows, protecting us both from our emotions and from a full realization of what has transpired. When we are ready, we will gradually shed this denial and accept the changes in our lives. If we are unable to break through denial after a long time, however, we may lose access to all our emotions.

The term "denial" is complex. Psychologists distinguish between avoidance, suppression, repression, dissociation, and denial. Technically, there is also a difference between denial and the numbness that stress can bring, especially early in an abortion experience. For our purposes here, though, we will call all the mental tricks that shield us from pain "denial."

HOW DENIAL FEELS

Denial about an abortion manifests in different ways. One's memory may be faulty, as is true for Yvette. Twenty-one-year-old Fritzi shares this experience. "I have such a good memory of things," she says, but where her abortion of two years ago is concerned, she notes, "I have blocked out a lot of it. I really don't remember a lot of dates." As Fritzi fields questions about her abortion experience, she sounds like a recalcitrant witness in a trial, although she clearly speaks the truth. When did she tell her new boyfriend about the abortion? "Gosh, I don't know when I told him." How did she get along with people in the weeks after the abortion? "I don't remember," she answers, and then laughs, "It must have been awful." Fritzi concludes, "I just blanked out a lot of it. It's scary," she says of this unfamiliar behavior. She likens it to another experience: "Sometimes if I told a little white lie, it's the same. I try to ignore it. It's something I put behind me and I don't look back at it. I separate it from myself." Fritzi accurately describes how we might deny a fact or experience. We push it away, disconnecting ourselves from the truth, or from our emotions about that truth. We now meet Becky, who has achieved this distance from her abortion.

Becky: "It Didn't Really Happen to Me"

Two months after her abortion, 25-year-old Becky finds it easy to forget that this event ever occurred. She explains, "A lot of times, I can say, 'It didn't really happen to me.' I can distance myself from it. There's still a lot of denial." Many aspects of an abortion make it easy for Becky to distance herself. First, when we have an abortion, the people in our lives may find the subject uncomfortable and pretend that it has not happened. Second, most of us never see the fetus, so we have no visual proof that the pregnancy even existed. Third, the idea behind an abortion is often to eliminate something that should never have been there. People therefore reason that, after an abortion, it is better to proceed as though the pregnancy never existed and to resume a pre-pregnancy life and focus.

This attitude suits Becky perfectly. When she interacts with others and the subject of abortion comes up, she is especially inclined to tell herself that it never happened. Once, when she and her uncle discussed abortion, she felt uncomfortable. "But then," she says, "I started to distance myself and say, 'Oh, it didn't really happen to me.'"

Becky has used denial throughout her experience. When she discovered her pregnancy, she recalls, "I was in a daze almost, like it wasn't really real. There was so much denial. Even till the last minute. I said to my mom, 'What if I'm not pregnant and they start doing the abortion?' I just felt like, 'how do they know? Maybe I'm not.'" She thought, "Maybe I'm just making up these symptoms and my period's going to come!" The procedure caused this denial to fall apart. Becky says, "After the abortion, I remember getting off the table and looking at the jar. I just saw it for a minute, but it looked like tissue. And then it hit me. I really was pregnant. There really was something in there."

Irene: "Keeping Busy and Not Thinking About It"

Another way to achieve distance from an abortion is to stay busy, occupying oneself constantly in order to ward off painful thoughts. Nineteen-year-old Irene approaches her abortion experience this way. Irene had an abortion two months ago, right before she returned to college for sophomore year. She laughs as she describes how she spends time lately: "I'm really busy! It's not just my schoolwork. I got a volunteer job, I'm in a women's group, and I go out. I'm with people all the time." She explains why she is so social: "It's another way of keeping busy and not thinking about it. 'Cause the way I've dealt with the whole thing is not to think about it. And the only time I can think about it is when I'm alone. So I just make damn sure that I'm not alone now much."

Irene has pushed away her feelings ever since she discovered her pregnancy. She recalls that prior to her abortion, "I didn't feel it the whole time beforehand. I just laughed it off." As the abortion occurred, however, she "didn't feel that disconnected." During the procedure and directly afterward, she had "a moment of hysteria." She used no denial at that moment. Now, she says, thinking about "the actual procedure" is "the only thing that really upsets me. I don't know if it's because that's the only part I couldn't really deny," she muses. Otherwise, Irene notes, "I just don't feel it. I don't let myself get like that."

When she received a flyer about contributing her abortion experience to this book, she recalls, it "freaked me out." She read about the project, thinking, "Oh, that's me." She muses, "I guess I had put it out of my mind and thought it didn't happen. For a second I started to get upset, and then I was like, 'Suppress, suppress, suppress!'"

"I'm afraid it's going to come out sooner or later," says Irene of her feelings. They have only a dull presence in her mind. She speculates that they will hit her later, explaining that her tendency is "to pretend even to myself that things don't bother me, to get through it. But then again," she reflects, "maybe it doesn't bother me that much." Is the emotional aspect of her abortion experience settled, then? "I'd like to think it is," Irene says. But she remains unsure. "I mean, I never actually let myself think about it."

Oriana: "I Put Myself in a Numbing State, So I Felt Disconnected"

Like Irene, many of us avoid thoughts about our abortions so we can continue to function. We may also numb all feelings about them. Thirty-two-year-old Oriana, who ended pregnancies at ages 18, 19, 25, and 30, has done this. Calling herself "emotionally unconscious" after the first two abortions, she says, "The only way I could have those abortions–I think it's true for most young women–is you just lock the doors, pull down the shades and say, 'I'm not at home.' You're just thinking about, 'When's it going to be over?'" Oriana experienced numbness less as a lack of feeling and more as a sense of drifting through events as if they weren't really happening.

For her, this sense of floating on top of the experience showed up as humor. She recalls, "The first time, there was elation. It was giggly. It was like, 'Gee, body knows how to work.' My partner and I were calling each other Ma and Pa. Or Mom and Dad. There was some joking to ease the tension. It was almost like, 'Gee, look what happened.' And, 'Look what bodies do. They make babies.' And not really a sense of connection."

She has seen the downside of this disconnection. After her first two abortions, she recalls, "I put myself in a numbing state, so I think I felt disconnected from people and things in general for a while." Ultimately, she felt detached from her abortions. She says, "I would wander around and see babies and feel confused about what I had done and what I should have done." This disconnection can cause overall numbness, as Oriana explains: "You have this hard time feeling like it's safe to connect back up to your feelings."

After both of her early abortions, the numbness eventually dissolved. She says, "Each time it went away in stages. It just took time for me to allow myself to experience feelings around it." She estimates that it took a few months each time.

Oriana sees two reasons for her disconnectedness. One is that such a reaction is common for young women. When she had abortions at ages 25 and 30, she approached them with much more awareness. The second reason for her disconnection is unresolved grief. "I'm one of those people who hates to cry," she says. This attitude may have prevented her from releasing her pain. Saying, "I never really had a good cry about what I've done," she adds, "Maybe that's why there was that disconnectedness." Afraid to get close to her grief, she had to distance herself from the whole experience.

Cassie: "I Didn't Want to Deal with It, So I Made a Big Joke out of It"

As for Oriana, humor was an integral part of 25-year-old Cassie's abortion experiences. She laughed her way through abortions at ages 22 and 24. This was not because she failed to see the seriousness of the situations. On the contrary, as she recalls her second pregnancy, she cries frequently. At the time, however, humor helped her ward off pain. "It was like armor for me," she says, adding, "I was putting up this huge front because, in my eyes, it reinforced my decision. That if I were really strong about this, and treated it as if it were light, there would be no reason for anyone to doubt what I did. And, in turn, no reason for me to doubt what I did." Raised in a family that regarded abortion as murder, Cassie had ample reason to doubt her choices. The "armor" prevented her family's voices from seeping into her brain as she carried out her decisions.

Aware that this humor served as a form of denial, Cassie says, "I dealt with it in a way that I knew how. And it got me through it." Cassie relied on this resource because, as she recalls, "I felt very vulnerable. I'm usually a really strong person and I have no problems telling anybody what I think and doing what I want to do. But both times I was pregnant, I prayed that there was not going to be a picket line there, because I would have lost it. Even though I knew what I was doing was right, I was so fragile."

The first time, in particular, Cassie treated her pregnancy "like a joke." She recalls, "I'd make jokes when we were in the supermarket: 'Pushing through. Lady with a baby.'" She explains, "I wanted to capitalize on how people treated pregnant women. They put pregnancy on this pedestal, like this is what women are for. And here I was saying, 'This is not what I want to do. This is what I think about all that.' I didn't want to deal with it so I made a big joke out of it." Cassie acknowledges that her pregnancy seemed unreal and too strange to be actually happening; this unreality added to her laughter.

During her first abortion procedure, she laughed the whole time, both to lighten the mood and out of nervousness. She recalls, "When the doctor stuck his finger up my vagina, I laughed hysterically, and he told me he wouldn't continue until I stopped. And I couldn't stop laughing." Cassie has dealt with other situations the same way. She notes, "If get into a fight with my husband, sometimes, I'll start laughing at really inappropriate times." As awkward as this can be, she values the way this defense helped her through her abortions, saying, "I'm glad there was something there for me to fall back on."

USING DENIAL IN EACH STAGE OF THE EXPERIENCE

Throughout an abortion experience, denial can protect us from facing things we are not yet ready to face. Here are various stages in which denial might arise:

Before Conception:

> As we engage in sex, many of us block out the possibility of pregnancy. If we're fully aware of sex's dangers, we would probably be unable to enjoy ourselves in bed. We often think of unplanned pregnancy as something that can happen to others, but from which we are personally protected. The following comment illustrates this mindset.
>
> When I became sexually active, if you'd asked me what I would do if I got pregnant, I would have answered, "I won't get pregnant." It didn't enter my mind I could get pregnant. Until I did. Even then, I was like, "This can't be." (Toni, age 23, who had abortions at ages 21, 22, and four months ago)

If we feel shielded from the threat of unplanned pregnancy, we will be unable to imagine ourselves as candidates for abortion. We will deny this possibility even more if we have been raised in antiabortion religions or families. The next quotation exemplifies this attitude.

> All of my life I have been pro-life and was disgusted with the idea of abortion. An unwanted pregnancy would never happen to me. Obviously, I was wrong. (Evelyn, age 18, who had an abortion ten days ago)

Before a Pregnancy Test:

After we conceive an unwanted pregnancy, we might put off recognizing its symptoms, attributing missed periods to stress, choosing not to see our engorged breasts, or thinking that swelling abdomens are the result of overeating, not pregnancy. The following comments illustrate such denial of pregnancy symptoms.

> [On her first terminated pregnancy] About five weeks before our wedding, I noticed my period was late. I imagined it was the excitement of prenuptial planning and details. (Beth, age 41, who had abortions at ages 27 and 40)

> [On her first terminated pregnancy] The abortion occurred when I was fifteen weeks pregnant. I was dealing with a lot of stuff with my parents. I was like, "God, I still haven't gotten my period. Well, I'm around my folks and I'm so tense." (Wanda, age 23, who had abortions at ages 19 and 22)

At a Pregnancy Test:

Many of us discover that we are pregnant by using a home pregnancy test. This can be quite a jolt. What seems even more shocking is to hear the news from a health care worker. The next two comments describe the denial we may use as we learn of our pregnancy in that way.

> [With her first pregnancy] I saw a gynecologist. I remember politely but insistently challenging his credentials, education, and professional ability, in spite of his obvious twenty years' experience. He humored me, but held onto his observation that I was ten to eleven weeks pregnant. (Gabriella, age 38, who had abortions at ages 22, 24, and 26)

> You couldn't tell me nothing. I thought it was a false pregnancy. Even after I called Kaiser, I acted like I didn't hear it, like I didn't know. (Ricki, age 20, six weeks after her abortion)

While Making a Decision:

Once we hear that we are pregnant, we might find the news so hard to take that we put it out of our minds. Teenagers, especially, tend to do this, and often end up having late abortions. The next comments show how three people dealt with the news of their pregnancies when they were in or just beyond their teen years.

> [On being pregnant 16 weeks before her second abortion] The rational part of me knew I needed to make some decision. But the emotional side of me overrode my logic, so all I did was beat myself up for becoming pregnant. I let myself get caught in a standing pool of shame and fear until it was almost too late to do anything but keep the baby. (Abigail, age 24, who had abortions at ages 19 and 20)

> [On how her boyfriend prodded her to schedule an abortion] He would call and remind me that I was pregnant. He was like, "When are you going to call a clinic?" I said, "Let me get off the phone. I'll do it right now." And I wouldn't do it. He had to force me to do it. I was just like, "I can't fit it into my busy schedule." He's like, "Well, you're going to have to do it before the baby comes!" (Ricki, age 20, six weeks after her abortion)

> I said to myself that I was going to keep it, name it, teach it how to swim, how my friend would be known as "auntie."

All that, and at the same time, I knew what I had to do. (Blair, age 17, one year after her abortion)

At an Abortion:

At the procedure, we may need to be as unemotional as possible. Fearing that we will change our minds if we pause to consider our actions, we may steel ourselves. Others of us proceed numbly because surgery seems so frightening; we need to grit our teeth and forge through the challenges. While it is difficult to deny the events taking place at an abortion, we may try to block out what we are feeling. To protect ourselves from scary emotions, we may find ourselves cracking jokes and being flippant, as the following speakers did.

They wheeled me up on the cart. I was singing, "They're coming to take me away!" My doctor came in. And I said, "This drug is really good, doctor!" (Daphne, age 44, who has had three abortions since her twenties)

The nurse was playing polkas. The uum-pah, uum-pah struck my sedated brain as tremendously funny and I started to giggle. The woman next to me looked at me with contempt for my lack of seriousness in the face of where we were and why. (Melinda, age 42, who had abortions at ages 20 and 25)

The sedatives probably made both of these women giddy, but it would seem that they were also trying to distract themselves from the procedure's solemnity.

Immediately After an Abortion:

It is hard to believe that we could go through an operation and put it out of our minds afterward, but many of us do just this. General anesthesia adds a dreamlike quality to the experience. Whatever type of anesthetic we have, we may find it odd to return from the surgery to a world where people go about their business, most not knowing about our abortions. The experience may feel so isolated from our daily lives that on some level, we tell ourselves that it never occurred. A month after her abortion, one 24 year old recalls, "The first week was the most intense–I went in and out of realizing I had an abortion." A 25 year old reports that something similar happened the day after she had an abortion a year ago: "I forgot it all until the next week, when I got an infection."

We might put off dealing with our emotions. It might seem too painful or frightening to think about how we feel, so we try to block it out and reimmerse ourselves in our lives. As one 20 year old comments, six weeks after her abortion, "I try to stuff things into the closet. It's there, but you don't think about it." The feelings may demand to be noticed, however, and may surface in a delayed reaction. As numbness wears off, our true emotions can come forward. Some significant event or stress can also cause the blocked feelings to flow. This happened to one 20 year old who ended a pregnancy two years ago. She recalls, "After the abortion, it took several months for me to react. When I did, I also found out I was pregnant again and miscarried, and that's when I felt my life was falling apart."

A Few Months or More After an Abortion:

Much of the denial we might have about our abortion wears off with time, as we gain the courage to look at our experience more closely. If denial persists long after an abortion, however, it can create problems, crystallizing into a sort of lie that we cannot dismantle with ease. The following comments illustrate long-term denial:

> I try to pretend it never happened. I wish I could forget it, but it will always be there. (Hilary, age 18, two years after her abortion)

> I remember almost nothing from my second abortion. I must have blocked the experience out. I have tried to remember, but nothing comes. . . . The second one is a mystery and I don't like to think about it. It was a very bad

> part of my life. (Ilsa, age 29, who had abortions at ages 14, 19, and 27)

After an abortion, the cycle of denial can begin all over again. Many of us find it hard to contemplate the possibility of another unplanned pregnancy; as we resume our sex lives, we may block out thoughts about conceiving against our will. While such denial is normal, it can present problems if we fully deny the possibility of another pregnancy and use no birth control. The next quotation illustrates this mindset.

> [On speaking to nurses after her third abortion and her second IUD failure] They said, "What is your choice of birth control?" I said, "Oh, I really like the IUD. I'm happy with it." They said, "I don't think it works for you. I think you'd better get something else." And I went, "Oh." I just thought that would be one in a trillion if it happened again. (Daphne, age 44, who has had three abortions since her twenties)

Clearly, denial can occur in every stage of an abortion experience. Now we will meet Meredith and see how she used denial throughout her abortions.

Meredith: "I Knew I Was Pregnant; I Basically Tried to Deny It"

Meredith, who is Caucasian, seems older than her 21 years. In a rich, deep voice filled with self-assurance, she speaks of the painful things she has done and seen. The way her parents divorced when she was young and Meredith moved in with her grandparents. The way her mother ran off, never to be seen again, and her grandfather molested her. The way she dropped out of high school and slipped into alcoholism and heavy substance use at 19, when she had her third abortion. She cries several times during her interview, suddenly looking young, frightened, and very much in need of love. Then she resumes a tough exterior, snapping when she finds a question insulting, intent on maintaining her dignity.

Meredith certainly needed this toughness when she was 17. "I was in a lot of trouble at that time," she recalls. "I was sent to an

Outward Bound course called Youth at Risk. And I was pregnant." On some level, says Meredith, "I knew I was pregnant, although I avoided pursuing a test; I basically tried to deny it for the longest time." Being scrappy, she evaded the required medical tests that would have revealed her condition. She simply told her doctor that she didn't need a urine test, and he complied.

Things stopped being so easy once she faced the program's rigors. She recalls, "It really started to be a problem when I got dizzy a lot. Just the normal symptoms of pregnancy that really didn't go with a survival training course! Nausea, dizziness. And my equilibrium was totally thrown off by hormones. I was just way out there."

She continues, "My period hadn't come, but I was lying to myself, 'This is not happening.' But at one point, we did rock climbing and rappelling. At that point, I really could not deny that I was pregnant, because I had a little belly. I had to tie this harness around my waist. It was like, 'Hmm, I don't know,'" she says. "But," notes Meredith, it wasn't "at that point that I had to really face it." That moment came three months into her pregnancy, when she fell and the group leaders took her to a hospital, worried that she might have a concussion. Meredith recalls, "The nurse just looked at me and said, 'You need a pregnancy test.'"

Suddenly, her private pregnancy became very public. The course leaders called Meredith's dad and stepmother, who cut short their trip in Europe. Meredith had to tell them about the pregnancy, which was embarrassing, because of how she had concealed the pregnancy from her doctor. She explains, "It should never have happened because their regulations state you have to have a test before you come. I really fucked everything up." What was even more humiliating was that Meredith's father and stepmother assumed full authority over her pregnancy. Meredith recalls, "My parents didn't even ask me. They told me that I was getting an abortion."

Meredith had an abortion, but her denial helped her feel little emotion about it. Because she avoided recognizing her pregnancy for so long, she felt no connection to the fetus. She says, "During the whole time I was pregnant, it was like this alien thing. I just tried to deny it, what was happening to my body, what I was thinking." Meredith explains that this abortion and the two she had over the next three years "had certain pain for me," and says that the "emotions come up from time to time," but notes that she managed to remain calm during each procedure. She says, "I always seemed to handle it as if I knew everything I was doing." Meredith explains how with her latter two abortions, she would "come to a decision and just do it. It surprises me," she comments, "because I'm a very emotional person." Particularly with her last abortion, she recalls, "I just did my thing once again. I was looking forward to going home and sleeping it off. It felt very mechanical."

After her abortions, she maintained the same lack of emotion. Rather than wringing her hands about the past, Meredith says, "I plunged myself back into whatever my life was at the time. I just kept going." Meredith thinks it unwise to dwell on an abortion, especially with thoughts about the fetus. She notes, "If you really want to screw yourself up, you could play with a bunch of ideas about boy or girl, what it would look like, la la la. I learned that first time that that was not how one survives one of these things. You just put it behind you." Meredith adds sardonically, "At that time, I put it behind me by drinking."

BREAKING THROUGH DENIAL

Meredith's last comment touches on an essential point: the more one wants to avoid thinking about an abortion, the more energy one must put into denial or into activities such as drinking. In the long run, this can be more exhausting than facing intense emotions. We now meet Amelia, who is trying to break through denial and let those feelings emerge.

Amelia: "I Had No Idea It Was All of an Inch Big Already"

Twenty-seven-year-old Amelia, who is Caucasian, used denial almost from the beginning of her experience. She recalls that when she discovered she was pregnant two and a half weeks ago, she "didn't really believe it." Immediately, she took abortive herbs. Amelia explains, "In taking the herbs, I felt like I would just have a natural miscarriage. It would be like getting my period again, as if I were never pregnant. I went through this la la land and thought I wouldn't have to actually resort to abortion." After herbs did not work, Amelia tried acupuncture, which also failed. She calls such attempts "total denial," which seems untrue. Total denial would mean that she became immobile, unwilling to recognize that she was pregnant, and therefore unable to take action. Amelia only hoped for a more "natural" method than surgery and wished, it seems, to keep her abortion private. With no medical record of her abortion, she could forget these undocumented facts.

Lacking alternatives to surgical abortion, Amelia enlisted a clinic's help. The clinicians did a sonogram to locate the fetus and Amelia says, "I actually got to look at it on the screen. The doctor showed me its heart and it was beating fast. I had no idea it was all of an inch big already. As the doctor told me, that was probably including the sac and placenta, but still! I thought it was a microscopic dot, or so I kept telling myself." Until then, Amelia had no positive regard for the fetus. Saying she "felt no maternal feelings for it," she adds, "I also felt mad at the baby for forcing this on me." Aside from her anger, Amelia felt numb about the pregnancy. "I detached myself from it," she says, "knowing it would end." She pretended it was just a tiny egg. "I think I was only telling myself that to make it easier," she says, adding, "I don't think I wanted to know." In what Amelia calls a "blind illusion," she "tried not thinking about it."

Seeing the fetus on the screen ripped through that illusion. She explains, "After I learned how big it was and saw its heart beating, I grew loving toward the baby." She cried hard the night after the sonogram. Amelia says, "I started measuring how big it was (an inch) on my stomach with my finger and thumb, imagining it inside. This made it more emotional and intense for me to abort." She notes, however, that she also wanted the abortion "over with right away to avoid any more growth and attachment."

She ended the pregnancy a few days later and felt numb again right before and after the procedure. She recalls, "I was in a very strange mood, as if in a daze." Afterward, she felt "happy and relieved." The relief lasted only one day. Then, grief crashed in. The day after her abortion, she wrote, "Now, feelings that I have killed a baby go through my head–*my* baby. That hurts, and it hurts to have seen that heart beating so fast and strong." As emotions pummel her, she says, "I have been running from thoughts and emotions, because I don't want to look at it. I feel really awful when I start thinking how irresponsible I was and how I could have gotten the morning-after pill or used birth control. I never thought abortion would happen to me." Amelia is looking at every aspect of her experience at once, stripping away denial.

As Amelia wrestles with guilt and grief, she fears her feelings. She says, "I'm seeing how much I run from emotions and how they catch up and haunt me. I try not to feel it all, but I have to." Amelia notes, "I have been wanting to escape in any way I can, and have been wanting to drink." But she has not done this. Nor has she shut off her feelings. Despite all the denial she mentions, she tries to open herself to the tides of unexpected emotions. Amelia says simply, "I just feel. I feel a lot of things and I don't think I have felt the extent of these emotions yet. I feel loss today, when yesterday I was relieved. Tears are coming to my eyes now, and I think I've got a lot to deal with here." Because she is trying to let feelings move through her, Amelia will likely shake off any remnants of denial and resolve her guilt and grief.

ARRIVING AT THE TRUTH

Amelia has begun to uncover painful truths about fetal development and about what the fetus means to her. But these feelings may not be the "truth" for everyone. Other women have seen the same images and have had different reactions, either feeling relieved that the fetus was still so small and formless, or appreciating this chance to break through denial.

Twenty-five-year-old Florence reacted the second way when she ended a pregnancy four years ago. She says that when she saw a sonogram, "It really hit home that there was a baby inside. I realized it was a person in there. I wanted that realization of humanness, because it would be irresponsible of me not to have it. I need to know the facts. It would be childish of me to ignore it." Florence, who had her first abortion at age 18, did not always find it easy to acknowledge that fetuses have a physical reality. During her first pregnancy, she dreamed about "rocks" in her "tummy." Thinking of "something solid" in there evoked fear and shock. It took some time for her to want to face the reality.

Many of us share this fear of knowing exactly what we remove in an abortion. Not knowing helps us get through the act. The danger in such denial is that we may feel shaken if we come across pictures of fetuses or information about fetal development. Some pro-life literature claims that first-trimester fetuses are larger or more developed than they actually are; knowing the facts can protect us against such falsehoods. While it can make us uneasy to think about fetal development, we may find ourselves on more solid ground if we look at abortion with as little denial as possible. One could argue that much of the denial in the abortion experience comes from avoiding this central issue, and that looking at it more closely could help us dissolve other denial in the experience.

Chapter 7

A New Self Emerges

With well-scrubbed skin, a chestnut braid, and sturdy hips, Fritzi, who is white and 21, looks like she just stepped out of a Land O' Lakes commercial. Indeed, she comes from the Midwest, although she now attends a stellar college on the East Coast. Looking at Fritzi and listening to her describe her abortion forces one to examine stereotypes about who has abortions. Can that group include farm-fresh women like Fritzi?

Aware that the public has a narrow answer to this question, Fritzi hesitates to tell people about the abortion she had two years ago. She senses that their idea of who she is does not match the image of who ends unplanned pregnancies. For instance, her high school peers see her as nearly perfect. In high school, Fritzi explains, "I graduated at the top of my class. I got all these honors." She worries that her abortion would diminish her excellence in her peers' eyes. "I think of the abortion as a mistake," she says, before correcting herself. "Not the abortion, but the pregnancy. Any blemish like that is hard to announce to someone who has seen this other side of you."

Fritzi never thought she would have an abortion. "I was one of these people who always fully believed in choice," she says. At the same time, she "knew" she would not conceive unintentionally. She explains, "I would have birth control, I would know what to do, and I would certainly have some safety net." Unfortunately, says Fritzi, things "didn't really happen that way." Despite her careful use of a diaphragm, Fritzi conceived two years ago and ended the pregnancy. "One thing that struck me," she notes, "is that a lot of people who end up getting abortions don't expect that they're going to have them."

She is absolutely right. While we may view abortion as a backup in case we conceive unhappily, few of us envision that abortion will touch our lives. One 25 year old felt this way when she discovered her pregnancy seven years ago. She says, "I was surprised that I was actually pregnant–a teenaged statistic. Things like STDs, car accidents, rapes, and abortions exist in society, but they'd never existed *for me*. It felt strange not to be on the 'other' side–for once, I wasn't looking in at the victim; I was looking out from the cage." Long after an abortion, it can be jarring to realize that this event has touched our lives. Fritzi feels this way whenever she goes for a doctor's appointment. She muses, "It's all on the records. You can look it up and see I've had one pregnancy."

Fritzi must figure out how to integrate this fact into her idea of who she is. She needs to answer the question, Who am I to have had an abortion? How can she accept that this unthinkable event has happened to her? One way is to frame her abortion as something that meshes with the rest of her life. Fritzi has done this. "My mom always teases me," she says, "because my brother and sister have all these medical problems." In fact, her siblings have been disabled from birth. In contrast, Fritzi's medical problems "are all accidents." Fritzi continues, "I've tried to put it as much as I could in that category" of accidents. She also sees the pregnancy and abortion as enormously helpful growth experiences. Looking back on that time in her college career, she says that those events stand out as being like "a class," a time of great learning and maturing. Fritzi comments, "I wouldn't be who I am now without" that experience. "Two years ago, I wasn't the same. It's part of me."

The other large question that has arisen for Fritzi is, How do I feel about myself now that I have had a unplanned pregnancy and abortion? Before the pregnancy, Fritzi felt terrific. She ranked second on her sports team in tests of strength and endurance. Fritzi says, "I felt good about that. And I let that go to pot after I got my abortion." The reason? She says, "I didn't feel great about myself." Her self-esteem dropped so dramatically that in the summer after her abortion, she began dating a man she did not like. She observes, "I know I must not have been feeling too good about myself to go out with this guy."

That fall, Fritzi's self-esteem began to improve. She went to Europe on an exchange program and "was very far from everything." In Europe, she excelled academically. "I think grades helped," she notes, in assessing how she began to feel good about herself again. What helped even more was that Fritzi brought high self-esteem into her experiences with pregnancy and abortion. Fritzi acknowledges that she has a lot of self-confidence, "which is what enabled me to have things like the abortion, and which has enabled me to continue to be premed and to get Cs and C+s and decide to go through with it. It think it's the same kind of confidence that says, 'You may not be great in this area, you made this mistake then, but there's so much more inside you that you can do.'" That confidence also allows her to take pride in her efforts, no matter what the outcome. When she reflects back on the term she was pregnant, Fritzi recalls, "I took two science courses. I had two labs, I had sports practice every day, I had a work/study job, and I was pregnant. I look at my transcript and I see a C+, a C, and a B. And I think, 'How did I not fail out? I am so proud of those three grades!'" Fritzi's solid base of self-esteem helped her endure a difficult experience and emerge with a new, and ultimately more positive, sense of self.

HOW DO I FEEL ABOUT MYSELF NOW?

As Fritzi's story illustrates, after an abortion, women need to find a place for this experience in their sense of who they are and what their lives entail; we will look at these issues later in the chapter. First, we examine the matter of self-esteem. Frequently, an abortion experience causes self-esteem to waver a bit. Because many of us consider unplanned pregnancies to be mistakes, we are likely to feel badly about ourselves after a positive pregnancy test. This feeling may arise even if we used birth control, and even if sex was not consensual. When we decide on abortion and follow through with this decision, it can foster a sense of competence, mending self-esteem or even taking it to new heights. As one 39 year old says of the abortion she had four years ago, "Being able to make the decision and follow through with having an abortion actually increased my self-esteem because it was an empowering decision." We now meet Deirdre, whose abortion made her feel wonderful about herself–better, in fact, than she ever felt.

Deirdre: "The Abortion Was a Way to Say I Believe in Myself"

Deirdre, who is Caucasian, calls her abortion experience "such a relief and a real reality check." She explains, "I was doing badly in school and in a bad relationship. It was my first step toward independence and it was a way to say, 'I believe in myself and I deserve to be happy.' I became motivated and applied to college and dumped my lame boyfriend! I am a truly happy person today and I see the abortion as the beginning of that." She adds, "I feel sorry for the old me, a sad 17 year old. Five years later, I am proud of who I have become. I am strong, bold, know who I am, what I want, and how to get it." She praises herself for handling her first adult crisis competently. Deirdre puts it this way: "I applaud my young self and say to her: 'You did it. You are strong. I love you.'"

Because Deirdre feels so good about herself now, it is painful for her to remember being 17, pregnant, in a bad relationship, and devoid of confidence. "Looking back," she says, "what is hardest to deal with is that I was so weak. It sickens me to think I didn't have enough self-esteem to tell that guy to fuck off. It's hard to understand where my faith in myself went during my teen years and I worry for other young women—teen years are so hard. Why do young women lose self-esteem? These are questions that hurt."

Deirdre describes how badly she felt about herself when she conceived: "I was very insecure, had a hard time communicating with my parents (they hated my boyfriend), and didn't know how to take control of my life." She had dated Saul for one year and says, "I remember being very depressed at the time, unhappy in my relationship. I'd tried to break up with him, but he begged me to go back to him and I eventually gave in." Deirdre has little compassion for her own flipflopping. She says, "I was weak—didn't trust myself." When she broke up with him, she went off the pill to "prove" to both of them that the relationship was over. She did not, however, go back on it when they reunited; perhaps taking the pill again would mean admitting her change of heart. She thought, "Oh hell, it's too late," as if after going back to him, she had no energy left for birth control. When she conceived, she was not surprised. She recalls, "I was expecting it and just felt verified and dark. I felt covered in a fog. Now I had a real reason to feel bad. Sort of hopeless–but not like I saw no way out–more like I'd reached my bottom and it was a wake-up call."

Deirdre decided on abortion and had to cope with several practical details in order to obtain one. She recalls, "I didn't want to tell my parents and had no money. I had to get Medicare–stand in lines at the welfare place–all things I'd never done before. But it really forced me to grow and learn I can do it and feel like a adult." Jumping these hurdles made Deirdre see her own strengths. She says, "I know I can survive a stressful, difficult, scary experience and rebound as a stronger person." Deirdre exults in having exercised power in her own life. She says exuberantly, "I feel in control, definitely. I know what I want and I know I can get through hard times. I believe in myself and in my ability to make decisions and to survive. After my abortion, I began to trust myself more, believe in myself more."

Armed with new self-confidence, she broke up with Saul within a year. Deirdre explains, "It was a bad relationship and I finally trusted myself enough to leave him." Since then, she says, "I found a man who isn't afraid of my power and sexuality." Now, Deirdre approaches gender issues differently. She observes, "I have become more of a feminist, or it's more that I'm living my beliefs. I feel girls need to be raised to have sexual and social power and taught that they don't need men to be happy." This is a lesson Deirdre has learned on her own. She says, "I don't need a man to be happy, because I love myself."

Deirdre's words resound with the energy of a convert. They may be so forceful because she does not want to return to that earlier, depressed state. Her vigor may also come from her despair that young women often share her previously low self-esteem, and that it can take something as drastic as a pregnancy and abortion for them to climb out of that place.

Peggy: "I Didn't Like Myself for Doing What I Did"

Unlike Deirdre, Peggy has seen her self-esteem plummet since her abortion. A 26-year-old African American with perfect hair and makeup, Peggy looks like she might feel terrific about herself.

Although she is beginning to approve of herself more now, nothing could have been further from the truth right after her abortion.

Peggy's low self-esteem stems, in part, from her dissatisfaction with her life. As she surveys her achievements to date, she concludes that she is "not where I thought I would be. I always thought by now I'd have a house and two cars and three kids and a husband." Instead, she has a 7 year old by a gang member and has had two recent abortions. Peggy is not even pro-choice. "I always thought abortion was wrong," she says. As a teenager, she saw her friends have six or more abortions. Peggy recalls, "I felt so sorry for them. Like, 'How could you let yourself go through this? How could you do this to your body? How could you let men do this to you?'" She could not identify with them, and explains, "I never thought I would get in a situation where I would even think about having an abortion." She had one abortion six months ago, however, and another six weeks ago. She feels fine about ending her first pregnancy, but regards her second choice as a terrible mistake, and blames herself for failing her baby. She comments, "I'm starting to like myself again. But I didn't, because I was mad at myself for doing what I did."

On top of that, her self-esteem is particularly low right now because she just lost her boyfriend. Charles grew distant right after her second abortion. When she confronted him, she learned that he had lost his job and become an escort, selling his time to keep afloat financially. This rejection has made her doubt her worth. She laments, "Ever since I was young, I wanted to be married. And I've never been able to find that with anybody." She now feels, "I'm not worthy of loving, not worth having a relationship with, and nobody wants me." Soon after Peggy found out about Charles's problems, she was laid off herself. Because so may losses have occurred at once, it can be hard to sort out which feeling comes from which trauma, or how much Peggy's feeling of worthlessness precedes her troubles. She acknowledges, "I've always sensed that I had low self-esteem. It had a little bit to do with my upbringing and my relationship with my father." The troubles she has experienced only dissolved her shaky self-esteem a bit more.

Even so, she sees that the second abortion and Charles's rejection have enhanced her sense of self in a way. She explains, "I feel like

I've changed. I have become stronger and I've grown from it." She says her pain from the abortion and from Charles's cruelty "makes me see things differently." So differently that she believes she would no longer be drawn to Charles. Peggy muses, "If I were to go back to the man who just left me, I probably wouldn't want him." In addition, she thinks Charles "would not be attracted to me anymore." This statement comes, not from a sense of being unattractive, but from Peggy's feeling that she has transformed for the better, even in other people's eyes.

WHO AM I, NOW THAT I HAVE HAD AN ABORTION?

Since their abortions, Deirdre and Peggy have evaluated how they feel about themselves. As they examine this issue, they also consider the matter of who they have become. Both cite growth and new strengths. After an abortion, we may feel changed in many ways. One 38 year old describes how she struggled to accept her altered identity before she ended a pregnancy fourteen years ago. She recalls, "I walked in the park, through the zoo, by the lake. Crying. Saying 'Gravida 1, para 0.'" Using medical terminology, she expressed her new identity: she would become a woman with one pregnancy in her history (gravida 1) and no deliveries to show for it (para 0). The pregnancy and abortion made her someone she had never been before. She faced the question that many of us tackle after an unplanned pregnancy and abortion: Who am I, now that these experiences have entered my life?

Sabine: "I Always Look at Things Cynically Now"

Sabine begins answering that question by describing how she used to approach life. She is a 23-year-old African American who tucks her hair up into a baseball cap; the lines of her face are stark with anger and pain over the abortion she had two years ago. "I looked at the world through rose-colored glasses before it happened," she says. "Now I don't. A lot of that has to do with the abortion. It's not all easy as pie. Life isn't a fairytale. Experiences like that make it really clear that things don't always work out as you want them to. That makes me feel a little bit more cynical about people, a little more bitter."

Sabine and her boyfriend Frank lived together and were very much in love when she conceived. After she discovered the pregnancy, they felt delighted and planned to marry and have the baby. Sabine shared the news with her mom, although they had always had a difficult relationship. Sabine explains, "I thought it was a good thing I was pregnant and Mom should be happy. I'm her daughter, so any decision I made would be okay with her. And she'd love me anyway." Sabine's mother did not take the news well, however. "She completely freaked out," Sabine recalls. "She said I was a slut and that it was going to ruin my life and that she ought to know–she had two kids and it ruined her life. It was awful. I couldn't handle it. My mother had just lost it, and so did I." Sabine began to doubt her own judgment. She notes, "I made a mistake thinking that Mom would be supportive of this. It made me think that all I made were mistakes." Sabine figured that if she could not cope with her mother's outburst, she was not ready to face the challenges of parenthood, so she decided on abortion. Sabine recalls, "I was distraught because I didn't want to do it." She went through the abortion numbly, taking painkillers for several days afterward to sedate her emotions. Once the numbness wore off, she was filled with regret about her decision. Now, she no longer thinks of the abortion as a mistake and is glad of her choice. Still, she has sorrow about ending a pregnancy she wanted to keep.

Added to this trauma, her relations with Frank deteriorated soon after the procedure. Sabine attributes 90 percent of the change to the abortion. She explains, "We couldn't talk about the abortion, because it was very painful for me and I don't think he thought about it a lot. I got mad at him" for not feeling much. Sabine does not know if Frank realized how much pain she felt about her abortion. Recalling that time now, she begins to cry, saying, "He thought things went back to normal. But they never did for me."

Sabine still wanted to marry during the year and a half in which they continued to date, but Frank lost interest in this idea. He began to see other women and to lie about it. Sabine moved out to shore up a dwindling sense of self, but they continued to see each other.

Some months later, he claimed he had married another woman. He put Sabine's belongings in garbage bags and left them outside his home for her to retrieve. It turned out he had never married after all, although he was, indeed, involved with someone new.

These losses and disappointments have taken their toll on Sabine's optimism. She muses, "I always thought of myself as young and innocent about life. But," she says, "I stopped being that way. I always look at things cynically now." She criticizes herself for the way she approached her abortion, saying, "I just thought I would walk into this office and it would be over with. Maybe it was a little naive of me to think that I wouldn't feel anything." At that time, she trusted people like Frank and her mother. Sabine recalls, "I always thought people were good, no matter what. That even if someone did something bad, it didn't mean they were a bad person." She now reviles this trust, saying, "I was naive in the sense that I could believe in this person, that I could believe that my decision, no matter which one I made, would be okay, that I could have believed in all the things I believed in, and that they turned out so wrong."

Sabine says she lost not only her optimism, but also "all the stuff that went with" the pregnancy: "the way I felt about it, people and ideas that I used to have, and the way I used to look at things." She notes, it "wasn't just about losing a baby. It was about losing a part of myself." Sabine thinks joy eludes her now and regrets that she isn't as "carefree or spontaneously happy" as before, that she can't get back to that person she used to be.

She views these changes as permanent, and she doesn't see herself as the only person transformed by an abortion. She declares, "No woman comes out exactly the same as when she went in. In a little way, she's changed." This may not, in fact, be true. Many women regard an abortion as a way to return to their pre-pregnancy selves and they pick up right where they left off after the surgery. But others do indeed feel as Sabine does, that "Once you've been through it, you know that you can't do it and be the same ever again."

Her transformation comes from going through such large experiences all at once. How could they not change her or the way she sees the world? Her loss of happiness is tragic, but the other changes are somewhat positive. We all have to lose innocence at some point, and Sabine feels ambivalent about her earlier innocence anyway. Her new wisdom will prevent her from making choices that she considers naive in the future.

What happens if a pregnancy or abortion conflicts with a treasured part of oneself? Does one stop believing in that aspect of one's personality? We now meet Annika, who has grappled with this issue.

Annika: "I Felt That I Wasn't Me"

After Annika, age 31, had an abortion five years ago, she says, "I felt that I wasn't sure who I was anymore." The abortion conflicted "so drastically" with ideas she embraced about herself that she questioned her "whole identity." She says the abortion "really pushed me to look at who I was and what I believed in and what I didn't believe in. No other experience had ever asked me to do that to that extent." The unplanned pregnancy and abortion presented her with new information about herself that she had trouble accepting.

Annika could not understand how, as someone with her act together, she could neglect to use birth control. A petite woman in a business suit, she tousles her thin, blond hair as she recalls this conflict: "I felt so irresponsible. I could have avoided this huge trauma. How could I have been so stupid to even set myself up for the possibility? It just felt so unlike me, too. I still can't understand it." There are many possible reasons Annika avoided using birth control. We will discuss such issues in Chapter 11. What is relevant here is the way Annika's actions conflicted with her sense of self.

Using no birth control was just the tip of the iceberg. Even contemplating abortion astonished her. Annika grew up in a European country where abortion is largely illegal, so she never imagined having one. Knowing that her peers at home did not have her luxury of choice made her feel guilty. In addition, she had finished her education and had a boyfriend ready to marry her and start a family. There were many problems in their relationship, however, ones that triggered huge doubts for Annika about having a child together.

She reluctantly chose to end the pregnancy and recalls that when she made this decision, "Part of me was shocked that I was able to do it. If somebody had told me, 'In the fall, you're going to have an abortion,' I would have said, 'You're crazy. I'll never do such a thing.' I really believed that of myself." After her abortion, Annika still had trouble accepting that she had ended a pregnancy. A practicing Catholic, Annika thought she "had done something so awful, so much against my moral values" that she felt quite guilty. "I was extremely hard on myself," she recalls. Feeling like "a bad person," she forbade herself to attend church, thinking she no longer belonged among the devout.

Annika also felt badly about ending her pregnancy because she perceives herself as compassionate and as having a great maternal capacity. Saying the abortion "was against the way I saw myself as a woman," she explains, "That was hard for me to integrate, that I was capable of doing that." Unable to weave this action into her sense of self, she began to doubt who she was. She recalls, "I felt that I wasn't me. I felt like if I looked in the mirror, I was going to go, 'Who's this? Who is this person that could do something as terrible as that?'" The abortion, Annika says, "really started a huge identity crisis for me."

Five years have passed since her abortion. She still does not know what she thinks of it morally, but has managed to accept her abortion by going through therapy and looking closely at herself. "I have become much more accepting of myself," she notes, adding, "Having the abortion has changed me." She calls these changes positive and enriching, saying, "It has opened up depth to me. Depth of experience and depth of pain that I wasn't even sure I was capable of feeling. And I feel that I can be much more empathic to people's trauma. I think that sometimes with the biggest pain, the biggest growth happens."

Simone: "Not to Help Form Life Was Somehow Nonmaternal"

Like Annika, Simone has felt a conflict between her abortion and her values. Whereas Annika has questioned her whole identity, however, Simone has only felt a rift within one part of herself. After Simone, age 39, had an abortion a year ago, she hesitated to tell her friends the news. She cannot understand this reluctance, because many of her friends have ended pregnancies and several are abortion rights activists. She recalls, "I was very sensitive to how I thought people would react." As she speaks, the blond hair she has probably worn long and straight since the 1970s falls softly against her face. She continues, "I felt ashamed of it, because I was a mother already. So to be a mother and do that, to be a mother and not to help form life, it was somehow nonmaternal."

Simone conceived during an incredibly hectic time, when her and her husband's careers were in turmoil. She did not feel she could give sufficient attention to a new child. Moreover, she wanted to devote herself to the 17-month-old son she already had. Her abortion solved her practical problems, but raised some troubling issues about how she could be a mother and end a potential life. In a voice filled with passion and pain, she says, "I think mothers have a special relationship to the whole nurturing of life." She stresses that by "mothers" she does not mean "women." Instead, she means, "people who are maternal and who take on that maternal role." Such people "have a special relationship" to life, "so it seems counter-intuitive not to want to nurture life at any cost."

Her qualms about ending life make her oppose war. She sees abortion as conflicting with this philosophy, and muses, "I think abortion is a really violent solution to certain very natural problems. I don't want to see myself as implicated in murder of innocents, since I see myself as a pacifist. And that's where the sense of shame comes in."

Simone's shame about acting in a nonmaternal way has roots not only in her social values, but also in her personal life. She is a successful professional, who has spent years nurturing her career. When she had her first child at 37, she felt doubts about how good a mother she could be, given her continuing commitment to her work. She explains, "Because I was a professional before I was a mother, my professional image is much stronger than my maternal image." It galls her that, "As professionals, we have these children and then we don't spend any time with them." Simone spends time in the evening playing with her daughter, but her mind is still at her desk. She wants to "be in a balanced situation," but notes, "I'm so conditioned by my previous lifetime as a professional that it's hard to give that all up and put it into perspective." Simone's anxiety about her maternal capacity may exacerbate her feelings about her abortion. She is currently five months into a third pregnancy, and might have renewed concerns about how she can be a good mother to a second child, especially while her daughter is still so young. As she watches for signs of life within her, her current pregnancy may also intensify her doubts about her abortion.

To cope with these doubts, Simone reminds herself that her pro-choice beliefs are just as valid as her objections to abortion, if not more so. While she feels it is "counterintuitive not to want to nurture life at any cost," it also piques her "social conscience" to see unwanted children brought into the world. It is "a horror," she says, "to have children born into unhappy relationships, or to drug-addicted mothers, or alcoholic parents, or parents who don't want them." She adds, "I have that sense of children saying, 'Why was I even born?' It must be so horrible to be a child who feels abandoned, either in a physical or an emotional sense, that it's probably better that they're not born." She also appeases her maternal conscience by expressing concerns about overpopulation. "You can't just go on reproducing like chickens!" she exclaims. "There have got to be better forms of birth control. I don't think we have them. So women are pushed to using abortion."

Simone and Annika have taken on the large moral issues of abortion that grip our country, issues that seem to defy simple resolution on a social or personal level. To ease the discord between their abortions and their identities, the two women have taken different routes: Annika has changed her idea of who she is, whereas Simone has examined the social aspects of abortion. Both have found it difficult to attain easy answers.

Veronica: "I've Redefined My Idea of Whom This Can Happen to"

Like Annika and Simone, Veronica has faced a conflict between abortion and her self-image. Veronica, however, has resolved the conflict fairly easily. Her task has been simpler, because she does not harbor moral doubts about abortion. Instead, issues have arisen for Veronica as she has confronted stereotypes about people who have abortions.

A 21-year-old Latina, Veronica seems easygoing, laughing frequently, tossing her dark, curly hair behind her shoulders. But behind her wire glasses, her eyes have a steely determination.

Veronica plans to be a doctor and drives herself hard to get there. She had not expected any deviations along the way, especially not an abortion. "I had these really naive misconceptions that it didn't happen to people like me," she says. "I wasn't supposed to get pregnant in the first place. It was like, I don't sleep around, which is a really stupid way to think. But that's how I thought in the beginning." Veronica believed she would not have an unplanned pregnancy both because she had slept with only a few men and because she has always used birth control. She recalls her pre-pregnancy attitude: "Just not thinking about it carefully enough to realize that accidents could happen. You think accidents happen to other people. They must not have been careful."

Veronica turned out to be one of those people. A year ago, a condom failure led to conception. A counselor reassured her that this can happen, saying, "There could be a leak in the condom." Veronica had trouble taking in this news. "I blamed myself in the beginning," she recalls. It seemed easier to take out her anger on herself than to blame a condom. As her disappointment about the birth control failure subsided, however, she accepted that it was "bad luck" and "just an accident." She notes, "I wasn't irresponsible."

Veronica also tackled her previous notions that only women who sleep around or who are careless have abortions. Because she felt that abortion affected these groups, ones with which she did not wish to identify, she says her abortion made her "want to turn away from myself." She thought, "I'm a really bad person." Then, Veronica "redefined" her "idea of a person that this can happen to," and concluded, "It can happen to anybody." Once she realized this, she says she didn't have to "change how I felt about myself." Instead, she has altered how she views other people. Veronica says her new perspective has "strengthened my sense of sisterhood. I can look at people on the street and go, 'She looks really normal. She could have had an abortion.'" With abortion so prevalent in our society and with the way it has helped so many women keep their lives on course, Veronica is probably right. Normal, successful, and happy women are quite likely to have had abortions. Having such a positive picture of the typical woman who has had an abortion makes it much easier to accept an abortion into one's self-image.

When It Is Easy to Weave an Abortion into One's Sense of Self

It may sound from the preceding stories as if an abortion must conflict with one's self-image. This is not always the case. For some women, abortion confirms or even enhances a valued part of themselves. This is true in the following examples:

Maternal Identity

Whereas Simone saw an automatic conflict in being a mother and having an abortion, 35-year-old Charlene sees the two as a natural fit. She says, "I feel very proud to be a mother" and raises her children full time. Eight months ago, when her second child was only five months old, Charlene found herself pregnant again. She quickly decided on abortion for the sake of her other children. Now, she says, "I give the abortion very little thought. I bless the child that was to be. I was/am not ready emotionally for one more." Charlene's decision has helped her "feel like a more responsible mother and individual." She explains, "Other women struggle with three or four children. There doesn't seem to be any pleasure or grace in their motherhood. That, I have."

Wanting to Stay Child-Free

Sally says that when she conceived at age 40, "I had been pretty sure that I did not want children and did not want to become a single parent. The pregnancy allowed me to confirm that feeling." Now, twelve years later, she notes, "Not only do I have no regrets about terminating that pregnancy, I have had no desire to become a parent since then. I also am lucky that I've never gotten pressure to be a mother." She feels sorry for infertile friends who are desperate to have kids, but who refuse to adopt, simply because society says they are "supposed to be mothers." Her view of motherhood? Sally says, "Do it if you want; be good at it. Don't do it; be good at that. Self-esteem has to do with being good at or at peace with who you are."

Seeing Oneself as Radical

Sylvia, age 49, views herself as one who defies society's norms. This makes it easy for her to accept the abortion she had twenty years ago. She explains, "I've always been out on the edge. I moved to California after college, to the surprise of my family. I moved in with a man! (Remember, this is 1968.) I had a child out of wedlock. Later, I did a stint as a lesbian. Having an abortion was another part of riding the edge." Sylvia adds, "I tend to give myself a wide range of experiences and this was another one." She notes, however, "I'm speaking from a twenty-year-old and very philosophical perspective. I'm pretty sure I didn't think about it that way at the time."

Expecting Oneself to Have an Abortion

Elissa, age 24, says, "I always knew I would have an abortion. I remember being thirteen, a virgin, never having even kissed a boy, and recommending to my best friend that every few months we put aside money for some sort of emergency abortion fund." This rare point of view means that Elissa did not have to break through the same "it wasn't supposed to happen to me" attitude that many of us confront with an unplanned pregnancy. She was one step further along when she had this experience five months ago; it did not conflict with her sense of self or with her life plan.

Unlike Elissa, some women do have to readjust their ideas of their lives after a abortion. We now see how other women have grappled with this issue.

HOW DOES AN ABORTION FIT INTO MY LIFE?

Just as we all have an image of ourselves and struggle to make various events mesh with our idea of who we are, many of us have a vision of our life. This may involve where life has taken us in the past, the life decisions we face now, or the path we chart for our futures. After a unplanned pregnancy, we must accommodate this new event in our lives. Some of us feel that an abortion mars our life record. Others accept that life does not always turn out the way we plan. We may see the experience as yet another deviation, or even welcome it as an opportunity to reevaluate our lives.

Donna: Facing "The Time After Childbearing"

Donna, who is white and 42, confronted this issue in midlife, when she had two unplanned pregnancies after age 40. Pregnancy has colored Donna's life for the past two decades. At 22, she became pregnant and had an abortion. She married at age 25 and had a son ten years later. At age 38, she had twin boys. Two years later, when she found herself pregnant again, Donna considered carrying the pregnancy to term.

She wrote in her journal, "I have been tempted to throw myself in the path of this fate, to give up all our plans, our control, our sense of our family and work and life as we know it, and let it all become something else. It would mean abandoning my work at this stage. It would mean bowing to circumstance, to physical and emotional hardship. It would mean giving myself over to my reproductive capacity–in some sense, relinquishing choice. Barry has not once felt this temptation," she wrote, referring to her husband.

While Donna felt a slim desire to have the child, she also saw this as unrealistic. She thought, "I am too tired, too old, too stretched by the children I have, to do this." Donna decided on abortion, and tried to come to terms with this choice.

Two years later, she conceived again. She had another abortion and Barry had a vasectomy. Now, two weeks afterward, Donna faces several losses at once. First, she says she feels "piercing sadness" that "I will never see the face of another child we make together." She writes, "I am left with this intermittent, inconsolable longing" to see "a new person who bears my features and Barry's and some star-drawn physicality all its own."

Beyond the loss of the fetus, Donna says she now confronts "what I thought I had already come to terms with: I will never have a daughter." She has to accept that her childbearing years have drawn to a close. This means entering unfamiliar territory. She writes, "Back to normal life. But it is not the life I have known. It is a new time, the time after childbearing, the time after the period that has been the richest, most surprising, most benevolent and blessed. We have chosen, consciously and with pain, to end that time, partly because we could see that it would end itself before too long, and the risks of drawing it out would be too messy, perhaps too hard on those of us who are here now."

Donna finds it difficult to enter this new phase. She surveys the terrain ahead of her, observing, "This is plain old midlife, isn't it? Menopause, disease, death: those are the things it's most easy to foresee. I can't tell whether this is a failure of the imagination or prescient clarity. I don't ordinarily insist on knowing the future, and I don't now either. It's just that it's hard to see what I ought to do, what's worthy and compelling."

As she searches for a new path, a friend has offered guidance. Knowing that Donna struggles to feel worthwhile, she tells Donna, "Now you get to take up the work you were doing when you decided to have children: the work of believing in your own goodness." Donna mulls over this statement and concludes, "In some ways, childbearing moved that project forward, gave me a irrevocable and profound affirmation of my worth. In another sense, though, the time devoted to reproduction was a hiatus in the struggle. I now have to face–once again and in a new way–the task of caring for myself."

Mariel: "I Needed the Pregnancy to Make Me Look at My Life"

While Donna's abortion prompted her to question her future, an unplanned pregnancy and abortion made 25-year-old Mariel, who is white, examine her past. Ten months ago, her life was in a perilous condition. Mariel conceived with her friend's lover. "I had tried to stop sleeping with him before," she recalls, "but I would always end up doing it again and I would really hate myself for it. I was suicidal off and on during this time." She explains how their relationship was further complicated: "We also had threesomes with his girlfriend and she and I slept together, too. She never knew he and I were having an affair," Mariel says, probably meaning that the friend didn't realize Mariel and this man met without including her. This betrayal caused Mariel to feel horrible about herself. She says, "I felt like such a failure and a loser because of the whole thing." On top of this betrayal, Mariel had a boyfriend of her own and assailed herself for cheating on him.

"In general," Mariel says, "I was out of control in all areas of my life. I was drinking way too much, smoking too much pot. I was bulimic." She adds, "I was into numbing my body and I was very alienated from what I was really feeling. I was sleeping with a lot of people. I had tried to change this, but I was having trouble changing."

Rather than just viewing the pregnancy as one more stressor, Mariel embraced the chance it provided to reevaluate her life. She says, "I needed something like the pregnancy and abortion to make me look at my life." This experience was "a huge reality check." She says that having to "take responsibility" for her behavior "was a turning point for me. It helped me get clear on who I was and what I was doing."

Mariel's life did not turn around instantly. She first mourned for the fetus and for her old self. She explains, "I was letting go of who I was before the abortion." Although she felt deep grief about the abortion, she has no regrets. Instead, Mariel notes, "I do have regrets about my behavior that set the stage for my getting pregnant and having to have the abortion." She says she felt sad that "I had let things in my life get so out of control."

Gradually, Mariel began to reconstruct her life. First, she told her friend's lover that she had been pregnant and had an abortion. Next, she worked up the courage to tell her boyfriend that she had slept with someone else and conceived. "I dreaded telling him," she says, "but knew I had to, because I couldn't keep it a secret from him. Plus, he was leaving for a month-long trip the week after the abortion was scheduled." Telling him made her confront her behavior again. She recalls, "I felt like such an asshole for cheating on him and getting pregnant." She and her boyfriend had just begun to date after a lapse in their relationship, so her news came at an especially bad time. Despite the tense circumstances, he reacted well. Mariel says, "He was actually very supportive and understanding. I was so amazed that he could 'forgive' me. He was wonderful through the whole thing, which was very important for me, since I had a lot of feelings that lingered after the procedure." His compassion may have helped her forgive herself for the way she acted.

Mariel then began to build a better relationship with herself. "The abortion was a watershed of sorts," she muses. "It helped me reconnect with my body and live in a more authentic and healthy way with myself and other people." Mariel concludes, "It's been positive to integrate this experience into my life. Even though it sucked, I am a much stronger and happier person and I have a perspective I wouldn't otherwise have."

Chapter 8

Feeling Sure of the Decision

A year after she ended her pregnancy, Simone, who is 39 and white, says, "I was surprised how difficult the decision to have an abortion was. I thought I would say, 'This is terrible, but I'm going to have the abortion and it's not going to be this soul-searching crisis.' But it was an absolute crisis." Simone struggled to make a decision about her pregnancy. She knew that her life was too hectic to accommodate another child. Her 17 month old consumed much of her energy. Plus, both Simone and her husband faced turbulence in their careers. He clearly did not want Simone to carry to term; he felt that another baby at that time would plunge the family into a deep depression. On the other hand, they very much wanted another child and had planned to conceive later.

This desire made the decision much more difficult. Simone also had trouble thinking about abortion because she had already given birth once. She could envision the fetus as a baby, and says, "It was hard already having a child, because I knew what it meant to go through the whole process" of giving birth. "And I knew what the outcome was. So even though I really don't believe that it's life yet, that it certainly can't sustain itself out of my body, I knew what would happen if it went along a little way." Feeling protective of the fetus, Simone notes, "I was amazed at how much I was in sympathy with the pro-life argument. I really thought, 'I wish there was some other thing I could do.'"

These words may seem surprising in light of the fact that Simone has long been an abortion rights activist. But Simone wisely notes that politics and emotions do not always agree. As she puts it, "I believe intellectually and politically that it's my right to do it. But to say it's your right doesn't cover the emotional stuff about what your responsibilities are."

Simone weighed these issues as she tried to make a decision. Finally, after a week of feeling tormented, she chose abortion, not because she had achieved any clarity on the issue, but simply because she had to choose one thing over the other. Simone recalls that the situation then became a little easier. She says, "Once I decided to do it, the procedure was like an afterthought. It was as if I had signed off on it." Saying, "I remember always being at the edge of panic," she adds that she didn't let herself question the decision again. She kept the matter at arm's length and ended the pregnancy.

Since her abortion, though, she has not felt so sure of her choice. Her uncertainty manifests as fears of retribution. Simone intentionally conceived seven months after her abortion and worried that God would make her miscarry. She explains, "I thought I was going to be punished. That my body was going to punish me for the abortion." Fearfully, she imagines how her body, "or whoever is speaking through the body," views her reproductive choices: "You didn't want to do it that time, and we were all set up to go. You think you can control it, so I'm going to show you that you don't have control." She notes, "It would be too fortunate just to have the baby, a simple replacement."

These ideas about punishment do not concur either with Simone's feminism or with her form of Judaism, and she finds them "disturbing." Simone's ideas about punishment probably stem from doubts about her choice. She was able to reconcile herself to the abortion by planning to have a child later. Conceiving again has, in fact, helped her accept the abortion, but if she had truly accepted her decision, she would not need this other event to make her feel resolved. Simone made her decision in a muddied, frantic way, seizing on abortion, but trying not to keep sifting through her thoughts. She could not accommodate indecision at that point; she had to act quickly. She closed the file on the issue without working through her uncertainty. As a result, she is unsure if she made the right decision.

Such uncertainty is not inherent in having an abortion, as many people think. Instead, doubt about the choice often results from the way one decides to have an abortion. We will now see how feeling forced into an abortion can result in even more misgivings.

Olivia: "Making a Decision That I Didn't Want to Make"

Olivia is a 46-year-old African American who had an abortion two decades ago. The years have helped her realize that she felt unsure about her abortion because she did not make that choice clearly and freely. Instead, she felt pressured into her decision.

When Olivia discovered her pregnancy, she felt "ambivalent." She explains, "I didn't see any reason not to have a baby, since we were married. While I would not have planned it" at that time "I'm not sure that I ever would have planned getting pregnant." Olivia thought she really wanted to have this child. She and her husband had just earned graduate degrees and she felt that the world lie at their feet. She recalls, "I was in fantasy land. It just seemed that I could do anything and that if this was the time to have a baby, then I would have a baby." Her husband felt otherwise. She says, "The idea of a baby cutting down his options" bothered him intensely. "He was insistent right from the beginning that there be an abortion," Olivia says, adding that he saw "too many opportunities in front of him."

Olivia recalls feeling "very upset that he didn't want to have a baby with me," but dared not express her anger directly. She had become submissive with him, though she was not always this way. Olivia explains, "Once I married, I fell into a more passive role that had not been so of my first twenty-four years." She describes how her passivity and her husband's dominance had affected their life so far: "I remember wanting him to decide where we were going to live. He decided we were going to stay in Boston. I worked on getting this job in Boston. Got this wonderful job. And he decided at the last minute to move." Olivia felt angry, but moved and found yet another job. At that point, she learned she was pregnant, which became another source of contention between Olivia and her husband.

Once again, Olivia gave in. She "made the decision reluctantly" to have an abortion, but held him responsible for the choice. She says, "I remember immediately afterward feeling empty and very angry at my husband. That was the beginning of the end in the marriage. Within a few months, he got another job opportunity and we went to a foreign country." Moving to Africa angered her. Not only had he uprooted her again, but they had moved to a place where she did not feel free to discuss her abortion. She recalls, "I really had a very difficult time in the aftermath around my feelings about the abortion. The whole sense of feeling bad, guilty, ashamed, and therefore depressed stayed with me for about a year. It was very hard to shake it off." She says this pain was "related to my making a decision that I didn't want to make. And then blaming him for making that decision."

She began to long for a child. She remembers, "In my sense of helplessness, I began to notice babies and say, 'Why can't I have a baby?'" Olivia now sees that her desire for a baby "was an impulsive response to having had a choice and feeling that it was made for me." She adds that her desire for a child "was again not based on reality."

When some months passed, Olivia began to realize the role she had played in the abortion. She says, "I had to come to terms with the fact that I could have left my husband. I'm a very independent person. I could have said, 'Fuck you. I'm going to have this baby.' And I didn't. It got to be better when I realized that I wasn't a victim, but it was in my own ambivalence that I made a decision to have an abortion." What Olivia means is that she did not have to let her husband make the decision. She refers to her "ambivalence." She must have felt torn about giving birth, but could not admit this to herself. Olivia solved this problem by having an abortion and then blaming the decision on her husband. That way, she could have what she wanted without taking responsibility for the choice.

Olivia realized that she had weighed her husband's opinion too heavily and given him control somewhere along the way. The fact that she never considered walking out with the pregnancy showed her how "disempowered" she was. She saw, too, that, as she says, "I had to assume responsibility for my life and decision making." Olivia left her husband. She says, "We were in Africa less than a year and I just walked out of the house."

Over the years, Olivia continues to see the abortion and walking out as pivotal in her life. She notes, "The abortion became symbolic for my own sense of dependency and helplessness. What was empowering was getting into a position where I was responsible for my life." Of course, she says she did not realize at the time that "that was my moment of empowerment. I don't know that I could have said that two or five or seven years later. But looking back twenty years, I think this is pretty evident that that was an important milestone in my life." Since that time, Olivia has earned a doctorate, had a child, married and divorced again, and attained a powerful position in a prestigious organization. Only she calls the shots in her life now. Being able to "own" her decisions, or take responsibility for them, Olivia no longer lets others force her into decisions or blames others for her actions.

Fern: "It Was My Moral Responsibility to Be Very Conscious"

Unlike Olivia, Fern decided by herself to have an abortion and wanted to take full responsibility for the choice. Fern is a 45-year-old Caucasian who had an unplanned pregnancy thirteen years ago. Several obstacles to having a child jumped out at her immediately. She didn't feel she had the money. In addition, she didn't like the man with whom she conceived and didn't want a lifelong tie to him. Finally, she says, she "thought that the life of the child wouldn't be what I would want it to be." Those reasons seemed solid, but to Fern, reviewing the facts was not the same as making a decision. She wanted to explore the issue thoroughly because she says she realized "that it was my moral responsibility to be very conscious about the process on every level."

She put her full attention on the pregnancy for two weeks. Fern recalls, "It was absolutely the most important thing in my reality for that period." She turned to her therapist, who used psychic and psychological tools to help Fern explore her feelings. Fern recalls, "I did guided imagery to try to decide what was the right thing to do." She says she also prayed, meditated, and had "a dialogue with what I felt was the soul of the fetus."

This dialogue with the fetus paid off. Fern felt like she "worked through the relationship" and said "an appropriate goodbye" to the fetus. Fern believes she faced a legitimate choice, made that choice, and feels "fine" that "that being went back to wherever it came from." By the time of the abortion, she had "resolved any sense of guilt or unfinished business." Thirteen years later, she still feels fine. She says, "I don't have any lingering feelings about, 'Did I do the right thing? Did I hurt a being?'" Fern entered into the abortion consciously, working through anything that might have bothered her later.

These three stories show that the ways in which we decide to have an abortion greatly affect how doubtful we will or will not feel afterward. If we make a choice without clarity or conviction, as Simone did, we will often feel lingering uncertainty. If we feel forced into a decision, as Olivia did, we will feel full of blame and guilt, unable to accept our own actions. In contrast, if we approach the matter in Fern's conscious way, we may work through any doubts before we even have the procedure. It is not always easy to know what to be conscious of when one makes a decision concerning a pregnancy. Because there is relatively little time in which to make a choice, it helps to have a high level of self-awareness before ever conceiving. The more we know about our values, beliefs, and psychological makeup, the easier it will be for us to resolve our feelings about the abortion.

DOES ABORTION HAVE MORAL CONSIDERATIONS?

The abortion issue might appear to us to have only practical, not ethical, considerations. In that case, we may have no doubts afterward. We now meet a woman who felt this way.

Abortion as a Good, Amoral Decision

Bernice, a 41-year-old Caucasian who had abortions at ages 18 and 20, feels a lack of moral conflict about her abortions. She says, "I really expected to have to grapple with the questions of life and is this right or wrong? For it to be really complicated morally. But both times that it actually came to that decision, there was nothing like that there." Bernice has probed herself for negative feelings about her abortions. Occasionally, she thinks, "Is there something wrong with me? Shouldn't I have had this nervous breakdown?" But she says she has "never questioned whether what I did at both those times was right for me or not. It was almost as if there were no decision to be made." Bernice notes that her attitude toward abortion made her experiences "easier for me, because I didn't go through a long period of questioning, wracking myself with guilt."

She formed her opinions on abortion early. Although her mother was a pro-life leader in their community, insisting along with the church that abortion was a sin, Bernice says, "I never bought into that." As a teen, she notes, "I had already started questioning the church." She adds that at 15, "I was completely of the opinion that you do what you want to with your body, probably because that was the first year *Ms.* magazine came out."

Solidly pro-choice, she resented the pressure she received to feel guilty about her abortions. Much of this came from the clinics in which she ended her pregnancies. She recalls, "They wanted me to talk to a counselor. I was like, 'No, I just need the operation. I don't have any doubts or questions. I don't need whatever you're trying to give me.'" Bernice adds, "People at times made me feel strange because I wasn't questioning myself, because I wasn't saying, 'Is it a life? Should I do this?' I was just, 'I'm pregnant. I need an abortion.'" Bernice says slowly, "I think I'm supposed to feel guilty and horrified, like I'm bad. But I don't feel that way, because what was right for me was having an abortion."

Abortion as an Immoral Choice

Some of us do not regard abortion as an amoral issue, but as being loaded with ethical considerations. Now that we have been through the procedure, we may be filled with guilt and remorse, feeling that abortion is a bad thing to do. We may be angry at ourselves for breaking our moral code, for preventing the fetus from having a life, or for getting out of a tough situation in what we consider an easy way. If so, we might expect to be punished for our actions. For instance, one 23 year old felt uneasy six months ago, after her second abortion went smoothly. Insurance paid for the whole procedure. Feeling that she "should have paid a higher price somehow," she decided to punish herself. She made a donation to Planned Parenthood for the amount her doctor billed the insurance company. She explains, "I felt like something bad should have to happen to me for doing this."

She is not alone in feeling that she should be punished for conceiving or ending a pregnancy. Such attitudes permeate our society and show up in the phrases, "You reap what you sow," "You made your bed. Now you have to lie in it," or "What goes around comes around." These ungenerous sayings imply that we were "asking" to get pregnant by having sex and deserve to suffer the consequences. They indicate that an unplanned pregnancy reflects an irresponsible or flawed character and that being forced to raise a child would remedy this defect. In the corners of our minds, we may harbor such attitudes about unplanned pregnancy, ourselves, though they may only arise when we feel vulnerable. One young woman found that she held such punitive ideas and decided to eradicate them.

Abigail is a white 24 year old who had her first abortion at age 19. She went into that experience pro-choice, mostly because that's what she was taught to be, rather than out of her own conviction. When she had her first abortion, she felt "fairly comfortable" with her decision, but "the security" of her belief was "tested." Abigail began exploring her views of abortion. She faced "issues such as whether it's wrong or right, moral or immoral, copping out or exercising my power as a woman."

This first time, the decision was hard to make, but "acceptance was easy." Abigail explains that the choice concurred with her self-image: "It confirmed me as a liberal-minded woman who was capable of making choices." When she conceived again at age 20 and had another abortion, "Acceptance was a little harder to get to." She comments, "I had images of myself as a feminist who had done things to help label herself as a feminist, but things that one only needed to do once, like have an abortion. I had two, and it conflicted." She "felt guilty for stretching the unspoken limit of one abortion." Abigail continues, "I had conflicts over my image as a good, loving human being" versus "that of a cold-hearted baby killer who could do it more than once." She also doubted the morality of her decision and says, "It is not as though I wanted to destroy the fetus, but I had to think of the impact a child would have on my life," as well as her inability to support a child.

What helped her "cope with a hefty amount of guilt," especially after the second abortion, was returning to the abortion facility for post-op checkups. She explains, "It enabled me to be in a safe, pro-choice environment, if only for those few hours." At other times, when she heard "even the slightest hint of antichoice sentiment expressed in any way," her guilt sprang back to life and made her "overly defensive." She notes, "After the second experience, seeing a mother and child would sharply remind me that I had had an abortion, and mixed feelings of guilt and wonder would emerge." Even bleeding after her abortions sparked "sad or guilt feelings over where the blood was coming from and why."

Abigail's guilt often showed up as fears about divine retribution. She did not feel this way after the first abortion because she thought that in God's eyes, "It was an understandable experience." Her second abortion, however, made her "fearful" that she "had committed a severely punishable sin." Abigail comments now, "I find it funny that God comes into the picture, because I don't think of myself as religious. I have always been spiritual without concepts of a god or a devil, and yet abortion brought all that out."

Shocked to find herself having such thoughts, Abigail says she "had to reconsider my beliefs." She adds that she "evaluated how much I wanted to buy into a fear-driven religious system that seemed to have invaded my mind without my being conscious of it." She eventually succeeded in removing these ideas from her mind and says, "I now do not consider abortion a sin and feel sorry for those who torment themselves by that thought. I think the whole punishment ideology professed by a religious right is so manipulative and unneeded, considering everything else stressful that is caused by abortion."

Now, Abigail feels more at peace about her choices to have abortions. In fact, she is glad for the chance to take "such a good look" at herself and her beliefs. She considers herself more pro-choice than ever, and feels that this conviction comes from within, rather than being a received opinion. She explains, "I have had to give thought to it more than once, and this has led me to deepen my understanding of what abortion means to me."

Pro-Choice Women's Doubts About Abortion's Morality

Several women fall somewhere in between Abigail's earlier conviction that she was wrong to have an abortion and her later acceptance. Some of us have lingering doubts about whether our choice was right and whether we should question any aspects of our decisions. We often feel that abortion was the best choice, especially as we observe the positive effects on our lives, but some part of us may believe abortion is immoral. We may not even be aware that we have such attitudes, but our words reveal our reservations.

Becky, a 25 year old whose abortion occurred two months ago, says, "I feel a little guilty maybe that I caused this fetus pain. Maybe I destroyed a life. Even though I wasn't far along." Becky had the abortion at about six weeks. As to her first worry, some doctors feel that one cannot cause a fetus pain during a first-trimester abortion. A fetus's brain and nervous system are not developed enough at twelve weeks to feel pain, as doctors have determined conclusively. They are unsure when a fetus begins to feel pain, but some believe that this occurs after twenty-four weeks. Did Becky take a life? This question has no answer and will always be a matter of interpretation and debate.

There are incontestable facts, of course, about fetal development, and Becky was well aware of these, which only fueled her guilt. She says, "I've taken an embryology class. So I couldn't really deny that it was a life. I remember learning that the heart starts beating at twenty-one days." Actually, a leading obstetrics textbook says that the heart begins beating much later. According to *Obstetrics: Normal and Problem Pregnancies*, by Steven G. Gabbe, Jennifer R. Niebyl, and Joe Leigh Simpson, the heart beats five to six weeks after conception, or seven to eight weeks after the last menstrual period.

When Becky took the class, she felt uncertain about the morality of abortion. Adding to her uncertainty, her teacher was very pro-life and proclaimed, "Life begins at conception." She says his viewpoint made her "more ambivalent, because I felt like, oh my gosh, he's this PhD in biology." Becky assumed that because her professor had a fancy degree, he had more authority on the abortion debate than she. He may well have known every fact about when a fetus develops which features, but his opinion about when life begins and how we should treat this developing life holds no more validity than anyone else's.

Twenty-two-year-old Vivian does not share Becky's concerns over whether abortion is moral or whether she has hurt a fetus. Instead, Vivian worries about whether her reasons for choosing abortion a year ago were worthy. She had an abortion in the spring of her senior year at a top-notch university. Vivian muses, "Is it because I didn't really feel it was right to have a baby, or is it because it would be embarrassing? Is it just that I don't want to be any different from everybody else in my social circle?" Vivian feels that she let social norms dictate her choice and says, "I felt a little bit as if the decision had been taken away from me, because in my whole circle, people don't have babies. In the high school I went to, people had babies. But at this college, you know people are getting pregnant right and left. There's nobody actually having children." Vivian now questions this cultural attitude. She says, "I felt a little bit uncomfortable with the idea that this was a routine thing. If you get pregnant, you don't have children. It's stupid. You're too smart."

Vivian regards pregnancy with a certain reverence, and worries about how casually her friends treat abortion. She says, "It's something I've thought about with horror." Even so, she approached her abortion with the attitude, "Let's just get this done." She now wishes that she had given herself "more time to think about it" while she was pregnant. She does not know what would have changed if she had spent more time, but regrets deciding so casually. That fact, more than the abortion itself, gives her moral qualms.

Becky and Vivian have grappled with doubts about the morality of their abortions, seemingly without hope of resolution. This need not be the case. We now meet a woman who has wrestled with the issue and feels certain that abortion can be a moral choice.

Abortion as a Conscious, Moral Choice

Heidi, who is white and 42, approaches the issue of abortion's morality as a Buddhist, although she was raised Catholic. When Heidi had her abortion at age 24, she was an atheist and did not have quite the same concerns with morality as she does now. Still, until recent years, she has seen the abortion as incongruous with the rest of her principles. Heidi explains, "I want to act responsibly in the world and not just be self-indulgent." She adds, "Part of my trouble was that my decision was on behalf of myself."

She stood by her reasons and did not have a strong sense of guilt, but the abortion conflicted with her sense of who she was. She says, "I didn't know how to frame it within my ideas of myself as a good person who does the right thing." Heidi says that the conflict between being a good person and having had an abortion only troubled her in a latent way for many years; it was not in the forefront of her mind. Heidi did not know how to view the abortion, how much importance to give it in her history. As years passed, she "wanted it to carry the weight of what it really was. No more, no less." Heidi comments, "I never experienced it as this guilty, horrible yoke around my neck. But I didn't want to treat it like it was getting your teeth cleaned either. There was some way in which I wanted to say, 'It really was as big a deal as it was. And I accept the responsibility for that.'"

The issue of how much weight to give abortion arose right when she ended her pregnancy. At that time, in the 1970s, Heidi lived on a commune, where people treated sex, relationships, pregnancy, and abortion very lightly. She had a different attitude. Heidi recalls, "I was a prude for those times. I really believed that you had to love someone and have a connection to them before you had sex with them. Everyone I knew was jumping into bed randomly with people just because they felt like it at that given moment." Heidi knew people who had five and six abortions without batting an eye. As Heidi observed her peers, she felt different. She notes, "I do think that I couldn't take it casually. I've had other gynecological surgery. I've had thyroids and polyps and endometriosis, and to me there's a difference between the surgery I had for those things and having an abortion."

Heidi also feels alienated from reproductive rights activists, whom she feels treat abortion too casually. She says, "I find myself not being a great supporter of the pro-choice movement. When I ask myself why that is, since I believe in the right to choose, what comes back as my answer is that it is something you are killing. You are killing a child." Heidi laments that so much of the pro-choice side "tries to pretend that's not true. These are just a collection of cells and da-da-da-da-da." She feels uncomfortable that pro-choicers say "it's just a medical operation" and it's not about "the taking of, at least, a potential life."

Feeling set apart from this mentality, Heidi has struggled to form her own ideas of what abortion involves. She says, "Where I have come down is that it is a life and you are taking it and that that's okay under certain circumstances. Each person has to decide what those circumstances are." Heidi advocates entering into abortion as consciously as possible. She thinks one should say, "I am taking a life, and it's okay that I am doing this." Heidi feel that this approach would remedy "a lot of the feelings of guilt, loss, and sorrow," which "come from not acknowledging that you are taking a life." For Heidi, acknowledging this truth makes her actions and beliefs seem much more integrated. She feels at peace about how she could have had an abortion and still be a good person.

GUILT ABOUT OUR ROLE AS WOMEN

Concerns about morality are probably the largest reason for guilt after an abortion. We may also harbor guilt for reasons that have nothing to do with ethics. Heidi thinks simply being a woman causes much guilt. She says, "There's a way in which women like to beat themselves up. We love too much; we don't love enough. If anything goes wrong," we blame ourselves. In terms of pregnancy and abortion, Heidi feels this is especially true.

Many of us do lash out at ourselves for conceiving pregnancies that we did not cause by ourselves. Moreover, we often compare our abortion decisions unfavorably to those of friends who have given birth. In making such comparisons, we may not take all factors into account. For instance, we ignore that the other women may have wanted a child much more than we do, or that they have more financial and emotional support.

It can be difficult to live in this pronatalist society and not to give birth. Heidi points out that if we choose never to reproduce, we defy cultural conditioning from the millennia in which women have had babies without much of a choice. She says, "Throughout history, what has women's function been, but to give birth?" Choosing to "step outside" this societal norm by having an abortion can make us feel that we have done something wrong.

Society has not only assumed that all women should become mothers, but also defined a saintly maternal role that is impossible for any woman to achieve. One of the ideals ascribed to women is that they are all-nurturing–that they should care for any being who crosses their path and needs protection. Women often feel guilty for turning away from the maternal role, either by having abortions or by having no kids. Those who do have kids may feel guilty if they ever put their own interests first.

Heidi not only wrestled with issues about women's responsibility to children, but also felt guilty about another type of responsibility involved in her pregnancy; she lambasted herself for using no birth control. She says, "I felt terrible that I hadn't put my diaphragm in." Heidi worried about her possible motivations in using no birth control. She may have unconsciously wanted her boyfriend to commit to her and says, "I felt guilty, like, had I done this on purpose to try to lure this person closer to me?" Even if we used birth control when we conceived, we may have guilty thoughts that we could have used it more carefully. Most people look to women, not men, to prevent pregnancy, so guilt about the use of birth control reflects another way in which being a woman brings us more guilt.

After we discover an unwanted pregnancy, some of us feel guilty about having had sex in the first place. Sex may seem self-indulgent, particularly in light of a serious consequence, such as pregnancy and abortion. If sex is relatively new to us, we are more likely to have this reaction than is a woman who has had sex for twenty-five years. Having sex outside of marriage might also seem blameworthy to us; although we may have felt all right about engaging in premarital sex before the pregnancy, "getting caught" may cast a new light on the matter. Many women refer to unplanned pregnancies as "mistakes," or as "stupid," even if they were using birth control at the time. It is doubtful that they refer to other instances of sex as mistakes if those episodes did not cause them to conceive.

We may think ourselves too modern for such sexual guilt, but we may be listening to societal messages that reinforce such guilt. Many people in our culture still condemn those who have sex with no intention of reproducing. Others accept sex for pleasure, unless it has consequences, such as a sexually transmitted disease or pregnancy. Then, those people see pregnancy or disease as apt punishments for hedonistic sex. The idea that women can have sex voluntarily and pleasurably and then not carry every pregnancy to term devastates some people who are uncomfortable with the idea of women's freedom. Those ideas might trickle into our consciousness and emerge when we feel vulnerable.

In addition to feeling uncomfortable about sex, we may also feel guilty for becoming pregnant, especially if we are young and there has been a lot of pressure from our parents not to let this happen before we are ready. Pregnancy might have come to represent a negative thing, a fate that we should have done everything to avoid. If we have received such messages, we may feel stupid, as if we have been warned many times and have fallen into the trap anyway. The following two comments reflect guilt about conceptions; coincidentally, they both come from young, college-educated, Latina women.

> I felt more guilty about getting pregnant than I felt about the abortion. I've always been told growing up that it's not supposed to happen to you like that. That's a precious thing. That's something that you're supposed to share with your husband. It's something that you don't take for granted. (Veronica, age 21, twelve months after her abortion)

> I felt so guilty for becoming pregnant. I thought, "Here I am with a college education and I help the stereotype that Latina women are always pregnant, that all they know how to do is reproduce." I felt I let other Latina women down, but I don't feel that way anymore. Now I feel I'm a Latina woman who had an abortion and who supports anyone who chooses to do the same. (Rosita, age 23, nineteen months after her abortion)

Just as people often see pregnancy as a proper punishment for premarital sex, many people believe that carrying to term is a appropriate penalty for becoming pregnant out of wedlock. People forget the male role in pregnancy and judge young, unmarried, pregnant women harshly; they think girls who have premarital sex are bad, and those who get caught are even worse. If any of these opinions run through our minds, we may feel incompetent. It may seem that while everyone else has sex, we are the only ones who end up pregnant.

There is one more type of female guilt that we may feel when we have abortions. If we have had any pain about our abortion experiences, and if we identify strongly with the pro-choice cause, we may feel that we have betrayed our ideological sisters with our negative emotions. Abortion is something many of us have fought for; how can we have any ambivalence now? One 22-year-old liberal feels this way a year after her abortion. She comments, "It's a little odd that I feel unfaithful to my feminist beliefs. But still somehow I feel really guilty for feeling bad. I feel guilty like I hurt someone." We might ignore any pain about our abortions, preventing ourselves from exploring our feelings because they seem politically incorrect. As chapter 4 shows, guilt about betraying feminism can inhibit mourning, making it difficult to resolve feelings about an abortion.

RESOLVING GUILT

How does one deal with all this guilt? Is it just a matter of waiting for time to soften doubts? People work through guilt in different ways. We now meet some young women who have coped with their guilt by taking action.

Acting on Guilt

After 26-year-old Josie had an abortion two years ago, she felt guilty and "sure that God would have some horrible fate in store" for her. Josie's guilt did not stem from her religion; she says, "God's too busy to care about my little uterus." Still, she felt guilty about "throwing away what might have been a beautiful and brilliant child." Then, Josie saw an ad seeking ovum donors. Josie rejoiced that "This was the perfect way to ease some of the guilt I had." She explains, "I could give my healthy eggs to people who really wanted and needed them." Josie donated some eggs and says, "The first donation cycle was such a positive experience that I decided to do it again. I've donated three times and I'm scheduled for a fourth." Josie's gifts have dissipated her guilt. She says, "I've given life to two other couples, so I feel like I've fulfilled my karmic debt, and then some."

Like Josie, 22-year-old Kendra has felt guilty about the abortions she had at age 17 and three months ago. She recalls, "After my first one, I felt like a murderer." To ease her guilt, she has helped other women care for their children. She links the abortions to this generosity, saying, "That experience motivated me to help friends who end up in hard times trying to raise their children. I've given free child care to mothers who can't afford baby-sitters. I even lived with a friend of mine, helping her out with child care, transportation, and money" for eighteen months. Kendra's actions have assuaged her guilt. She says, "I always hoped that my favors might be a karmic undoing of my abortion."

Contributing something to the world can counter feelings of having done something harmful, of being a "bad person." Such actions should not be carried out, however, in a self-lacerating way. A healthy attitude would be to do some good, to give where we feel we have taken, perhaps to fill a void or pay a debt. An unhealthy approach would treat this payback as never-ending, as a well-deserved punishment.

Annika: "I Was Searching to Feel Forgiveness"

Because of her background, guilt was in the cards for Annika when she had an abortion five years ago. She is a 31-year-old white Catholic from a European country where abortion is illegal. After her abortion, she felt so guilty that she stopped going to church. Throughout her pregnancy, Annika felt ambivalent about having an abortion and recalls, "It was intolerable, because I felt like I hadn't really made a decision. I was just going through something that I wasn't really ready for." As we have seen, such muddied decision making leaves plenty of room for guilt to accrue. Annika felt guilty not only because she never fully embraced her decision, but also because she questioned the morality of abortion. During her pregnancy, she lamented that the fetus was "not being consulted here at all. There was this little life that depended on me to grow. And I was just going to toss it. The fragility and helplessness and dependency really were making it problematic for me."

Afterward, Annika felt like a "bad person" who had done something "against God's will" by having an abortion. She thought, "Maybe God had a reason for me to be pregnant." Wondering what her defiance would mean, she asked, "Does this mean that a child will be taken from me? What if I am never able to have other children?"

Annika not only feared God's punishment, but also forbade herself to go to church. She felt that given how Catholics view abortion, she didn't belong there. Plus, she felt God was angry with her for having an abortion. She says, "I always thought of God as loving and forgiving." She sought forgiveness through prayer, saying, "I always felt like if I intensely pray about something, I'm going to know the answer. And there was just complete silence. I felt like if I don't get a response, this means that I'm not forgiven."

One Saturday night three years ago, as Annika lay in bed, she heard "a gentle voice." She explains, "It was clear to me that it was Jesus. All it said was, 'Come to me.' I started crying." She fell asleep and woke up Sunday morning to find the same thing again.

She took Jesus' words at face value and returned to church that day. She was unsure whether she belonged there, but she says, "It seemed like everything was geared toward my experience." The priest said, "I want to welcome any newcomers" and "the first song was about how nothing can be that bad that it can't be forgiven." Annika recalls that because of these good signs, "I felt accepted and I felt like He really wanted me to be there." When it came time to go to communion, she hesitated, thinking, "I can't do this." Then, the same voice that steered her to church told her, "It's going to be okay. Just do it." She did. Looking back on that day, Annika says, "That gave me a lot of peace" with the abortion. She is not completely guilt-free and still does not know if abortion is moral. Nor is she sure of God's plan for her pregnancy. Now, however, Annika has a looser idea of God's plan for her life. She can even entertain the idea that God wanted her to have an abortion to enhance the understanding she brings to her work as a therapist.

Curbing Guilt

Beth, age 44, has also wondered about God's role in her pregnancy history, but she limits such questions. At age 27, she had an abortion. In her thirties, she lost three planned pregnancies. Four years ago, she conceived accidentally. Losing three planned pregnancies had taken such a toll on her body, mind, and marriage that she could not face another possible disappointment. As painful as it was to turn away from this last chance to give birth, she knew what she could and could not handle. Beth had another abortion.

Her pregnancy history is ripe for provoking guilt. When her first planned pregnancy ended in a stillbirth, she considered whether it could be a result of her abortion. Beth also started wondering for the first time, "What if I hadn't had an abortion? Would I have had a healthy baby?" Beth's later tragedies complicate the fact that she ended her first pregnancy. She notes, "I think it would have been easier for me emotionally if I didn't have that piece of history that I had to work into all these pregnancy losses."

Beth does not wish to torment herself with guilt or regret, however. She could say, "maybe" and "what if?", but says, "I have to stay away from these words and not try to speculate on how things might have worked out. I can't second-guess what my life would have been like had I not had an abortion." "No way to look backward with a crystal ball," Beth philosophizes. "I decided that I couldn't look at it that way." Beth also refuses to see a punitive connection between her first abortion and her later inability to carry to term. She says, "I didn't want to buy into this idea that I was being punished for what I did then."

Emotionally, too, she has accepted the legacy of her abortions. Beth wisely concludes, "Even if you make the best decision you can, there is still pain that can be associated with it. Difficult decisions aren't pain-free. Nor does it mean if you feel pain that you made the wrong decision. I always believed that the right decisions made you feel good. I now understand that life is not that simple–especially for women."

Beth's approach makes sense for several reasons. There is no need to see the events in one's pregnancy history as connected. It is unlikely that an earlier abortion has anything to do with later pregnancy losses or even infertility, so why provoke unnecessary guilt by insisting that there must be a connection? Nor is there a need for us to torment ourselves by regretting earlier abortions in light of later childbearing disappointments. A woman named Melanie has a very sensible outlook on this matter. Melanie says, "I am forty-three and have pretty much given up the idea of having children–for many reasons. I have regrets about not having children, but not regrets about the abortion. It was not the right time to have a child." If Melanie had carried her pregnancy to term at age 24, it would not have solved her current regrets, for she may well have had an unsatisfying life. Perhaps she couldn't have pursued career goals. Plus, she had later opportunities to conceive–just as many of us do–and does not need to pin her lack of children on that one decision to have an abortion. As she says, "Over the years I've had intensely ambivalent feelings about motherhood–intense yearning and intense fear." Melanie realizes that the decision to have children always remained in her power. As long as she has had some say over her abortion, and takes responsibility for that choice, regret and guilt need not enter the picture.

For whatever reason doubts and guilt appear, whether because of unclear decision making, concerns about abortion's morality, or because we are women, this logical way of thinking may help curb guilt about our abortions. At some point, we may need to put aside our concerns about the past and move on, knowing we have done the best we can.

Chapter 9

In the Mind's Eye: What the Fetus, Pregnancy, and Abortion Mean to Us

Before Marilyn, age 28, became pregnant a year ago, she and her fiance had long and wonderful talks about their plans to have kids. She recalls, "We had speculated about children and we talked about what we would name a child." Because they had fantasized in this way and their thoughts had become very real to them, when Marilyn conceived accidentally, they saw the fetus "as a baby with a name, who would have lived in a certain city." In their minds, there was more than a fetus in her uterus. Marilyn explains, "In the technical sense, it was a fetus. But in the fabric of life, I really was deciding whether or not to have a baby, not whether or not to abort a fetus." Before her pregnancy, Marilyn says, "I did believe that it's just a fetus." After she conceived, she "didn't believe that anymore. I became less politically correct about it. It wasn't just a fetus. It was a baby. It was a life." Marilyn has not changed her political stripes. She remains pro-choice, saying, "I don't think it's anybody's business but my own." The difference is not how she approaches the matter politically, but how it feels emotionally. She notes, "It had become a real person."

We each perceive the contents of our uterus differently during a pregnancy. Because we cannot see the fetus while it is inside us–at least not without technological intervention–we see it with our mind's eye, conjuring up images of the fetus. These images may have little to do with the facts of embryology. We might fantasize about how the fetus would look in the future and feel loving toward it, or resent its intrusion and envision it as a tumor or parasite. The way we view the fetus will affect how we feel about our abortion. It's all a matter of perspective. One woman expresses this idea in the following way: "I didn't think of it as a baby. More like I could choose to make it a baby if I decided to keep it, but if I were going to abort, it was something that I needed to get rid of."

A woman might feel nothing about an abortion if she has known about her pregnancy for only two days; the same woman might feel quite emotional if she was aware of the pregnancy for three weeks. Even if the two abortions were identical physically, they might be worlds apart emotionally. Her consciousness of the pregnancy and the meaning it has for her make all the difference. When she thinks of the fetus, she might envision an 18-year-old son with blue eyes and a sheepish grin. The fetus might symbolize the happiness she shares with her husband; she may be unable to picture the fetus without also seeing her husband cradling an infant in his arms. Alternatively, the fetus might seem to her like a creature that threatens to strangle her and cut off her livelihood. It may seem like an infection, a growth that she needs to eradicate. These images will affect how she responds to her abortion. She may feel sad, as if she has lost her handsome, teenaged son. She may feel relieved to have slain the creature and to proceed with her life, free of its threat. Her perceptions of the fetus, as well as of pregnancy and abortion, make all the difference.

HOW WE SEE THE FETUS

The way we describe the fetus reveals a great deal about our attitude toward the pregnancy. If we paint an unappealing picture, we have likely resented and resisted the pregnancy.

The Fetus as an Intruder

Many of us see an unwanted fetus as a growth that threatens to overtake our bodies and endanger our way of life. One 37 year old who had an abortion sixteen years ago felt this way about the fetus: "It was awful to carry. I felt like it was a cancer growing inside me. It was a very helpless feeling." Another woman, age 39, is of like mind after five abortions. She comments, "I felt no attachment to the clump of cells in my body. In fact, it felt like a cancerous growth–I wanted to get rid of it and be back to normal."

Many of us are hostile toward the fetus, feeling angry that it has invaded our uterus against our will and lodged there so obstinately. Having an unwanted fetus take root in our body can seem as undesirable as having someone despicable move into our home. One 28 year old who had her second abortion three months ago conveys this disgust in the following way: "It was really awful for me to imagine that there was something growing inside me. I didn't want to look at my stomach. I was really grossed out by my body–just totally disgusted with its ability to make this thing."

The most unappealing part of an unwanted pregnancy may be that the fetus depends on us to fulfill its needs, which can make us feel like incubators. We might feel that pregnancy reduces us to our basest biological functions–providing a womb, blood, and food to a fetus. Some of us express resentment about the fetus's dependence by comparing it to a parasite. Two years after her abortion, a 26 year old says, "I couldn't stand the feeling that there was some parasitic thing inside of me that was making me act and think differently. I wanted the baby out of me as quickly as I could get it out."

Some of us stop short of describing the fetus as a tumor or parasite, because we do not necessarily view it with hostility. Like the previous speakers, however, we may regard the fetus as an organic substance that lacks consciousness; it grows, but has no self-awareness. Some of us have used the following words to describe what was inside us: a pea; blood and mucus; tissue; an amoeba-like organism; dividing cells, not a life unto itself. For some of us, the fetus's lack of consciousness makes all the difference in the abortion debate. The operation seems ethical because in some doctors' opinions, an undeveloped fetus cannot feel pain. We may see the fetus as part of our body and feel that we are entitled to make decisions about it, as we would about any other anatomical part.

In our minds, the fetus might resemble an animal that isn't terribly cute, like a fish. This was true for one 23 year old when she ended her first pregnancy four years ago. She says she pictured the fetus as "a little baby chicken when it's still in the egg. It's got one gigantic blue eye and it's like a blob." It may make abortion seem more acceptable if we envision the fetus as an animal, particularly one that humans frequently kill.

We may be unable to picture anything at all if we want to avoid focusing on what we are removing from our uteri. We might need to believe that our uteruses are virtually empty, or try to push away images of developing fetuses. As one 27 year old says two years after her abortion, "I didn't want to picture any baby down there, because I wanted to have an abortion. I didn't want to make myself feel worse about it. I was trying to do everything in my power to make it so it wouldn't feel so bad. Blocking out things." A 37 year old felt similarly when she ended a pregnancy fifteen years ago. She says, "I was curious–'what if' thoughts–but I couldn't let myself make contact with the experience. I had to push away any positive feelings because I knew I had to give it up. I tried not to let myself get emotionally connected to any urge to continue the pregnancy."

To reinforce the decision to end the pregnancy, we may tell ourselves that the fetus has negative attributes. One 22 year old who ended a pregnancy eight months ago found it easier to envision the fetus as having an undesirable gender. She says, "I think it would have been a boy. With blue eyes and curly hair. Definitely male. Without a doubt. I know it." She does not know why she is so sure, but says, "I'd rather have a little girl."

Similarly, we may choose to believe that the fetus is deformed. Some of us even try to damage the fetus in order to make sure of this. A 22 year old recalls how she did this two years ago when she was pregnant: "I did not want the baby inside me at all. I smoked a lot more to reassure myself that even if I had the baby, it would probably be deformed. I smoked defiantly." Treating our bodies badly may be a way of reasserting control over our bodies. We might be telling the fetus or the world that we do not intend to care for this fetus, no matter what anyone expects. After feeling that a fetus has usurped control, we may take pleasure in having the ultimate say over what goes on in our uterus.

Whether or not we try to damage the fetus, the strength of our hostility will certainly affect how we feel about our abortion. If we are angry that a fetus has implanted itself in our uterus, we will likely feel great relief after the procedure. Stress and anxiety will probably subside after we end the pregnancy. If we feel as hostile toward the fetus as the previous speakers have, we will likely feel clear about our decision after the abortion.

Of course, human emotions are more complex than a simple cause-and-effect relationship. We cannot isolate variables and predict what factors will cause which effects, because pregnancies come into full, complex lives with rich histories. Some of the women quoted above had turmoil after their abortions. In a few cases, they took a different view of the fetus once they shed the denial that they used during the pregnancy. Going through an abortion under local anesthesia, listening to the sounds the machine makes, and feeling the machine's tugging motion in one's body can make the fetus seem more real than it ever did during the pregnancy. We may feel differently about the fetus once it is gone and no longer presents an problem. In the big picture, however, hostile feelings toward the fetus tend to mean that there will be much less conflict after an abortion.

Thinking About the Fetus with Love and Sadness

Not every woman who has an abortion feels negatively about the fetus she has carried. In fact, some of us feel loving toward any fetus inside us. We may develop a bond, no matter what a pregnancy's outcome. As one 22 year old says of the pregnancy she ended three years ago, "I felt very connected to that baby. I felt very in love and I had [chosen] a name."

We might take pleasure in fantasizing about how the fetus would develop or how it would appear after birth. One 21 year old, who ambivalently ended a pregnancy eighteen months ago, explains how she visualizes that fetus: "I just see a baby. If it were a boy, maybe it would have looked like him. We both have green eyes. Maybe the baby would have had green eyes. I was imagining the final baby product." This woman sees the fetus as a physical link between her and her boyfriend, a joint product of their genes. Similarly, we may see the fetus as the embodiment of our romance. Giving up that fetus may feel like losing part of our relationship. A 31 year old who had an abortion five years ago recalls, "I was very much in love with the man. To think of this life inside me as being partly him and partly me, it was just painful." This may have been even more acute for her because her romance ended soon after the abortion. Her feelings about the man and fetus may have become tightly bound together.

Our grief about losing the pregnancy may be so strong that it influences our image of the fetus. In some cases, we grieve the lost potential; after three abortions, one 38 year old thinks of a fetus as having "the bittersweet beauty of a rosebud that you know will never bloom." We may feel sad that the fetus will remain unknown to us in a physical way. One 19 year old who had an abortion eighteen months ago expresses her grief in this way: "People think that if I could have an abortion, I don't feel anything, that grieving isn't even an option. I did grieve, though. I was sad that I created something that never could be, that I was never going to know anything more about. It made me very sad when I would wonder what sex it would have been, what color eyes, tall, short. . . ."

Sometimes, feelings of loss manifest as concerns about the fetus's gender. Just as one woman wants a girl, and envisioned a male fetus to make the abortion easier, we may believe that the fetus is the son or daughter we long to have, and feel sad to lose a child of this favored gender. Even with no preference about the gender, we may have a strong sense of the fetus's sex as we carry the pregnancy, making the fetus more real in our minds and making us sadder after the abortion. This was true for a 23 year old who ended a pregnancy two years ago. She says, "I remember being upset, because I was convinced it was going to be a boy." This speaker has lost the boy she envisioned.

If we have positive feelings about the fetus, we may treat our bodies well during our pregnancies. We might refrain from using alcohol, cigarettes, caffeine, and drugs, and might eat and sleep in a healthy way. Some of us do this anyway, in case we change our mind about the abortion. Others of us feel that we ought to treat the fetus well for the short time it is inside us. One 22 year old who had an abortion eight months ago dropped unhealthy behaviors before she even knew she was pregnant. She says, "I just instinctually was not wanting to smoke marijuana or drink. It was totally unconscious. I was eating really well." She continued this behavior once she confirmed the pregnancy, and recalls, "I had an opportunity to get drunk and I chose not to," thinking it "too bizarre" to abuse something inside her. She could not see treating the fetus badly. She says, "Even if I'm planning to get rid of it, it would be sick to get drunk. It would be rude." She is not alone in this feeling. One 28 year old who had an abortion five months ago comments, "My instinctual reaction was to treat my child with the same love and attention that led to my decision to stop the pregnancy. I was concerned about what I ate. I abstained from coffee and alcohol. This change seemed very natural."

We may treat the fetus well simply because we feel confused about how we should act during our pregnancy. It can be very strange to live the life of a pregnant woman, feeling all the symptoms of pregnancy, but having a different agenda than women who plan to carry to term. We may refrain from consuming harmful substances out of a sense of disorientation; we might forget and then remember our situation. One 27 year old felt confused about this matter when she was pregnant two years ago. She recalls that when her boyfriend was smoking, she said to him, "I really wouldn't mind your smoking except now I'm pregnant, so why don't you stop smoking?" He went outside with his cigarette, and then she thought, "Oh, gee whiz. I'm not even going to have this baby."

The more positive our feelings are toward the fetus, the more likely it is that the abortion will give us emotional or moral challenges. These need not be insurmountable. Many of us feel that the abortion is for the sake of the fetus, who deserves a better life than we could provide right now. If we have such positive feelings about the fetus, it is likely that we have wrestled with ethical issues; we might feel guilty if we care about a fetus and prevent it from becoming a person. With positive feelings about the fetus, it is also likely that we will feel grief after the abortion, missing the baby we will never see or hold. Whatever we value about the fetus and pregnancy affects how we feel about the abortion.

The Fetus–Mini-Human or Amorphous Blob?

Whether or not we have positive feelings about the fetus, we may harbor concerns about how developed it is at the time of the abortion. At some point, we may see pictures of fetal development, especially if the clinicians do a sonogram, or if protesters hand us literature. The pictures protesters display may be inaccurate, but even if they are accurate, they can disturb us. If we think of the fetus as a microscopic egg or clump of cells, it can be shocking to learn that a fetus is more developed at the time of an abortion.

Thirty-one-year-old Annika felt this shock when she had an abortion five years ago. After she took a pregnancy test, she wanted to have an abortion quickly while her uterus contained "a formation of cells, rather than this fetus that was so developed." She could not have an abortion immediately, because it is hard for doctors to locate a small embryo during the procedure. Annika had to wait five weeks and calls this wait "complete torment for me, because with each week, I knew this child was growing." Waiting until it was "medically easier or safer to take this life" seemed "awful," "absolutely absurd," and "cruel" to her and to the fetus, given how much more developed it was going to be. During that wait, Annika looked at fetal pictures and concluded that it "looks like a little baby. It's completely developed and the heart beats." She thought, "Oh my God, I can't do this." Annika did have the abortion, in a state of distress, partly due to concerns about fetal development. She muses, "You feel bad being two months pregnant. You would not have felt quite as bad in the beginning, when you think of it as an accumulation of cells."

Like Annika, 23-year-old Toni has felt jarred upon seeing pictures of fetuses. She saw sonograms before her abortions at ages 21 and 22. Prior to her first abortion, Toni didn't think about the contents of her uterus. She explains that her pregnancy seemed intolerable to her, so she felt anxious to have the abortion. She adds, "I didn't feel guilty until I was in the clinic and I saw the sonogram, because it became a life to me. I hadn't seen it, hadn't thought about it; it wasn't moving, none of those things." She says the sonogram was "weird" to look at, but didn't upset her too much, because the image was very small. She recalls, "It was like a dark spot, because it's black and white. It's just a dark clump of tissue mass." She was eight weeks pregnant that first time.

A year later, Toni conceived again and discovered the pregnancy in the eighth week. She planned to have an abortion, but became sick and had to take antibiotics. The clinicians could not give her anesthesia while she was ill, so Toni had to wait until the twelfth week. She says that when she saw the sonogram that time, it "really freaked me out because of the size. It was almost as if I could visualize the whole thing all the way up to giving birth." She adds that the sonogram "bothered" her, "because the shape was different from the one I remembered before. It was really starting to form. I started to cry." Toni went through with the procedure, but feels quite guilty about both abortions.

Toni and Annika were both upset to see how developed the fetus was in the first trimester. Some women have looked at the same pictures and felt the opposite way. To them, the fetus has seemed very undeveloped, so they are relieved. When one 18 year old was pregnant a year ago, she looked at books to determine the fetus's size and appearance. She comments, "I knew I would abort at eight weeks and felt relieved that pictures of fetuses at eight weeks did not look very developed." Similarly, a 25 year old who had an abortion three years ago saw a sonogram before her abortion. This woman says, "The thing in my uterus just looked like a little blob." Her abortion occurred at six weeks; if she had seen a more developed image, she may have reacted differently.

One 46 year old has seen many first-trimester fetuses with her naked eye and does not think they are very developed either. Melba is a doctor who performed abortions for three years and who had an abortion after that, fourteen years ago. In her opinion, women who believe a seven-week-old fetus is the equivalent of a baby have been "fed a line of bull about the level of development of the child." She emphasizes, "It's simply not a baby." This distinction helped Melba go through her own abortion guiltlessly.

Melba's viewpoint is reassuring, because she has performed many abortions and has a lot of authority on the matter. We can all have legitimate opinions, however, about what fetal development means to us in terms of abortion. Presumably, all those quoted here about fetal development saw similar pictures, and yet they drew different conclusions. That situation is at the heart of the abortion debate; we can each be presented with the same facts and still have our own perceptions about the act of abortion.

Speaking with the Fetus's Spirit

Spirituality brings up even more differences; while some see a fetus biologically, others believe a fetus has a soul or a spirit, which affects the way we perceive pregnancy and abortion. Several of us have tried to speak with this spirit before or after our abortions.

We may talk to the fetus before an abortion in order to explain the decision and obtain the fetus's consent. One 42 year old, who had her third abortion two weeks ago, says, "I have spoken to the souls of the children I have refused. I have told them my regret that I have chosen against giving them life and flesh, I have thanked them for the honor of their desire to live through me, and I have wished them well. They have gone on." A 17 year old also spoke to her fetus when she was pregnant one year ago, but feels funny about having done so. She comments, "I did talk to Devon (the unborn) a lot. Does that sound crazy? I tried to explain to it that this was what I had to do. I explained to it that I was sorry for everything." Such conversations can occur even if we resent the fetus. One 22 year old spoke to the fetus before she ended her pregnancy five years ago. She recalls saying, "Sorry, but you're going to die so I can live my life the way I want." She comments, "I was very cold, though I'd also imagine what its face was like and wonder about its sex. It didn't seem real. I felt like I was acting on a TV show and talking to a stuffed animal, not a fetus." The danger in speaking with the fetus is that we may make promises we cannot keep. One young woman wrote a poem about breaking a promise to her fetus. Here is part of that poem: "I lay in the hot tub grown cold./I touched my belly and said,/'Don't be afraid./No one will hurt you.'/And then I killed it."

Some of us have sensed that the fetus's spirit has returned after the abortion. This devastated one 22 year old. The night after she had her abortion three months ago, she says, "I felt my baby's spirit come to visit me." She adds that the spirit "found its body gone. Then it disappeared. I was positive that's what happened and I cried like I never had before, sobbing and sobbing. The world seemed so empty, with nothing left to live for."

Another woman, however, felt happy and resolved after the spirit returned to her. Dana is a 27 year old who had an abortion at age 25. A few weeks ago, she envisioned the spirit. She says, "I pictured this little cupid spirit flying around. It said its name was Dixon." Dana explains that as a child, she had an imaginary friend named Dixon. She continues, "It said that it wasn't mad at me that I had an abortion, because it wasn't his time to come into the world." Dana adds, "It didn't talk. I just knew what it was saying."

Until Dana spoke with Dixon, she felt ill at ease about her abortion. She had grown up Catholic and always disapproved of abortion. When Dana conceived by accident, she wanted to have the baby, but this seemed impossible, due to her schooling, career, finances, and her boyfriend's wishes. After the abortion, Dana felt quite relieved, but was also sad and unsure of her choice. She wishes she could know more about who that child would have been and has gone back and forth about how she might have revamped her life to give birth. She always devises the same answer–on a practical level, having a baby simply wasn't possible. This line of thinking leaves her feeling unresolved.

"This spirit made me feel much better," Dana says. Seeing "such a little happy person" filled her with joy. Dixon's visit makes her feel that his spirit lives on. She finds further confirmation of this in astrology, which maintains that a soul enters a body at birth. Dana speculates that if this is true, perhaps the soul didn't come into the body before the abortion. She thinks that Dixon will enter the first baby she delivers.

Some women find it comforting to feel connected to the fetus's spirit and to maintain a relationship with it after the abortion. Peggy has done this. She is a 26 year old who had her first abortion six months ago and another one six weeks ago. Both times, she named the fetus, but only feels a strong connection to the second one, whom she named Terrell. Peggy is glad to feel this bond, saying, "I'd rather have some connection than not feel involved." Why does she want this connection? She explains, "Because it was real. It did happen. And because I did love it, for however long I loved it. It was in me. I keep envisioning that moment when it was sucked out of me and put in a bucket and I remember them carrying that bucket out of the room. It hurts my heart to think that my baby's in this bucket." Peggy, who is in so much pain that she regrets her abortion, believes that Terrell is now in heaven. This is partly why she named him. She explains, "I felt like I had to name it, because I should have never let it go. The child should have been a person. And I felt like if I did name it, then I could pray for the Lord to keep it safe. Instead of saying 'it,' like it was never real, I could just ask that Terrell be taken care of."

DIFFERENT VIEWS OF PREGNANCY

Part of the reason Peggy regrets her abortion is that she believes God wanted her to be pregnant. She says, "I definitely think the pregnancy was meant to be, because I have this connection with the Lord, fate, my purpose, and love all entwined into one." Peggy feels that at the moment she conceived, her heart was entwined with her lover's and with the Lord. "I think that the Higher Power was at work within me," she explains. She feels that by having an abortion, she went against what God wished for her. Because Peggy sees pregnancy as ordained by God, she is bound to have different feelings about ending a pregnancy than an atheist, who might see pregnancy as purely biological in origin. Another person may view pregnancy as the result of fate or karma. Our beliefs about the origin and meaning of pregnancy will certainly affect our choices and our feelings after abortions.

Elsa: Pregnancy as a Threat and Burden

Not everyone feels as positively as Peggy about conceiving against their will. For example, Elsa is a 40-year-old white "recovering Catholic" who had an abortion at age 18. She recalls how she felt about conceiving: "I was extremely disappointed and angry. I wanted it out–the sooner the better." She was mad not only that she conceived, but also that her boyfriend had falsely claimed to be sterile. Elsa felt "contaminated" by the pregnancy. She says, "Carrying a pregnancy I knew I was going to terminate felt burdensome."

Elsa has made it through many years without conceiving again, but still fears pregnancy as a threat to her freedom. She says, "I feel if I get pregnant, I'll no longer have a life of my own." Elsa feels so strongly about this that she says, "I drink so that I don't have to face getting pregnant." This feeling about pregnancy partly results from problems in her marriage. She says, "I feel all my husband married me for was to have children." His mother "endured" twelve pregnancies, which may have shaped his marital expectations. When Elsa's husband pressures her to have children, she feels "stressed." Their marriage is shaky and they are currently separated, so Elsa says she has no sex life anymore. Still, she worries about pregnancy and resents a society that expects her to reproduce. Elsa blames Catholicism in particular, saying, "I'm nobody's baby maker."

To Elsa, pregnancy represents far more than what happens biologically. It means losing autonomy and conceding to marital and cultural pressures to reproduce. Elsa's negative attitudes toward pregnancy made her abortion much easier. Afterward, she felt "a great relief," explaining, "I wasn't ready for that kind of responsibility, and I was happy it was over." In the years since then, she says, "I've often counted how many years old my child would have been, and whether it was a girl or boy, but for the most part, I feel nothing, as if the abortion was just a nuisance. The abortion never really affected me."

Rather than having Elsa's overarching rejection of pregnancy, we might have negative feelings only about certain pregnancies. Conceiving might bring us great joy at other times, but we might feel distraught about being pregnant against our will.

Pregnancy as Caused by Forces Beyond Biology

Even if we feel strongly about not wanting to carry to term, we may be amazed by the powers of pregnancy. Many of us feel wide-eyed about how the body changes and how pregnancy is a total body experience, not just the absence of menstruation. As we watch pregnancy transform us, we may feel a new respect for our body's power.

Gina, who is 28 and Caucasian, felt that way during the pregnancy she ended five months ago. From the moment she discovered her pregnancy, she was wonderstruck. Gina says, "I felt myself incapable of comprehending the enormity. My identity seemed impossible to merge with the concept of 'pregnant.' I found myself staring in the mirror, hands to my cheeks, repeating the awesome fact to my reflection."

Gina was most impressed with her biology. She says, "I was constantly in awe of the control my body seemed to be taking over my life." This statement could certainly have negative connotations; many women resent that their bodies can wrest control from them so quickly and thoroughly. Indeed, Gina felt that way before she conceived. The night she got pregnant was the one instance in her life she used no contraception "after years of conscientious behavior." She recalls "feeling exhausted, tired of the subject, and very weary of having to bear the burden of worry as the wearer of a female body."

If Gina still felt that way after she discovered her pregnancy, she does not say. Instead, pregnancy has lifted her to a new height. She comments, "The experience of being pregnant was one of the most fabulous I have ever encountered. Nothing in my life has more convinced me of the joy, beauty, and absolute mystery possible in life." She did not expect "the intense feelings of awe and reverence for life" that the experience of pregnancy gave her. Gina looked carefully into single parenthood, speaking to friends and the man who impregnated her, visiting day cares and maternity stores, and making lists of life goals. Ultimately, she chose to end the pregnancy, but her excitement over her new perspective continues. She says, "I went into the experience a rationalist agnostic, and I'm now finding myself in a spiritual quest for the meaning behind the concepts of God. I got a glance into another dimension, and I am deeply grateful for that look."

For Gina, seeing pregnancy as an event with spiritual ramifications is positive. She views pregnancy as a window to the spiritual world, maybe as a gift from God, as one woman puts it. Some people connect pregnancy with God, as Gina has, but it may seem less a gift and more a punishment, a payback for being sexually active or for not using contraception. One 28 year old alludes to this idea. Recently, she has had a strong urge to settle down with her boyfriend and start a family. She thinks this urge is the unconscious reason she has taken her birth control pills in the wrong order twice in the last year. She did not conceive the first time this happened, but says, "Whoever's upstairs didn't let me get away with it a second time." She may be speaking tongue-in-cheek here, but she implies that something beyond biological factors caused this pregnancy.

The more helpless we feel in conceiving against our wishes, the more we will be inclined to look to outside forces as the cause. To say that pregnancy is caused by forces outside biology is startling. How are we to control our bodies if other forces play a role? Such thinking is provocative, but dangerous. If we attribute pregnancy to God, spiritual forces, or the unconscious, we may overlook our power to prevent pregnancy. It is easy to become fatalistic and throw caution to the wind, figuring that we can't control what happens to us. This will probably be a self-fulfilling prophecy. Contraception does work a lot of the time. It is self-defeating to cast it aside and let other forces take over.

Oriana, a white 32 year old, has taken chances with contraception, partly because she feels that more is at stake in conception than just biology. Oriana has tried every birth control method, but has had five unplanned pregnancies since age 18. She ended the first four pregnancies and is currently carrying the fifth to term. Speculating on what contributed to her conceptions, she muses, "Part of me says, 'Oh, it was fate.' With this pregnancy, it really felt that way. Despite my best attempts at not conceiving, here I am." Oriana also thinks spirits "can follow you around" and cause conceptions. Before she conceived her last pregnancy, she felt that one was doing this, so she "gave it a real talking to." She used a diaphragm that month. When her period did not come, Oriana cramped to bring on a miscarriage. Oriana tried to miscarry not only with abdominal contractions, but also with her mind. She says, "I was psychologically making myself cramp." Oriana believes that the mind has some power over whether the body keeps a pregnancy and even over whether it will conceive. Whether she attributes her pregnancies to fate, spirits, or her unconscious mind, she keeps wondering whether her body controls her conceptions or whether some outside force plays a role. Oriana does not see these questions as fun ideas. She feels that until she finds some answers, she cannot know whether abortion is moral.

HOW WE SEE ABORTION

In her questioning, Oriana has come to see a fetus as having a life. She says she therefore feels guilty about ending "what I now perceive as four lives." She views abortion differently from the way she once did. Beginning with Oriana, we will now investigate how various women frame abortion and how this makes them feel about their abortions.

Feeling Troubled About the Spiritual Aspects of Abortion

Eighteen months ago, after her fourth abortion, Oriana had a spiritual crisis. She says this crisis was "like having a light shone on my past and on life." She entered a state of heightened awareness in which she began to pay attention to things we take for granted, such as the "natural flow" of life and cycles, childbirth, and motherhood.

A nightmare alerted Oriana to these topics. She dreamed that she miscarried a fetus and carried it in her hands to show her father. She watched the fetus grow into "this man who looked like Jesus Christ, which is very strange coming from a nice Jewish girl!" He then died in her arms and went through a bloody crucifixion. This dream shook Oriana up and stayed with her for a long time. She did not know whether to read it as a literal message about the son she might have had, or as a statement about the morality of abortion.

Ultimately, she read it the second way. The dream, she says, was "the wake-up call on abortion" for her. It left her doubtful about the choices she had made. She recalls, "That was the first time the issue of spirituality jumped on me and said, 'What are we talking about? Whose life is more important? And how can you make that decision?'" She began wondering, "What is this baby thing? Is it just this fish thing that's got potential for life? Is there a soul in there now?" She asked when life begins and how God feels about abortion. Can the fetus's soul "be born in another baby?" Is there a "second chance" for that soul?

With these questions came a large dollop of guilt. Oriana already felt selfish for not giving birth, especially the time she was 25 and married. After her fourth abortion, spiritual concerns heightened her occasional guilt. Oriana felt she had lost her right to have kids and that she "would have to become foster mother to the world's children," adopting or helping deprived kids. Oriana regarded this as her "duty."

When she conceived a fifth time, she could not decide about the pregnancy. She scheduled three abortions and canceled each one.

Finally, she opted to carry to term and felt that having this child was her new duty. Oriana recalls, "Despite my ego that was saying, 'I don't want to be fat, I don't want to give up my freedom, I don't want to make all these sacrifices,' something bigger than me was saying, 'Tough! Your play life, your single life, is over. It's time for the baby.'" She feels that this choice will help her evade punishment for her abortions. Oriana says, "I feel like I will be forgiven, because I'm overcoming huge fears about having a baby and being a mom and going through this whole process."

She now views her abortions not so much with guilt, but with a sense of conscience. She says, "I try not to obsess on the guilt aspects. But you really need to be able to confront it, both the life and death issues, and take responsibility for this unknown factor about it." Taking responsibility, she points out, does not mean saying, "I've done a bad thing," but trying to explore abortion's spiritual ramifications.

Feeling at Peace About Spiritual Aspects of Abortion

Not everyone who explores the spiritual aspects of abortion goes through the same anguish as Oriana. On the contrary, many of us have taken comfort in spiritual thoughts when we have had abortions. Some of us believe that the soul enters a body not at conception, but at birth. If so, we feel that we are not destroying a life through abortion, because that soul or spirit lives on outside the body. One woman, who has had six abortions, says, "I believe I didn't kill anything, but the souls materialized in the babies I gave birth to." Some of us think that the spirit goes to live in other people's babies, where it will be loved and cared for better. In this way, we feel we have done something similar to giving a child up for adoption. Still others of us believe in reincarnation and think that even if the soul dies through abortion, it may be reborn later. One 32 year old who had an abortion nine years ago says, "I believe in reincarnation, that souls come into the world in different vehicles, that we are each responsible for our lives, and that on some level, everything that happens is perfect. That belief enabled me to see the abortion as an okay thing, that the soul that attempted to come into the world in that pregnancy was not meant to, and would go back and could come in some other way that is right." She adds, "If there were a soul attempting to be born, perhaps this being picked me because it only wanted–or was only meant to have–a very short life, the period of time it was in me before it was aborted."

Whatever our spiritual beliefs are, it is comforting to realize that there are no set answers. Religion and spirituality seem wide open to interpretation. We can use these beliefs as springboards for further thinking about how abortion fits into our spiritual world.

Abortion as an Unnatural Act

We may approach abortion not from a spiritual perspective, but from a social and biological one. In this framework, abortion may seem an unnatural thing to do to our bodies. During a pregnancy, we may find that although we have intellectually decided to have an abortion, our body disagrees and wants to hold onto the pregnancy. Two years after her abortion, one 20 year old recalls, "Rationally, I was fine–I wasn't really angry at myself. But physiologically, I swear there were maternal instincts that told me I shouldn't do it." She adds, "I don't think that first-trimester fetuses have an independent right to live," but during pregnancy, "my body told me otherwise. It was like arguing with a Siamese twin for a month straight." A 22 year old felt similarly and refers to a "dissonance" between her mind and body before her abortion four years ago. She says her mind knew "this was what I wanted and needed to do," but her body felt a "motherly instinct."

If we have tried to live in harmony with our bodies, we may be uncomfortable stopping a powerful physiological process such as pregnancy. This is how 22-year-old Nora felt when she had an abortion eight months ago. One night in the first weeks after her abortion, she became upset about "having stopped something that was really natural." Nora tries to be natural in everything she does, down to the substances she puts in her body and her hair. After her abortion, it occurred to her that she had transgressed this value. She saw her abortion as something that would not have occurred in another era or another part of the world, and says, "I felt like I had done something that was very now, in the times." She had followed the societal dictates, "Be your own person. Have a career. Finish college." She comments, "I'd been really urban. I'd done the civilization-type thing." But Nora agrees that this modern approach to life is important, as well. She wants to have a college degree and to be financially self-sufficient. She realizes that when it came to her pregnancy, she could not be both natural and modern; she had to sacrifice one value for the sake of another. In the realm of reproduction, Nora still opts for having control over being natural. She feels vastly relieved that she doesn't have a child and would like to plan her next pregnancy, rather than having "something imposed" on her. She concludes, "There are conflicts" in leading a natural but controlled life.

It is nearly impossible to live naturally in an unnatural world. As far as our reproduction goes, very little is natural. Birth control is not natural, not even the rhythm method, because it requires thought and intervention. Many people do not have untouched full-term pregnancies. Instead, there are sonograms, amniocentesis, and prenatal exams. We do not give birth as wild animals do. We have hospitals, clinicians, medicines. Some of these things have reduced spontaneity and mechanized beautiful experiences. They have also helped us live happier, healthier lives that we can control a little better. There are tradeoffs. We may need to decide how important our conflicting values are in the balance.

Abortion as an Act of Responsibility

Other values can conflict during an unplanned pregnancy. If we are mothers, we may want to nurture another child, but might lack the financial or emotional means to do so. We may feel that if we add another child to the family, none of the children's needs will be met. Abortion may seem like the most responsible way to preserve the family.

Charlene, who is 35 and white, has felt this way. Maternity has played a central role in her life for several years. Before she and her husband ever had children, they moved hundreds of miles to a safe environment for kids. Seven years ago, they conceived, but lost the fetus at twenty-five weeks. They then had two healthy children. Eight months ago, when the kids were 3 and 19 months old, Charlene conceived again by accident.

She did not know what to do. On the one hand, she thought, "I love being a mom, I love babies, I love nursing. Maybe this being wants me to be its mom." Charlene's spiritual beliefs lent weight to that last thought. She wondered, "Was I obligated (especially after losing the first one)? Was I supposed to let this person come through me?" If so, would she be able to give enough time and attention to all three kids? Charlene did not think so. Money was a big issue, as well; their standard of living would decline with another child. Plus, having a third child would violate her beliefs about limiting population growth.

Charlene quickly decided on abortion and says, "It made the most sense." These words reveal her practical approach. Although she found her decision difficult, she kept in mind her responsibilities as a mother, as she advises other pregnant women to do. She says, "Do what is right intellectually. Are you ready for motherhood emotionally, financially? Are you secure in your love life? If not, don't bring a child into it." Charlene thinks people must make mindful decisions about reproduction and says, "Those who do not think first about having babies are very ignorant and will be accountable for their actions as parents in the long run." She adds, "I feel my decision was very responsible, not only to my own children, but to an overpopulated earth." Because she views abortion as a responsible act, she feels resolved and unemotional about her own choice.

To some people, the idea of abortion as an act of responsibility might be surprising. People frequently attribute abortion to selfishness, figuring that when a woman has an abortion, she has not stopped to consider the child's needs. On the contrary, many of us have abortions out of concern for the type of life a child might lead. We may fear we have damaged the fetus by smoking, drinking, or taking drugs before knowing we were pregnant. In our minds, it would be unfair to the child to cause this damage and then to give birth anyway. Due to financial or emotional limitations, we may feel unable to rear children as well as they deserve and view our decision as being on their behalf. We may worry that if we have unwanted children, they will pick up on our resentment and feel worthless. Several of us who grew up unhappily say how difficult it is for a child to grow up in such circumstances and feel that we never want to put a child in such situations.

One 25 year old who had an abortion seven years ago explains how she viewed parenthood at the time: "I believed that a woman knows her abilities best and if she's not ready to raise a child right, it would harm all parties involved if she had the baby." Her attitude made her abortion decision easy. She explains, "If I'd had a baby at eighteen, without financial security, without being in a loving, mature relationship, and with my own emotional maturity severely lacking, I would only succeed in ruining my life and my boyfriend's life and the child would never have a chance at a decent existence. Every child deserves to be happy, and I could not have provided that." She adds that abortion is not wrong; instead, having an unwanted child is "a terrible thing." Many women share this view and think it tragic or even sinful to bear a child one cannot nurture.

People often criticize women who have abortions for acting on their own behalf. This is often a misogynistic view, stemming from a belief that women should not exist except to facilitate others' lives. It is a positive step for women to care for themselves, to take responsibility for their own lives, securing a promising future. Abortion can be one way to do this, to draw limits on which duties they will assume. One 45 year old sees it that way. She had two abortions in her late twenties, two kids in her thirties, and had another abortion a year ago. She explains that when she confronts reproductive choices, she considers the responsibilities she already has and whether she is willing to take on more. Pointing to her uterus, she says emphatically, "I don't care what's in here. I don't care about that life. I care about the quality of my life. I tell my kids I chose them and I'm responsible for them. Anything else, I care much more about myself." We might each construe this responsibility to ourselves differently. Some of us say, "Enough is enough–I've done my share" after rearing two kids. Others of us plan to achieve certain goals before giving ourselves to kids. Alternatively, we may view our own growth and development as lifelong goals and never see children in the picture.

Whatever our plans, if we see abortion as being on our own behalf, we may have one of several reactions to ending pregnancies. We may feel sad that we put our own needs above those of a potential child. Some of us find it difficult to put ourselves first and may feel guilty about this, believing that our needs aren't important enough to take priority. Alternatively, we might be relieved when a pregnancy ends and allows us to move on with our lives. After an abortion, some of us value our schooling or careers even more because a pregnancy threatened to interfere with those plans. Now that we have had an abortion, we may feel clearer about what we want from life and more motivated to attain those goals.

IT IS ALL RELATIVE

Our society views the abortion debate simplistically, assuming that opinions depend on whether or not we think the fetus has a life. This chapter shows how those of us who have had abortions espouse a rich range of beliefs and perspectives. We may see a fetus, pregnancy, or abortion in practical, emotional, moral, spiritual, or biological terms. These views affect how we feel after our abortions, whether that means feeling guilty and aggrieved, or relieved, free, and motivated. We each react in our own way to ending a pregnancy that has a specific meaning to us and a certain role in our lives.

PART III: OUR BODIES– FRIENDS OR ENEMIES?

Chapter 10

Making Peace with Our Bodies

When 20-year-old Phoebe, a Latina, became pregnant two years ago, her life turned upside down. Calling that pregnancy "hell," she recalls, "I was so sick like I'd never been in my life." She felt so weak that she lacked the energy even to shower. Phoebe suffered from dehydration to the extent that her family rushed her to the emergency room twice; most likely, she became dehydrated because of continual vomiting. During her pregnancy, Phoebe remembers, "I let myself go. I was really active and always like to look good and dress up, but I couldn't anymore." Her boss did not understand this listlessness and fired her. Ultimately, Phoebe says, she "turned into a living vegetable."

She could not go on like this. Although she and her boyfriend had planned the pregnancy, she now felt unenthusiastic about carrying to term. She worried that her father, who did not know about the pregnancy, would be disappointed if she gave birth. Her mom did know, and kept telling Phoebe that she would have to marry if she had the baby. This pressure scared Phoebe and fueled her desire to end the pregnancy. Phoebe's boyfriend still wanted her to give birth, but she decided on abortion. She went to the clinic, entered the room "where the doctors were going to do the procedure, and let them take over."

When she conceived, Phoebe lost control of her life. Even though she planned the pregnancy, she felt that her body pushed her around. Like Phoebe, we may be discouraged to have an unintended pregnancy control our bodies, to feel sick and reduced to the concerns of our flesh. This may be all the more frustrating if we have never given much thought to our bodies and have not expected them to cause us any trouble. We become dependent on doctors to end this condition, just as Phoebe "let them take over."

Many of us resent the nausea, exhaustion, dizziness, and sore breasts that we feel during pregnancy. One 34 year old says that before she had her third abortion three months ago, "I hated being pregnant against my will. I hated my swollen breasts, and I resented being so sick. I wondered what I would have done if I had had a job." She had little energy for anything. Another woman, age 26, concurs that her pregnancy two years ago greatly disrupted her daily life. She was so uncomfortable with her pregnant body that she did not want to have sex. She "loathed being pregnant," and adds, "I was nauseous day and night, while simultaneously I was starving. I ate everything in sight and I was always having to nap. This double-confirmed my suspicions that this was not the right time for me to have a baby." Some people believe such negative symptoms come from being unhappy about a pregnancy, and that they largely disappear with excitement about a pregnancy. Other women find that any pregnancy will bring unpleasant side effects.

Even if we have negative feelings about the changes our bodies have undergone, they may also fascinate us. We may study our body parts with great curiosity. One woman examined her vagina with a mirror. Another took new interest in her breast size and veins and pored over *The New Our Bodies, Ourselves.*

Twenty-year-old Ricki, who is African American, was preoccupied with her body shape before she ended her pregnancy six weeks ago. She recalls, "As soon as I found out, I always had this fascination with the mirror and thought one day I was going to wake up and I'd be showing. I was like, 'Oh, no. People are going to know.'" She stared into her full-length mirror and thought, "Damn, I'm getting fat!" Ricki, who is slender and small-boned, figured she wasn't very far along and couldn't possibly be showing. Her boyfriend, however, egged on her "paranoia about showing." He would rub her abdomen and say, "Oh, you're going to start showing in a minute." With new doubts, Ricki returned to the mirror. She says she felt bigger, maybe wider. At her abortion, she learned that she was three and a half months along, so she very likely was growing larger.

Along with feeling intrigued by the changes, we may find it exciting to see our familiar bodies undergo a makeover. One 23 year old, who had an abortion two years ago, now has more respect for her body. She explains, "I don't think I knew how much being pregnant could change it. I just thought you got fat and didn't have your period for a while." Instead, her body changed dramatically and quickly, which amazed her.

We may love some of the changes. A 23 year old recalls, "I loved my big tits. Although I was only nine weeks pregnant, my breasts doubled in size and became round and beautiful. When I went for the abortion, I was tempted to say to the clinician, 'Can't I keep the breasts?' but that was decidedly inappropriate." The changes of pregnancy might make us feel feminine, as if we have achieved our biological potential. We may find our new softness and roundness appealing. One 24 year old, who had abortions at ages 19 and 20, says she felt more connected during each pregnancy to "the aspects of my body that make me a woman." She adds, "I marveled at the capabilities of my body, like milk production and the ability to grow another being inside my body." We may feel proud of these qualities, as well as attractive, radiant, and in bloom. Some of us are relieved to know that we are fertile and that our body parts function well.

When a 31 year old conceived five years ago, she says, "I was proud to be pregnant." She had no idea what to expect from her pregnancy, and comments, "I didn't know it would change the way I looked at myself as a woman." She thinks of herself as feminine, and pregnancy "hit home" by enhancing those feelings. She recalls, "It felt like this huge miracle that was happening." She was amazed by her body's transformation and says, "I noticed the change in my breasts right away. My skin was so clear and my eyes were really bright and I just felt wonderful. My appetite changed completely and I was craving protein and carbohydrates and I didn't want the sugar anymore. It was this natural thing going on with me. And there was something really beautiful about that." She responded to those changes as if she were carrying to term, which part of her really wanted to do. She recalls, "I'd still watch what I'd eat. I would pass up the wine at dinner, and I wouldn't eat any sweets. I felt really hungry and I'd eat a lot of good things." This response seemed natural to her, both because the whole process of pregnancy was so natural, and because she welcomed the changes her body underwent.

Whether we love the changes of pregnancy, observe them with fascination, or outright detest them, we may find that a pregnancy is only the start of a new relationship with our bodies. The abortion can spark feelings we have never known before.

THE PROCEDURE: INNOCUOUS OR INVASIVE?

During a pregnancy, if our bodies feel out of control, we may look forward to the time when we will no longer be pregnant. We might regard the procedure as the path back to normalcy, the event that will restore our control. Some of us do find that the abortion meets this need. We may tolerate any pain, knowing that the discomfort is worth the relief it will bring. After the abortion, we may feel that our bodies are ours again, not host to an unwanted element. One 22 year old wept joyfully after the procedure a year ago and explains, "I felt so in control of my body." Our bodies may feel emptier, lighter, freed.

Simone, a 39-year-old Caucasian, also came out of her abortion a year ago with a positive feeling about the procedure. Before the operation, she feared that it would be invasive and wished that she could simply swallow a pill like RU 486, rather than going through "this physical act." The idea of the procedure bothered her, because it made her have to face what she was doing. Simone muses, "You can't really wish it away. You literally have to go there and they have to do something to you." When she went through the abortion, however, she found it reassuringly benign. She says that the violence she feared "got put in context for me, because it really seemed rather innocuous." It felt especially tame compared with her earlier experience of amniocentesis, "which seemed really invasive and violent." Some women agree that the pain of an abortion is mild and that the surgery is quick. Several say that the procedure is no big deal. But not everyone shares this opinion.

While we often go into an abortion hoping to regain control over our bodies, we may feel even more out of control afterward. The very set-up of an abortion procedure can make us feel ill at ease. If we are awake for the operation, we lie on a table inactively, half-clothed in a gown, with our legs spread wide open. Others, who are fully dressed, walk around the room and peer at our private body parts. In this state of passivity, we may feel acted upon, as if we are objects. Already, we have been through several tests and may have begun to feel that our bodies are things to be measured, assessed, inspected, and probed. Adding to this feeling, the clinic workers may not speak to us much, focusing on one isolated part of our bodies. They may act rushed or impersonal, possibly to deemphasize the sexuality involved. We may begin to feel as though we are just another vagina and uterus to them, not a whole person. General anesthesia may be a good way to avoid these feelings, but it can also enhance our sense of passivity about the procedure. One 23 year old who was knocked out for her abortion four years ago dislikes that the clinic workers were "doing things" to her body and that she "didn't even know what they were doing."

Often, they hang a sheet over our abdomen, making the experience more blind for us. One woman in her mid-thirties comments on how "disconcerted" this aspect makes her feel at any gynecological exam. She says, "You put your feet in the stirrups and they stick a sheet on you and disconnect you from your body." She adds, "Conventional doctors use the sheet because they want to disconnect from you, to separate doctor from woman. There's no medical reason for the sheet." There may be emotional reasons, however. The sheet protects us from frightening sights of blood, the suction machine, and long needles. Her point about the effect is quite valid, though. We may feel as if we have been cut in half, torso rent from legs, mind detached from body. The message that sheet can give is, "Don't worry about what's going on down here. It doesn't concern you."

When the doctors insert their instruments and begin to suction, we may feel not only pain, but also a sense of invasion. The instruments penetrate deeply and may move ungently within our uterus. During a routine gynecological exam, doctors enter only the outermost parts of our reproductive system. During an abortion, however, it may feel as if they are pumping out the center of our torso. A 43 year old says of the abortion she had nineteen years ago, "The abortion itself was the worst part of the experience. I experienced it as a real violation, almost a rape." She has been raped before, so she does not make the analogy lightly. A 22 year old whose abortion occurred two years ago brings up similar images of pain and invasion. She says, "Having the abortion felt like one long scream. It was violent. I felt like a deer in a classroom. I did not want to be there. I kept trying to put myself somewhere far away." Another 22 year old's words concur with this description of discomfort. Four years after her abortion, she says, "I will not forget the sound of the vacuum and how horrible it sounded. The procedure was not painful, but very, very uncomfortable. It was like someone was ripping and sucking out my insides. I felt empty afterward." She still has trouble hearing the sound of a vacuum cleaner. One woman, age 24, recalls how she, too, felt violated by her abortion five months ago. She laments, "How bare and ripped I felt. Never before had I felt so absolutely lonely. My body on a cold, metal table. I screamed. Absolutely screamed. Tears everywhere. I felt empty. Completely barren. Like a desert."

Nora, who is white and 22, had a similar experience eight months ago. She went into the procedure filled with wonder about the miraculous changes of pregnancy, but feels that the surgery "took the wonderment away." Pregnancy no longer seemed like a "floating type thing," a surreal condition. The abortion was so jarring that it made her "realize that there was something in there." That in itself is not necessarily bad; her denial about what she was aborting had to end sometime. But Nora says the procedure left her feeling badly about "myself and my body and the way people manhandled me."

Calling the operation "not nice," Nora says, "I thought the machines were very unprofessional. It wasn't at all smooth." During the procedure, Nora felt like a piece of meat, as though she were merely a body being worked on, no longer a person. It did not help that the medical staff members seemed mechanized in their approach to abortion, as if they were "processing" her. She expected them to use rhetoric about abortion, commenting on "how great it is that this is a right and that we can have it in hospitals and not in trailers." Instead, the nurse lectured her about birth control, while the doctor left without speaking to her.

Afterward, Nora felt so weak that she couldn't even move. She says, "I thought I was going to die." Nora adds that, physically, "I had no idea it was going to take that much out of me. I just had this feeling I had been through this battle! I felt like I'd been beaten up, like something had torn me down. Every part of my body." Feeling "wracked" and "battered," she worried that she had done something completely unnatural to her body. She regards pregnancy as a wonderful process that takes the sperm and egg way beyond their original state, and sees the abortion as having taken out more than her boyfriend ever put into her body. Nora shakes her head, saying, "I feel like I did something really bad to my body. And I feel like I could have damaged it permanently." Medically, that is not likely. Abortion is one of the most commonly performed operations in the United States, and also one of the simplest. Complications are rare. Still, there is a difference between how the operation affected Nora biologically and how she feels emotionally. Currently, she feels as if she lost control of her body, because the abortion "disturbed the system."

One odd footnote to Nora's story is that she had her abortion performed at the same hospital as Simone, who found the procedure "rather innocuous" and not nearly as bad as she imagined. They even had the same doctor, who must have performed a similar procedure, although Nora was at the end of the first trimester, while Simone was only six weeks pregnant when she had her abortion. Is this one difference enough to account for the enormous gap in their experiences? Probably not. Here are some other disparities.

Nora expected the abortion to be trivial, clean, and precise. Because she anticipated a painless removal of a pregnancy that did not seem real, the abortion shocked her in its very physicality. Simone expected the act to be quite physical; she disliked that she couldn't wish the pregnancy away. Thinking the procedure would be as invasive as amniocentesis or perhaps as painful as birth, she instead found it quite bearable.

They decided to end their pregnancies in very different ways. Nora coasted through her pregnancy with little emotional difficulty, treating her decision as automatic, because she needed to finish college. Simone, who was already a mother, agonized over her choice and expected more emotional conflict to follow the procedure. Both thought the experience of surgery would be as easy or as hard as making that decision–and both were surprised.

Nora wanted the clinicians to reassure her about the political necessity of abortion. They did not address this, or treat her as a thinking human, which left her feeling that she and her body had been processed. In contrast, Simone asked the doctor about her views on abortion and was relieved when she said she was doing an important service. This answer may have helped Simone see the procedure as having integrity. The medical staff might have treated Simone with more respect because she is nearly twice Nora's age. They may also have found Simone a more sympathetic figure, because she was anguished over her choice, whereas they may have seen Nora as callous or cavalier.

Whatever the specifics of Nora's and Simone's stories, the larger point is that our expectations of the procedure may affect our experiences. The abortion may seem traumatic if we have not accepted that we have to go to some lengths to end our pregnancy. The level of anesthesia and the doctor's roughness or gentleness also matter a lot. In addition, we each tolerate pain differently. If we are tense during the operation, it might hurt more than if we are relaxed. Clearly, there can be some physical challenges to the surgery, but there are also emotional ones, namely, trying to retain our personhood through the operation. If we are involved and assertive during the abortion, feeling that the medical staff is responsive to our concerns, we will probably feel more in control of our bodies afterward. If, however, we are ignored or disrespected, we will tend to feel dehumanized.

HOW WE FEEL ABOUT THE BLEEDING

In the weeks that follow the abortion, our concerns about our body may increase as we begin to bleed. The blood is part of the uterus's healing process, not the remains of the pregnancy or a menstrual period. The bleeding lasts a different time for everyone. There might be little blood, or it may continue for weeks, followed by a period. We may react in different ways to this blood, depending on how long it lasts and what it means to us.

For Nora, the blood served as a "constant reminder" of her abortion. She felt that the abortion played a central role in her life as long as she bled. Nora found the bleeding "really annoying," because one cannot wear tampons after an abortion, as that might cause an infection. If one is unused to wearing sanitary pads, they may seem bulky and messy, making one more aware of the blood.

Nora comments on the inconvenience of this by saying, "There's nothing worse than when you're bleeding and you can't use tampons. You're just schlepping around. You feel like this woman who has no control over her body and can't go outside. You don't have the same mobility and freedom."

Nora, who woke up crying in the weeks after her abortion, attributes some of her unhappiness to the blood. She says, "I think that had a large effect on my freaking out. It's just this constant bleeding. I was getting up in the middle of the night to change my pad, because I was bleeding so much." The bloody deluge reinforced her feeling that she interrupted a natural process by having an abortion. As she faced the blood repeatedly, she thought, "I've done something horrible to my body." She began to feel better emotionally when the bleeding ceased and when she no longer had to abstain from sex. The sex isn't what made her happy so much as her thinking, "I'm no longer affected by this thing." The bleeding served as a limbo that prevented her from moving past the abortion.

Bleeding may be unpleasant because it forces us to keep facing what we have done. A 32 year old who had an abortion nine years ago recalls that bleeding was the worst part of her experience, because it was "hard to confront" that the blood was "related to a fetus." She even thought she passed the fetus at one point. She says, "I remember looking at this pad with this big glob of dark, red flesh and thinking maybe that was the fetus." Feeling uncertain, she consulted someone, who assured her that it could not have been the fetus, unless the abortion was incomplete. Still, having red discharge that was "clotty, ugly," and "different from menstrual blood" made her uncomfortable and repulsed.

One woman, age 35, did have an incomplete abortion six months ago, so she bled for two months. She normally enjoys all phases of her cycle, but two months felt excessive to her. She says, "Bleeding all the time is like being fall all the time. Fall is fine for fall. But if you're fall all the time, you get out of balance. You need spring, summer, winter, too." She says that in her constant state of bleeding, "I was the giant drain hole. I was the napkin queen. I was . . . oops! I think a giant clot is gushing out of me!" When the bleeding ended, she delighted in buying new, unstained underwear.

We may be put off by the smell of the blood. One 27 year old felt disgusted two years ago by the odors she produced when she was bleeding, and felt horrified that "what could have gone into a baby was now just smelling really bad." When she smelled the blood, she thought, "Oh God, how terrible that I had an abortion." It seems that for her, the decision appeared as disgusting as the odor, and that the two things became associated in her mind. If we feel guilty, as this woman did, we may interpret the bleeding as a punishment for having ended a pregnancy. Biologically, the bleeding is a normal, predictable response to the surgery and does not mean that a deity is at work.

For some of us, the bleeding sparks a feeling of loss. One 25 year old who had an abortion two months ago started crying when she saw the first blood. The bleeding itself was not painful or excessive, but she says, "It was the fact that I'm not pregnant anymore. It was hard to let go of." For her, pregnancy was special, something different from anything she had experienced. As she stared at her stained underwear, she thought, "Oh my God, I'm just going to go back to normal."

Bleeding may make us feel very alone in our experience, just as we may feel isolated and sad during a sickness. One 21 year old, who has had three abortions since age 17, resents that although she and her boyfriend conceived together, she is the one who has gone through abortions, emotional pain, and bleeding. The bleeding makes her sense this inequity the most. She notes, "It's painful and it's lonely." She would like to take a bloody pad and "shove" it in her boyfriend's face as proof of her pain.

Subsequent periods can also bring up strong feelings. If we menstruate right after the postabortion bleeding, we may feel frustrated that we now face several more days of dealing with blood. A menstrual cycle may also remind us of the abortion. One 25 year old whose abortion occurred ten months ago has had this experience. Bleeding immediately after the abortion made her feel "a little nostalgic about the pregnancy. It was very emotional and symbolic." She reacted the same way to her next four or five periods.

At the same time, her first period made her feel purged. Indeed, postabortion blood can feel cathartic, as if our body is freeing itself of the whole pregnancy and abortion experience. We may feel deeply relieved upon seeing the blood, because an absence of blood may have come to signify pregnancy; upon bleeding, we might feel that we are finally back to normal. The blood may also seem like proof of our emotional pain, a concrete sign that we really have been through something major.

DISLIKING OUR BODIES AFTER AN ABORTION

After we experience unplanned pregnancies and abortions, we may regard our bodies in a new way. Some of us are less enthusiastic about them. If we associate abortions with back alleys or cheapness, we may feel unclean. One 23 year old who has ended two pregnancies says, "I felt this need to cleanse my entire system after each abortion."

We may still have a sense of violation from the procedure. The day after her abortion, one 27 year old feels that way. She says, "I feel somehow maimed and not totally healthy and complete. I feel my body is mad at me and feels violated." As strong as this feeling can be, it will probably fade as we regain a sense of privacy and ownership over our organs. A 22 year old felt violated after her abortion four years ago, but no longer feels that way. She comments, "I used to feel that my uterus was dark and gloomy after my abortion, like some evil crime was committed there. Now I feel okay."

After an abortion, some of us feel unattractive. This feeling can start in pregnancy, if we feel bulkier or somewhat awkward with our enlarged breasts. Those of us who have never been pregnant before may doubt that pregnant women can be sexy. Models in magazines are light and carefree, not weighed down by pregnancy. If, on the contrary, pregnancy makes us feel ultrafeminine and beautiful, we may feel the opposite way when the pregnancy ends. We may believe that we have erased the radiant look we took on during pregnancy, as if we are a tree stripped of fruit, now dim and unspecial. One 23 year old who has had two abortions began feeling unattractive after the procedures, due to her guilt about ending the pregnancies. Believing that you are as beautiful as the things you do, this young woman comments, "I've done something that's not very pretty." If any part of the experience lowers our self-esteem, this decline may cause feelings of ugliness.

We might have gained weight during pregnancy and may feel unattractive for that reason. The excess weight may linger, because hormones can affect us for a long time after pregnancy ends. While we may accept the weight gain during pregnancy, we may have less patience later. Four months after her abortion, one 28 year old notes this distinction. She comments, "I feel overweight. When I was pregnant, I felt beautiful and healthy. I now find it difficult to look in the mirror." Weight may even have increased our desire to have an abortion. If we struggle with eating disorders or work hard to be thin, the idea of becoming huge with pregnancy may have seemed offputting.

This was true for 28-year-old Yvette, who had one abortion at age 16 and another one three months ago. Her mother weighs 300 pounds and Yvette has an eating disorder, so weight issues have played a central part in her life. Her mom blames her own weight problem on her pregnancies. Yvette finds this unrealistic, but because of her mother's words, she has "an ingrained fear that that's what happens to you" with pregnancy. She emphasizes that although this fear "wasn't a consideration in my decision to have an abortion," it did spring to mind often during pregnancy. Yvette, who says she was overweight before the pregnancy, has gained twenty-two pounds since she discovered the conception. She put on twelve pounds during the six weeks in which she knew about her pregnancy. The stress of the crisis made her overeat; she used food as a way to console herself. Yvette became caught in a cycle where self-destructive thoughts made her eat more and like herself less. Her self-esteem remains low right now because "it's so tied in with the eating." These self-esteem problems aren't "about the abortion." Yvette feels fine about having ended the pregnancy, but struggles to accept the way she now looks.

FEELING ALIENATED FROM OUR BODIES

Beyond disliking how our bodies appear after an abortion, many of us feel as if our bodies are now our enemies. While our mind resists pregnancy, our bodies have other ideas and agendas. It can feel like there is a split, a disunity of purpose.

For some of us, this alienation is nothing new. Before we ever conceive, we may feel that our body's processes don't concern us. We might mistreat our bodies with alcohol and drugs or by sleeping and eating improperly. Our minds may wander during sex.

Pregnancy can cut through this alienation and awaken us to the way our behavior affects our body. For example, one 25 year old, who had abortions at ages 22 and 24, was detached from her body until her first pregnancy. She was molested during childhood, so she learned to dissociate her brain from what her body experienced. Her mind and body seemed like two unrelated areas. She recalls, "I slept with quite a few men in college, most of it unprotected or semiprotected. I wasn't taking care of myself. I wasn't eating right. I wasn't treating myself like a human being." She says her first pregnancy alerted her to "the consequences of what I was doing," and notes, "I feel like I was being warned" by that conception. "All of a sudden," she adds, "here I was, constantly thinking about my abortion and my body." Now, she says, "I respect myself a hell of a lot more now than I did before. I take care of myself and I don't abuse my body."

Others of us, however, find that pregnancy makes bodily alienation worse. When we have symptoms of pregnancy, we may be so distant from our bodies that we do not even notice the changes. Once we are aware of the pregnancy, we may still feel dissociated, both because we can do nothing about the changes and because we know less than our body does about what's coming next. Twenty-three-year-old Darian, who had abortions at 20 and just six months ago, says that when she conceived, her body "felt like an alien's body." Suddenly, it "was doing something very strange and powerful." She notes, "I did not treat my body any differently while I was pregnant, but it treated me very differently." Darian adds, "At times my body was my enemy. Just when I thought I had my head screwed on straight, my body went this completely opposite direction."

Darian found it weird to sense her "role in the perpetuation of the species," as though her body made her stop being an individual and aligned her with age-old forces of reproduction. Indeed, during pregnancy, it is as if our body tells us, "Your feelings and plans don't matter. Only your biological functions do." This attitude echoes what many believe about pregnancy. People often act as if we are nothing more than containers for fetuses. Those who oppose abortion believe that we should let our bodies balloon for nine months, not minding it a bit. Ironically, we receive the opposite message at other times; we are expected to achieve ideal body shapes before and after pregnancy, which means caring about the way our bodies look. With such ideas rampant in our culture, it is no wonder that we often have problematic relationships with our bodies, especially during pregnancy.

We might find it intolerable that our bodies go against our wills, especially if we have strived to be in control of all areas of our life. Forty-three-year-old Patricia cannot accept this lack of control. In her twenties, she conceived twice on purpose, and felt pleased that she could have such control over her body. Then, at 30 and 36, she became pregnant after contraceptive failures and had two abortions. These unplanned conceptions reversed the sense of mastery she had felt in her twenties.

The first unplanned pregnancy was the hardest for Patricia. She explains, "I felt very betrayed by my body." She wondered, "Why is my body doing this to me?" Patricia resented that she had lost power over her body and that her IUD had failed her. Having an abortion could not erase that sense of betrayal. She comments that the abortion "would resolve the pregnancy, but it didn't resolve why I got pregnant to begin with."

Feeling that she lacked control over her fertility and her body, she began to see herself differently. Realizing that she wasn't "immune" to unplanned pregnancy, she started to align herself with other women who had trouble controlling their reproduction. Patricia has worked in women's health care for a long time, even serving as an abortion counselor in her twenties. It wasn't until her first unplanned pregnancy, however, that she realized that she was just as vulnerable to unintended conceptions as every other woman. She notes, "Even though I was very responsible about birth control, I still got pregnant. It gives me an appreciation for how complicated that is. It's complicated for an adult woman in a monogamous relationship who has access to good birth control," so it is even more challenging for women who lack these resources. Patricia says she now sees how complex "fertility issues are. It's not cut-and-dry. You can't control things."

In light of this situation, we might impose more controls on our body so that it does not "misbehave" again. This may mean employing three contraceptive methods at once so that our bodies can never "get us" again with an unplanned pregnancy. We might start taking birth control pills, even with reservations about how it can affect the body. If we do take pills despite doubts, our decision may feel akin to saying, "My body doesn't matter. I care more about controlling my body than about its health." We may, in effect, declare war on our reproductive system, alienating ourselves even further from our bodies.

TRYING TO CONNECT WITH OUR BODIES

Given that we can conceive against our will, is it possible to make peace with our bodies? One woman has tried to do this since her first abortion three years ago. Nicola is a white 25 year old who once had a terrible relationship with her body. She recalls that as a teen, "I was distrustful of my body. I was afraid of its capabilities and its power to rule my life." She feared an unwanted pregnancy, and explains, "I thought abortion would be the worst thing in the world. I went on the pill when I was fifteen, when I'd only had sex twice. Even on the pill, I was always afraid of getting pregnant."

Nicola points out that by the time she was 22, "My ideas about my body and abortion had changed completely." By this she means, "I didn't think that abortion should have to be a big deal. It seemed like all the negative things that were supposed to go along with abortion were social constructions–constructed in a society that enforced the oppression of women." Fearing abortion less, she went off the pill and tried to learn about her body's cycles. She not only felt unafraid of abortion, but actually was so curious about it that she wonders whether she conceived on purpose that year. She doesn't think she did, however. Nicola muses, "I was used to relying on the pill and hadn't really figured out how to make myself be careful. Plus, for some reason, I had this idea that I was infertile."

She was, in fact, quite fertile. After she learned that she was pregnant, Nicola tried to induce abortion by drinking tea made of abortive herbs. Although this action would seem to put her in control of her body's functions, she felt the opposite way. Nicola recalls, "Sometimes I'd feel really distant from what was going on inside of me."

During pregnancy, Nicola tried to improve her relationship with her body. She says, "I started to read up on how women's reproductive systems worked, and started to get a better understanding of my body." She says she felt stronger "knowing that my body was capable of creating new life and that I was able to choose not to carry a pregnancy."

The herbs failed to work, and Nicola had a surgical abortion. Emotionally, the experience wasn't difficult for her. After the abortion, she continued to read about the female body and reproductive system, "demystifying" these things. The abortion itself made her more aware of her body and more comfortable living inside it. She explains, "It was like having an abortion finally taught me that my body was mine, brought me into it, made my body real. Having an abortion and learning about my body have given me power. I know I can have an abortion and not be destroyed by it, which has given me confidence and strength and a sense of security in my body that I never had before."

Since Nicola knew she could have an abortion without being devastated, she felt free to experiment with contraceptive methods "that are safer but less effective than the pill." When she conceived a second time, just a few months ago, she used no protection at all. Nicola recalls, "I was drunk and with an ex-lover." She expected him to withdraw, but he didn't, and she conceived. She had another abortion. This abortion was also fairly easy emotionally, so she still feels that she does not need to be terrified of pregnancy.

At the same time, Nicola wants to do her part to prevent pregnancy. She is "horrible at talking about birth control," and attributes this to having been on the pill for so long and to seeing birth control as "a difficult and unsexy issue" to discuss. Her second abortion helped her with this matter. Nicola explains, "Having this abortion has gotten me talking to my friends about sex and contraception—and hopefully that will help me have safer sex in the future." In her mind, pregnancy and abortion are something to avoid, but nothing to fear. This attitude helps her strike a balance in her attempts to prevent pregnancy.

LIKING AND ACCEPTING OUR BODIES AFTER ABORTION

An important part of feeling good about our bodies is accepting that they can conceive, even against our will. One woman, age 22, makes this connection five years after her abortion. She says, "I love my body. I'm proud of what it can do and I also honor its abilities by not denying them. I know I can get pregnant–it's no myth–and I am careful not to." Rather than resisting our body's potential, we may exult in its capabilities. One woman who has had five abortions feels pleased that her body "works well" and "heals well." Another woman, age 38, feels similarly. She had abortions at ages 22, 24, and 26, and comments on those pregnancies almost beatifically: "My body was simply doing what it was biologically programmed to accomplish: procreate." She adds, "To complain about my body's natural function would be to complain that my lungs breathe oxygen, or that my heart beats every day." It may help to adopt this accepting attitude. This does not mean treating pregnancy as inevitable. We can make large efforts to prevent pregnancy, trying to find a balance between controlling our bodies and living in harmony with them. If we are like Nicola, we may not see unplanned pregnancy or abortion as the worst thing in the world. Then, we will feel comfortable using methods that are less effective than the pill, but which are not at all harmful. The challenge is to decide what we value most.

Chapter 11

Preventing Pregnancy, Preserving Pleasure

During her first twenty-five years, Cassie has traveled a long road. She came from a white, Pentecostal family in which sex and birth control were never discussed, had two abortions, and worked in a Planned Parenthood. Now that she has gained so much knowledge and experience, she looks back on her past and despairs at how little she knew.

A few years ago, she started reading voraciously about the female body. She explains, "I had no clue how my body worked." She had a vague idea where her uterus was located and knew what her period represented. But that was it. Cassie says, "I didn't know about cycles, and there were some forms of birth control I wasn't familiar with."

Cassie's lack of knowledge about her body is completely understandable, given her background. Her mother explained sex when Cassie was eight, but sent a confusing message. She said, "If you're married, it's a beautiful thing. But if you're not married, it's dirty and disgusting and it's a sin." Refusing to think that her daughters might have premarital sex, Cassie's mother did not discuss birth control with them. Cassie tried to make her mother discuss sex with a younger sister, but the mother responded, "She's a good girl. She doesn't do that." A year later, at age 16, Cassie's sister conceived and carried to term. Cassie blames her mother for that pregnancy and for avoiding the facts.

After being molested during childhood, Cassie began to have voluntary sex at 14. Once that year, she thought she was pregnant and shared her fears with her mother. The mother commanded her to be celibate. Cassie continued to have sex, but lacked information about contraception and used none. With "little or no birth control consideration," she notes, "I managed to make it to my twenty-second year before I got pregnant." Pregnancies and abortions were "not going to happen to me," she says. She knew how women conceived, but never thought she would.

In a state of denial, she believed that something would shield her from those undesirable outcomes. This is common. We may envision that a protective force encircles us, preventing anything unpleasant from coming our way. Many of us cling to this denial as we take risks in our daily life, telling ourselves when we drive through town or fly in an airplane that we are not in danger. It would be too difficult to proceed if we were always aware of risks. We would be frozen in terror, unable to overcome our fears. Similarly, as we enter the sexual danger zone, we may tell ourselves that we are immune to pregnancy. If we kept in mind all the possible negative outcomes of sex, how could we relax in bed?

Cassie's denial is in no way unusual, nor is her lack of knowledge about sexuality. It may be hard to believe that children can grow up these days without frank talks with their parents or sex education classes in schools. But Cassie has met many other young women even more confused than she was. Although she had "zero" knowledge about sex and birth control, she says, "I was the one everyone always came to." Because she became sexually active so early, her friends assumed she knew a lot. They would entreat her to explain orgasm and would inquire about birth control. After Cassie had her first abortion at 22, people inundated her with more questions. Cassie went to work at Planned Parenthood to help educate others and "make it easy for someone else like nobody did for me." To her horror, she found more confusion among the clients. She counseled scared, pregnant girls who knew little about their bodies. Cassie says, "They were not aware that sex led to pregnancy, and they didn't know how it worked in their systems."

Some of us do know about our bodies, but underestimate how fertile we are and therefore use no birth control. A doctor may have told us that we are unlikely to conceive. We might also believe we are infertile because of irregular or menopausal-type menstruation, or because we have had uncontracepted sex for years and have thus far not conceived. Even if we have no concrete reason to think we are infertile, some of us wonder if we are. We may stop using birth control as a way to test our fertility.

At Planned Parenthood, Cassie worked hard to teach others about birth control. Still, she had difficulty finding a contraceptive method that met her own needs. Because she was sexually abused, she says, "I have a real problem with putting things in my vagina, like diaphragms and sponges." The pill has also been problematic. She explains, "I've been on it three times. All three times, I ended up on antidepressants, because I just cannot handle the overload of hormones." After her first abortion, she and her boyfriend began using condoms diligently. They became less consistent after a while, though. She conceived again at age 24 and felt furious at herself for not having been careful, especially since she had instructed so many others about pregnancy prevention.

After a second abortion, Cassie and her partner began using condoms "religiously." He is very willing to wear them, but she worries about their effectiveness, and feels she should also use foam. Cassie is correct; condoms are only 90 percent effective, but become over 99 percent effective when used with foam. She is somewhat in danger of another pregnancy. She does, however, have two good weapons against an unintended conception: knowledge and a healthy fear of pregnancy. A lack of information and an inability to face the risk of conceiving are two reasons for unplanned pregnancies.

There are often psychological causes, as well. We do not always conceive terminated pregnancies unintentionally. To fulfill emotional needs, we may try to conceive. Having a baby might seem like a good way to stabilize our lives or to avoid big changes. If we discover that we are pregnant, however, other needs, especially financial or emotional ones, may suddenly seem more important.

Unwanted conceptions are not simple matters. People often assume that if we don't use birth control, it is because we lack access to contraception. They think that a ready supply of condoms will remedy the matter. That won't hurt, but it fails to address the complex reasons we might forgo birth control. People also think that most terminated pregnancies result from birth control failures. Contraceptive methods do fail quite often; many women who seek abortions have taken full precautions with birth control. But the majority of ended pregnancies result from the absence of contraception.

We may use no birth control if the methods present various problems. Many of us dislike the pill, both because of its side effects and because ingesting chemicals and altering our bodies can seem unsavory. We might fear that the pill will cause infertility or cancer. In fact, there is no connection between the pill and infertility. It has never been proven that the pill causes cancer, and research has shown that the pill protects against certain types of cancer. Besides having such concerns about the pill, some of us feel that barrier methods, such as diaphragms and condoms, can interfere with spontaneity. Obtaining birth control might also embarrass us. Finally, contraception can be expensive and may not seem worth the financial cost.

If we feel that birth control has drawbacks, we might decide to try our luck and use none. Several of us view this decision as a gamble, referring to it as playing with fire, testing fate, or pushing limits. Abstaining from birth control may feel thrilling. Risk taking makes our adrenaline surge, whether we skydive, speed, go to casinos, or call an old lover. The payoffs tantalize us—free-falling through space, feeling powerful as we dodge cars on the freeway, fattening our wallets, or learning that a former lover still wants us. It can pay to gamble. In the case of birth control, we may weigh countless instances of carefree sex against the one time we conceive, and decide that the risk is worthwhile, at least before a pregnancy. After a pregnancy, however, we may have a new perspective.

Mariel: "I Was in Denial About My Body and About the Affair"

Twenty-five-year-old Mariel, who is white, certainly views her risk taking differently now that she has had an unplanned pregnancy. Before conceiving last year, she sensed that her life was problematic, but couldn't seem to fix it. She had a boyfriend, but they had broken up temporarily. In the meantime, she began sleeping with Trevor, her friend Paloma's boyfriend. Mariel felt horrible about all aspects of her behavior. She says, "I was caught in this cycle of having sex without condoms, feeling like shit, and hating myself for being irresponsible, then making promises to myself,

'I'll never sleep with him again.'" Mariel inevitably returned to Trevor, feeling worse about herself each time. When Mariel discovered that she was pregnant, she felt dumb and guilty. Ten months after her abortion, she still feels that way. She comments, "If I had been using birth control and still got pregnant, I think I wouldn't feel this sense of stupidity." Like Cassie, Mariel has worked in women's clinics and as a health educator, so she believes that she ought to have known better.

She now understands why she refrained from using birth control and explains, "This was part of the denial of it. I was in denial about my body and about the affair." Feeling guilty about cheating on her boyfriend and deceiving Paloma, Mariel told herself that the relationship was off and refused to believe that she would have sex with Trevor again. Obtaining birth control would mean admitting that she was still sleeping with him.

Like Mariel, some of us cannot face that we are sexually active. Our reasons may not involve an illicit relationship like hers, but may concern our general feelings about sex. If we oppose premarital sex, find sex hedonistic, or fear pregnancy, we might need to deceive ourselves about planning to have more sex. Obtaining a diaphragm or taking the pill means that we expect to have sex. We may worry that if a man knows we have taken precautions, he will think us cheap, easy, or unspontaneous. As Mariel has done, we might swear off intercourse, at least with a certain lover.

We may choose to let our partner supply condoms, because that does not require us to prepare and allows us to pretend that sex has taken us by surprise. Unfortunately, this will not happen unless he cares about contraception or disease prevention. Using a condom also requires us to be able to communicate with our partner about the potentially awkward subject of birth control. We may feel unable to do this; trust, respect, and openness may be absent. For Mariel and Trevor, this was the situation. They had "little real communication."

At that time, Mariel also drank a lot and smoked pot frequently. These substances probably gave her even less control over decisions about birth control. The pot and alcohol may have made Mariel's life seem too fast to keep up with; she might have felt too overwhelmed to think about both contraception and sex. Even without using substances, some of us cannot summon the energy to attend to matters of birth control. Mariel may well have felt exhausted by the multitude of things going on at that time.

Another event, way back in Mariel's past, may also have worked against her use of birth control; her father sexually abused her. Those of us who were molested as children often have a difficult time asserting ourselves about birth control and sex as adults, because we grew up having no say over what happened to us sexually. Sex may now seem like a routine activity to us, rather than a way to be intimate. We may not know how to control our sexual choices. Before Mariel became involved with Trevor, she slept with many people indiscriminately.

Now, the pregnancy has helped her change her approach to sex and birth control. She says, "Casual sex without communication and without condoms isn't so great and makes me feel like shit." Because she knows she will hate herself if she uses no birth control, it's easier to be responsible about it. For her, pregnancy looms as a threat. She notes that after the abortion, she was "terrified of getting pregnant."

This is common; many of us fear pregnancy afterward. Mariel has a more complicated take on this issue, however. She fears pregnancy so much that she thinks she is pregnant all the time. When her period comes, she feels unexpectedly disappointed. This reaction confuses Mariel, but she has some insight into the matter. Because her pregnancy with Trevor was so miserable, and because she is now back with her boyfriend who respects her, she wants to conceive with him and repeat the experience "the 'right' way." By "right," she means that she would either carry to term or have an abortion, whichever seemed appropriate at the time. Mariel wants to "redo the whole thing," knowing what she now knows about pregnancy and abortion. She even wants to be using birth control when she conceives again. Mariel notes, "On one level, of course, I don't want another unwanted pregnancy. But in another way, I feel it could resolve some things."

What Mariel has described is a repetition compulsion. In this mindset, we feel unhappy about how a situation turned out, so we want to recreate it and see how we would act the next time. If we regret having had an abortion, we may try to conceive shortly after the procedure. Once we are pregnant, we may choose abortion again for the same reasons as before. Afterward, we may once more be unhappy with our choice and repeat the cycle.

Meredith: "I Thought It Would Be an Achievement to Have a Child"

Meredith, who is 21 and white, has also felt this desire to recreate the three pregnancies she has ended in the last four years. Because she has deeply loved the man with whom she conceived those pregnancies, she has wondered how it would be to have a child with him. Over the years, she has had feelings of "wanting to replace that first baby. Make it happen again and make it be right." These feelings sound like the ones Mariel has.

Unlike Mariel, however, Meredith really wants to have a baby. To Meredith, who comes from an unhappy family, and whose early years were filled with molestation, abandonment, struggles in school as a dyslexic, and heavy drug and alcohol use, pregnancy beckons as a comfort, a solution. She describes the allure it had for her before her third abortion: "I thought it would be an achievement to have a child." Believing that a family would bring her security, warmth, and unconditional love, Meredith fantasized about marrying her boyfriend and having a child together. Her boyfriend was thirty years older and she depended on him to give her much of the love her parents had neglected to supply. Those of us who feel as Meredith did may want to become pregnant in order to elicit a commitment or even a marriage proposal from our partner. Meredith recalls that during this time, she had accidents with birth control that "really weren't accidents." In a semiconscious way, she was trying to conceive and start the family she wanted.

When Meredith finally conceived a third time, she was thrilled. She began to carry her pregnancy to term, but realized that she might have damaged the fetus by using drugs and alcohol before knowing she was pregnant. Reluctantly and miserably, she terminated that pregnancy. Her relationship with her boyfriend ended around that time, too.

Now, Meredith lives with a new partner. Pregnancy still has a strong pull for her, but her boyfriend wants no children. Meredith sometimes overlooks this constraint and pays attention to her instinct to conceive. She explains that when one has a lover, one's drive to have a child with him is "extremely strong." Meredith adds, "I always found the prospect of fertility very exciting. I'm assuming it's this natural thing that brings men and women together in certain ways." She believes nature makes us want to reproduce with the men we love. This desire may make it challenging for Meredith to control her reproduction.

Vivian: "I Just Felt Too Insecure to Assert Myself"

Meredith's struggles to prevent pregnancy come from being in long-term relationships that appeal to her. Twenty-two-year-old Vivian, who is white, has had trouble for the opposite reason—the temporary nature of her sexual encounters. Vivian had several one-night stands with Owen, and found contraception difficult to use each time. A year ago, they made love again. Vivian recalls, "It was just this unexpected thing. Suddenly we were in the middle of it." Vivian feels that she did not have to proceed with unprotected sex that night. She could have stopped and said, "This isn't what I want." Unfortunately, she says, "I just felt too insecure to assert myself." Maybe if she made a fuss, he would lose interest.

What may have seemed most important that night was the passion and excitement that filled the room. They got together so infrequently that birth control might have appeared less essential than seizing the moment. During sex, pleasure may have priority over contraception, which can dampen the mood and pose an inconvenience. An unwanted pregnancy and abortion can make us rethink all this, however, as they did for Vivian after she discovered that her second night of making love to Owen caused her to conceive.

Soon after her abortion, Vivian met a new guy. They first slept together two months after the procedure. To her surprise, Vivian did not fear that initial instance of sex, because it was so different from the night she conceived. She explains, "I was sleeping with someone new and using birth control." This man altered the way Vivian began to approach contraception. Calling him "really affectionate" and "a lot more sexually experienced than I am," Vivian explains, "Birth control was his concern" as well as hers. She says he conveyed "a real respect for my body and my person." Although the relationship did not last long, she appreciated his attitude. Comparing his outlook to Owen's, Vivian says, "There wasn't this guy who didn't seem to want to deal with it."

Vivian was mentally prepared the next time Owen came into her life for more noncommittal sex. Once again, the issue of birth control arose. They had begun foreplay and Vivian had not yet put in her diaphragm. When she got "signals" from him that he didn't care whether they used birth control, his attitude challenged her. Vivian explains, "It put me in danger of saying, 'We just won't use anything. Forget about it.'" Vivian says she was "still a little bit willing to not assert myself," and was at risk of giving in to his casual approach. Fearing herself perhaps more than him, she confronted Owen.

Vivian told him she felt annoyed that he treated contraception as solely her responsibility. Why should she be the only one to think about preventing pregnancy? She added that "being in sync with somebody" by "using birth control and dealing with each other's bodies" is "every bit as sexy as the rest." Vivian finished by saying, "You just don't seem to want to deal with this." She felt angry that he wanted to ignore all the contraceptive concerns and skip right to the pleasurable parts. Owen retorted, "Actually I think you have the problem with it because you seem hesitant to get up and use it." In his mind, her reluctance to put in a diaphragm was the beginning and end of the issue. He did not seem to hear that birth control should be their joint responsibility. Although she is no longer involved with Owen, Vivian still resents his attitude. She adds, "I think he'd have been happier if I'd gone on the pill and he didn't have to deal with anything."

Some men do feel this way and make it even clearer than Owen. A man may refuse to wear condoms, claiming that they decrease his pleasure. He may not only shrug off his responsibility to prevent pregnancy, but even interfere with our efforts to use contraception. Several women have conceived because their partners have falsely claimed to be sterile. These women had sex unaware that they were not protected. In situations of rape, women have no say about having sex or using birth control. If we have enough experiences with men who take no contraceptive responsibility, we may begin to hate birth control on principle. We might figure that women shouldn't have to bear the burden of contraception when both men and women engage in sex. Unfortunately, that only hurts us in the end.

Vivian has adjusted differently to Owen's views about contraception. She has learned to assert herself in bed, both by insisting on birth control and by confronting her partners when she doesn't like their attitudes. Now that she has known someone who treated her body and contraception respectfully, she may choose partners who value her more than Owen did. Even more important, Vivian recognizes the role she played in abstaining from contraception and now takes responsibility for birth control.

USING BIRTH CONTROL DILIGENTLY AFTER AN ABORTION

For some of us, an unplanned pregnancy quickly changes our thinking about birth control. Whereas pregnancy may have seemed a distant possibility before, it now becomes a real threat. Cause and effect are glaringly clear; uncontracepted sex can easily lead to pregnancy. One 18 year old, who had an abortion ten days ago, declares that her views on birth control have turned around 180 degrees. She says, "I had gotten off the pill when I conceived, because I didn't like the side effects (weight gain, crankiness). Now I'm back on the pill and don't give a shit about side effects." She adds, "We are thinking of using condoms as an addition to the pill. I am afraid of getting pregnant again, so we are going to overdo it in the contraception department." Overdoing it might be what she needs to do to feel safe. Without that security, she might be unable to relax during sex.

After an abortion, we often make statements full of conviction about birth control, as this woman has. One 23 year old, who had her second abortion three months ago, says, "I'm now obsessive about taking my pills. Again. After the first abortion I was, too. Hopefully, this time I'll remember the pain and keep it up." Past abortions and the specter of future abortions motivate her. Another woman, age 25, has had this attitude for seven years since her abortion. She says, "Abortion has affected my mental life in a 'negative reinforcement' manner. It was stressful, expensive, and it hurt. I'm *totally* careful about condoms, plus additional methods now." Thinking about the detriments of an unplanned pregnancy might help us use contraception well, just as we might find it more effective during a diet to envision a fat self and to feel terrified, than to think about the benefits of eating healthy foods. Fear may be a better incentive than maintaining the status quo.

The "negative reinforcement" approach can have drawbacks, however. It may feel unnatural or unpleasant to be motivated by fear. One 22 year old has felt this way for the four years since she had an abortion. She finds her fear of pregnancy "a little uncomfortable," not "too healthy," and "driven." She feels controlled by fear, rather than freely choosing her approach to contraception. Compulsive feelings about using birth control can interfere with sex. One 24 year old, who had abortions at ages 19 and 20, has felt this way. She says, "Having sex again with the possibility of pregnancy caused apprehension. I was overly contracepting and it was difficult to fully relax." Now, however, this is not as much of a problem for her. She explains, "Over time, this has lessened and is not an issue when I have sex. I continue to use contraceptives and have upgraded my communication skills with my partners." Having made her partners more aware of her desire to avoid pregnancy, she may feel that she can let down her guard mentally and focus more on what she must do physically to prevent conceptions.

The challenge is to find a balance between vigilance and relaxation. If we are too uptight about contraception, we may not be able to enjoy sex. If we relax our standards too much, we might decide that having sex without a condom just once won't matter. Another challenge is to keep feeling motivated about birth control over time. While we may be hyperaware of our fertility after an unplanned pregnancy and might use contraception well for a few years, the threat of pregnancy may fade and birth control might seem less necessary. One 33 year old says that after her first abortion at age 20, she tried hard not to conceive for eight years. But, she says, "At some point in time, I almost stopped worrying, for it seemed as if I could not get pregnant, no matter how often I neglected to use condoms. Thus, my second pregnancy was rather unexpected." Ironically, we may guard against pregnancy so well that we begin to feel immune to conceiving.

THE FRUSTRATION OF BIRTH CONTROL FAILURES

Many of us have unplanned pregnancies because our contraception has failed. A birth control failure might not be hard to accept if we know our method is risky, or if we feel we haven't used the method correctly. If we have trusted a method and used it well, however, a pregnancy may shock us, destroy our faith in birth control, and feel most unfair.

One woman, age 39, had five birth control failures and abortions in fifteen years. When she was a teenager, her doctor told her not to use the pill because it gave her migraines. She recalls, "I felt angry that I couldn't take the pill, because I felt really carefree and safe on it." After that, she relied on less effective methods, which all failed. At ages 18 and 20, she conceived using diaphragms. At age 28, a cervical cap proved ineffective. When she was ages 31 and 33, she used a sponge and condom, which failed. Declaring, "Contraception is practically a myth. I feel cheated," she bridles that birth control has let her down, though she has used it faithfully. She lambastes "the ineffectiveness of birth control" and "the false sense of security it can convey."

She has good cause to be angry. It is bad enough that the burden of contraception so often falls on women and that only women can conceive. To make matters worse, no method is 100 percent effective. Oral contraceptives, the best method other than sterilization, can have unpleasant side effects and can endanger our health.

How can we cope with this state of affairs? Maybe our anger will bring about some changes. Perhaps if enough of us complain to those in charge, more medical research funds will go toward inventing foolproof, safe, easy-to-use methods. One 23 year old who conceived on birth control pills and ended that pregnancy six months ago has considered voicing her anger. Feeling "disgruntled" with modern medicine, she intended to write an accusing letter to the company that produced those pills. She changed her mind, deciding, "This is probably not going to accomplish anything." She felt, too, that she was partly responsible, because she took the pills at irregular times during a camping trip. She now takes a pill with a higher dosage and says, "I am religious about when I take it."

Ultimately, she had to refocus her energies on her own contraception use. That is the best way to avoid unwanted pregnancies. As one woman comments after three unplanned pregnancies and abortions, these experiences have "made me take an active role in preventing pregnancy. It is up to me to prevent it, rather than thinking that the man is going to be responsible for that. I wish that more young girls realize this fact before they become pregnant." We have every right to be angry about the paltry contraceptive options available to us, but as this speaker notes, in the end it is our responsibility to prevent pregnancies.

SEX AND THE FEAR OF PREGNANCY AFTER ABORTION

If we have had a birth control failure, we may fear sex after an abortion. The woman we have just met who had a pill failure says that even though she has a higher dosage, she still feels anxious about sex occasionally. Some days she thinks, "The doctor knows what he's doing. It'll be fine." Other days, she wants to tell her boyfriend, "Don't come near me with that thing!" Overall, though, she trusts her doctor and feels pretty comfortable with the pill. Others of us may not resolve the matter so easily. This has been the case for Frieda.

Frieda: "My Fear of Pregnancy Affects Our Sex Life"

Frieda is a white 32 year old who conceived nine years ago because she and her partner used no contraception. Soon after the abortion, the relationship ended. Frieda then had relationships with both men and women. During that time, she says she began to feel "angry with men for not dealing with the risk of getting pregnant, for proceeding with sex without addressing that I might get pregnant." Eventually, she married a man. At 30, she had a planned conception and delivered a son. Her second pregnancy changed her views on her abortion. Whereas she had blocked out the idea of fetal development during her terminated pregnancy, and thought of the fetus as "just some tissue," she looked for "evidence of life" during the second. Frieda comments, "You want to know it's a person, a being in there. You imagine it as a person in the future." After "investing personality and sacredness in this unborn thing," she thinks she would have trouble "flushing another one." Frieda believes that if she conceived again by accident, she would give birth.

That would be fine, except for two things. First, Frieda says, "I don't want another baby now." Second, her husband is "adamant" about not wanting another child. He tells her, "With your next husband, you can have another one." This leaves Frieda in a bind. If their condoms fail, both birth and abortion will seem very unappealing to her. Not wanting to make that choice, she feels "determined" to be very careful and has taken few chances.

She explains that her fear of pregnancy "affects our sex life a lot. I don't even like intercourse much lately." She prefers manual stimulation or oral sex and began to avoid intercourse soon after her abortion. Frieda says, "I still have intercourse, but it's not a major focus of my sex life." She thinks that women can combat a fear of pregnancy by using "other types of sexual stimulation besides intercourse." This way, they can "have their sex life be gratifying without risking pregnancy." Frieda looks forward to the time after menopause when she can have sex without fear.

There is a happy postscript to Frieda's story. A few weeks after she wrote down these feelings, she realized that she had "run off" some of her "emotional charge" about the topic and doesn't "feel so upset about those things now." After reflecting on the challenges of her situation, she is more optimistic. She says, "I think if I did get pregnant and wanted to have a baby, my husband would end up supporting me. I'm also going to start using the pill, which seems like a safer bet than condoms." Although Frieda has placed more faith in her husband's flexibility, she has acted independently of him to shore up her own contraceptive security. Now, perhaps, she can enjoy intercourse with less fear.

If Sexual Guilt Interferes with Lovemaking After Abortion

What we believe to be a fear of pregnancy may be another fear in disguise. We may feel uncomfortable during intercourse or whenever we think about sex, and may interpret such feelings as anxiety about conceiving again. In reality, our uneasiness may have more to do with the idea of sex. Perhaps we grew up thinking that sex is sinful, especially if it occurs outside of marriage or if pleasure, not procreation, is the goal. We may see it as shameful or unnecessary to indulge our libidos. Many types of pleasure make us feel guilty, such as eating chocolate or taking an afternoon nap. Sex may evoke that sort of guilt. We may also associate intercourse with bad things, such as STDs, or earlier traumas, such as sexual abuse or rape. Sex may seem to ruin things, such as a relationship or one's character. If we felt at all guilty or fearful about being sexually active before an unplanned pregnancy, we are likely to feel even more strongly about this after an abortion.

In our culture, it is hard to admit such feelings. Sex is supposed to be the ultimate thrill. If we do not feel that way, it may be hard to acknowledge that, even to ourselves. This feeling can show up as a fear of pregnancy. Our anxiety may be keenest during intercourse, because it might assuage our guilt to have a miserable time in bed. We may think that if we don't allow sex to be fun, we are not blameworthy for making love. If we hold back sexually, we may want to examine the source of our fears. Are we more worried about conceiving or about having sex? Perhaps one fear is masquerading as another.

OVERCOMING FEARS OF PREGNANCY AND ENJOYING SEX

If we do fear pregnancy after an abortion, it is possible to allay these worries. For instance, a 19 year old named Virginia, who is white, black, and Native American, had an abortion eighteen months ago and now feels secure during sex. She explains that she has not always felt this way. She conceived after a condom broke. At first, Virginia felt angry at herself that this had happened, "irrational" though that response seems to her today. She comments, "I never blamed my boyfriend. I knew he didn't want it to happen and he didn't refuse to wear condoms." Now, she blames nobody and says, "I have to take responsibility for what I do, and a condom breaking is one of those things that happens."

Virginia had an abortion and went on the pill. Her partner used condoms as well. She became extremely careful, because, as she says, she was now "more aware that I could get pregnant again. It's no longer a distant reality." Even with all this protection, she feared pregnancy, and disliked sex. Virginia explains, "For about a month after the abortion I would either push my boyfriend away, or I wouldn't enjoy sex. Sex and my abortion were too closely linked." Seven months after the abortion, she and her boyfriend broke up.

Virginia currently has a new partner, and says, "Now that my boyfriend and I are together, sex has never been better, because I feel safer." Her contraceptive approach has remained the same. In fact, she still does not completely trust her birth control methods. She comments, "Even though I use two forms of contraceptives, I'm still afraid of getting pregnant, but I just ensure that I take all the precautions necessary." If she still fears pregnancy and distrusts her birth control, but feels safer during sex, the difference between sex with these two men may be that Virginia feels emotionally safer with her new boyfriend. The way we feel about our partners can affect how secure we feel during sex.

For some of us, trusting our method may be the key to approaching sex fearlessly. One 29 year old who conceived at age 18 with a diaphragm now steers clear of that method and warns friends to do the same. She says, "It's a tricky method and a sloppy one and I simply do not trust it anymore." Instead, she puts her faith in oral contraceptives. She says, "On the occasion when I've skipped a pill, I've been very responsible in using condoms as a backup." She can be both relaxed and cautious and notes, "I'm more conscientious about birth control than I used to be, but I consider that a good thing." Being careful does not feel compulsive to her. Nor does it interfere with sex. She says, "I enjoy sex too much to worry about pregnancy." She also engages in "other modes of sexual satisfaction that carry absolutely no risk of pregnancy at all." Her trust in her method, her responsible use of birth control, her love of sex, and her other means of feeling sexually satisfied have made sex pleasurable for her in the eleven years since her abortion.

When she says she enjoys sex too much to worry about pregnancy, her meaning is not entirely clear. We can like sex, but also fret about conceiving. She may mean that the pleasure she derives from sex outweighs her worries. It is also possible that she never fears pregnancy. If we cannot achieve that carefree state, the next best thing may be to disconnect our anxieties about pregnancy from the act of sex. A 30 year old who had an abortion six years ago has achieved this. While she says, "I'm always afraid I'm going to get pregnant," and adds that she was afraid even before her abortion, she also says that this fear "doesn't seem to curb my sexual activity." Somehow, she is able to keep fear and pleasure separate. This could be dangerous, because separating cause and effect–sex and pregnancy–is the form of denial that led many of us to conceive in the first place. But if we have protected ourselves well, perhaps we can see our fears as unproductive and can put them aside during sex. Their only use is to prompt us to be conscientious.

What if we don't trust our method enough to relax? If we're using anything less effective than the pill, we may have reason to worry. Then we might think about installing a backup plan. Condoms are a great match for any contraceptive. Combining condoms with another method will ensure that our partner takes equal responsibility and will protect against disease. If we fear that our method has failed, or have had uncontracepted sex, we can still prevent pregnancy with the morning-after pill. This is an underused safety net.

There is a more certain way to alleviate our fears. Many couples find relief in tubal ligations or vasectomies. One couple took this path after an IUD failure caused the woman to conceive at age 39. The failed IUD made her "very distrustful of all contraception," so they decided on a vasectomy. The operation met their needs. Nineteen years later, she comments, "After my husband's vasectomy, sex was more relaxed and enjoyable."

Ultimately, we should do whatever makes us feel safe. We may need to identify why we feel unsafe. Perhaps our partner frightens us, not our method. We may fear pregnancy because we feel guilty about having sex and want to limit our pleasure. We could address the constraints in our life that make having a baby impossible. If we examine what needs we have tried to meet through sex and through our approach to birth control, we can have a firmer handle on our decisions about sex, contraception, and pregnancy.

Chapter 12

Ending More Than One Pregnancy

Brittany, a 22-year-old Caucasian, has had abortions at ages 19 and 20. Although they were only a year apart, there was a world of difference between them. They were also distinct from her first unplanned pregnancy; Brittany gave birth at 18 after conceiving with her boyfriend, Dean. At the time, she viewed birth as a better outcome than abortion, and felt superior to high school friends who chose abortion over birth.

When she conceived again a year later, Brittany longed to give birth, but felt that having another child wouldn't be fair to her baby, Courtney. Brittany and Dean agreed on abortion. She was shocked to find herself ending a pregnancy and comments, "It wasn't really something that I expected to go through, especially after having become a mother." She felt disappointed not only that she wouldn't meet this child, but also that she would choose abortion at all. This turn of events showed her that she wasn't "a better person" than her peers simply because she had brought her first pregnancy to term. She stopped judging her friends, but was still hard on herself.

After her first abortion, Brittany felt isolated. She says that back then, "I didn't nearly have the community that I have now. I could spend whole days with just me and Courtney." In her isolation, she dwelled on her abortion. She explains that she didn't have "many opportunities to get my mind off of it. To enjoy my life and think about it when I needed to." Brittany not only had little contact with others, but was also unhappy with the few connections she did have. She notes that at that time in her life, "I was walking around, like most people do, waiting for someone else to pay attention to my problems."

Brittany and Dean broke up, but made love one afternoon. When Brittany discovered that she was pregnant, she wanted to carry to term. She also hoped that she and Dean might reunite and care for their children together. But Dean let Brittany know in no uncertain terms that he would not be responsible for another child. Eventually, Brittany understood his feelings and decided to end the pregnancy.

Brittany felt disappointed not to give birth, but was not as down on herself as before. There was a little of that; Brittany says that with both of the pregnancies she ended, she felt "disappointed in myself for being in the situation I was in." But when she decided on abortion the second time, she says, "I didn't feel so much like a failure." The difference was that Brittany had come to accept what she perceived as her imperfections. She can now say, "I make lots of mistakes. Tons of mistakes all the time." She adds, "By not being as hard on myself, I'm able to apologize more quickly and figure out what I need to do to repair things." She also feels more willing to make those mistakes, which she says lets her "move forward in my life in ways that I never thought were possible." She frames each ended pregnancy as "one of those mistakes that I've really grown from."

After her second abortion, Brittany found that she had more people to support her than before. Her social contacts have multiplied, so that she and Courtney visit at least five or six people a day. Her last abortion made her realize that she has "a full life." Brittany also feels more fulfilled because she can connect with these people in a satisfying way. She says, "I don't go around waiting for people to be the perfect friend. I put a lot more of my attention on being there for them." In addition, Brittany comments, "I have figured out how to say pretty clearly to someone, 'All I want is for you to listen to me for five minutes while I cry about this.' If I can set it up like that, as opposed to waiting for someone to give me permission to do it, it works really well." These resources help her deal with her feelings and prevent them from ruling her life. While she felt a deep sense of grief about her second abortion, that sadness dissipated more quickly.

Although Brittany had a larger community to help her deal with her feelings about her second abortion, Dean was not in her life to offer support. The second abortion decision had created a great deal of tension between them, showing them places where they had to "struggle to feel connected." The second abortion prompted them to start talking about these problems. They eventually sorted through issues that had accumulated over the last few years and decided to give their relationship another try.

Brittany's story illustrates some of the reasons two abortions might be different for the same person. Because she grew between her abortions and had better support, she had more resources to help her meet her emotional needs the second time. Since her relationship with Dean was more conflictual the second time, she also had more obstacles to overcome. As circumstances in our lives change, so will our experiences of abortion. We cannot assume that a later abortion will be like an earlier one.

Peggy: More Love and Less Anesthesia the Second Time

Peggy's story illustrates how two abortions can differ greatly, even if little time separates them. She is a 26-year-old African American who had an abortion six months ago, and another just six weeks back. These two abortions were like night and day for her.

With the first, she was certain that she did not want to give birth. She had conceived with Tyrone, her 6-year-old daughter's father. A gang member who had neglected Peggy during her full-term pregnancy, Tyrone had only come back into her life as a way to escape his own troubles. Peggy says that when she conceived with him six months ago, "I no longer wanted him in my life. I knew that I couldn't have another child at the time. So, it was a really simple choice." During that pregnancy, Peggy says she treated her body "like I knew I wasn't going to keep the baby." That abortion occurred at six weeks, and she notes, "I wasn't even really feeling like I was pregnant."

Peggy had that abortion under general anesthesia. She comments that from "the moment I was knocked out to the moment I woke up, I had no idea what happened. It was easier in that sense." Noting, "It was like nothing happened to me," she adds, "It was like a doctor visit. No emotion." If anything, she felt relief; "I was glad I did it," Peggy says.

Six months later, Tyrone was out of her life and Peggy had fallen in love with Charles. When Peggy discovered that she and Charles had conceived, she wanted to marry him and have his child.

Because she had such strong feelings for him, she says, "I wanted another child. I felt emotionally ready." Having a child with Charles seemed wonderful to her, whereas the same situation with Tyrone had seemed impossible and completely undesirable six months before. Charles, however, did not think having a child was such a great idea. He already had two children and two other women in his life. Plus, he had been laid off and had become an escort, or a male prostitute, to make money. He strongly urged Peggy to have an abortion.

Peggy consented, believing he would leave her if she carried to term. She explains, "I wasn't thinking about my needs and myself. I was thinking about him. Worrying about losing him or keeping him. Do what will make him happy." She carried the pregnancy until the eighth week. During that pregnancy, she treated her body well and says, "I was more conscious of what I was putting in, still knowing that I was going to have an abortion." Because she loved Charles so much, she cherished her pregnancy and felt connected to the fetus. The man and the pregnancy were connected together in her positive feelings.

The second abortion occurred under a local anesthetic, and was quite painful physically. Being awake, Peggy had to cope with clinicians, whom she felt treated her insensitively. The procedure lasted two days; she had to go home with a dilator in her cervix and return the next day for the actual abortion. This set-up required Peggy to be conscious of what she was doing for hours and caused her to wrestle with feelings about ending the pregnancy. She refers to that abortion as traumatic, because of its physical and emotional challenges.

Making it more traumatic, Charles dumped her right after the abortion without even telling Peggy why. Because she was abandoned and because she had so many positive feelings about that pregnancy, Peggy has been in great emotional pain since her abortion. She believes that ending the pregnancy was a mistake. The issue is not simply that she wants to have a child, because she still feels good about the first abortion decision, but that the second pregnancy situation appealed to her more. She wants to retrieve the happiness that came with that pregnancy. Peggy does not want Charles back. She cannot respect a man who would become an escort. Plus, she says, "I hate the fact that he didn't help me keep my baby." In time, she may feel better about the second abortion. Currently, however, the two abortions occupy very different places in her heart.

Iris: "By the Time I Faced My Third Abortion, I Had Really Mixed Feelings"

Iris also found later abortions more difficult. She is a 32-year-old African American who had abortions at ages 18, 19, and 20. Her first abortion was fairly straightforward. She says, "I did what I thought was the right thing at the time. I was a second-year college student with no means or experience to care for a child. The thought of disappointing my family was too much to bear. I felt that I was being responsible for doing something irresponsible."

In the next year, her grandmother found out about Iris's abortion. Iris explains, "It had a devastating effect on my grandmother, who literally could not speak about it to me. I had hurt her so much without realizing it." Iris soon learned why. When she was five, her mother died. For thirteen years, nobody told Iris the reason, or talked about it among themselves. Now, she discovered that when her mother was 23 years old, unmarried, and pregnant for the second time, she had an illegal abortion. The next day, she did not report to work. Iris's grandmother found her unconscious. She died of an infection from the abortion. This death devastated the family and shamed them into silence all those years.

When Iris became pregnant at age 19 after a cervical cap failure, she was in a quandary. She explains, "I was now facing the truth about my mother's death. I wasn't sure what to do." Because of what she had learned about her mom, Iris associated abortion with danger. She comments, "It was hard to decide to have another one, knowing that you could die." Of course, Iris's mother probably died because her illegal abortion was not sanitary and because she could not seek help for her infection, as that would have revealed her secret. Today's legal abortions pose very little medical danger. Still, Iris's fears are understandable, given her emotional tumult. Iris also worried that multiple abortions would damage her chance to have a baby later. There is no immediate cause for alarm about this. Some doctors believe that we are at risk only if we have fifteen or so abortions. Iris ultimately decided that giving birth wasn't realistic at that time. She says, "I braved the fears I had and made the decision to have a second abortion."

A year later, Iris conceived again after her cervical cap failed a second time. This decision was the hardest. Iris comments, "By the time I had to face my third abortion, I had really mixed feelings. I kept getting pregnant and was beginning to think maybe I should just have the baby. I had the support of my boyfriend, but we both knew we may not have had the support of our parents. Up until the day of the abortion, I was trying to make a decision. I really wanted to keep the baby, but the timing was all wrong. I hadn't finished school; my boyfriend wasn't finished either. It was just confusion." Iris had moral qualms about abortion by then. She says, "I felt I was destroying a life, but it was a life I couldn't support." She very much wanted to discuss the decision with her grandmother. Iris explains, "I needed a woman to talk to about what I was going through." Secrecy only added to her stress, but she did not tell her grandmother for fear of hurting her again.

Iris finally decided to have an abortion and headed for the clinic. There, she changed her mind again, right before the procedure. She had some last-minute counseling. Iris recalls, "The decision for me seemed to be the hardest thing in the world. Back and forth we went over the possibilities. Ultimately, I decided to go ahead. Halfway through the procedure, I wanted them to stop. Stop and save my baby. The pain was too much to bear. Not only the pain, but hearing the machine at work and watching the look on my boyfriend's face while the doctors were at work. I vowed I would never do anything like that again. If I got pregnant again, that was it. I was having the baby."

Fortunately, Iris has never had an unplanned pregnancy since that time; she went on the pill after her third abortion. She says the abortions made her wait until she was financially secure and married to the right man before having a child. At 29, when she had attained those goals, she had a baby. Iris comments, "I'm glad I waited, because even now that I am financially able, it is really hard to raise a child. It would have been too hard for me when I was younger." Iris adds, "I am comfortable with the decisions I made because when I look in the mirror, I see a college-educated, professional mother and a good provider." She acknowledges having "guilty feelings about terminating a life" and thinks about how old her children would be now, but also keeps in mind where she would be today with her "schooling, career, and life in general" if she had given birth.

Besides occasional guilt, the only thing Iris has struggled with is the idea of herself as someone who has had three unplanned pregnancies. She says, "I consider myself a smart and bright person who would know what to do not to get pregnant." Iris believes that if her grandmother had told her what happened to her mother earlier, she would have paid more attention to preventing unplanned pregnancies. Instead, Iris gained knowledge through her experiences. From her first three pregnancies and abortions, Iris learned the truth about her mother's death, the importance of preventing unwanted conceptions by using birth control, and the need to improve her life before having children.

Wanda: "I Didn't Feel Like I'd Gone in with My Eyes Closed"

Unlike Iris, 23-year-old Wanda found her later abortion easier than her earlier one. Wanda, who is white and who had abortions at ages 19 and 22, went into the second experience determined to get right what she felt she had done wrong before.

When she found herself pregnant the first time, she told herself matter-of-factly, "I can't have this child. I'm nineteen years old. I'll have an abortion." She comments, "I didn't really think about it, unfortunately." She had no positive feelings about the pregnancy, thinking only, "What a drag." Wanda delayed having the abortion until the fifteenth week. The second-trimester procedure, which occurred in a cold, unsupportive clinic, was expensive and physically taxing. It lasted two days and caused Wanda to have contractions the first night, which was frightening and painful. She had no support; her brother felt awkward about looking in on her and her boyfriend abandoned her. Wanda was a physical wreck after fifteen weeks of pregnancy. She was also stunned at how guilty, aggrieved, lonely, and angry she felt. She spent a lot of time by herself crying. Her pain didn't stop there. Wanda says the abortion kept "rearing its head." She recalls, "Every six months I'd get really upset. About nothing. I don't even know what would set it off."

Wanda conceived again at age 22 when her birth control pills failed. She decided to have another abortion and said to herself, "Now I know what I'm doing. I'm going to think more." Wanda did more than just reflect on her feelings. She knew she had a week to spend with this pregnancy. She begins to cry as she recalls saying to the fetus, "Okay, you little person-thing. You can't stay here. And I'm really sorry that you can't. But it's not the right time for you. So for the next five or six days, we're going to hang out together. But that's going to be it." Wanda remembers asking the fetus, "What do you want to do? For these five days, I'm your mommy. Whatever you say goes."

Wanda kept up with this pledge every day of the pregnancy. Each night as she went to bed, she would remind the fetus how many days they still had. Wanda says, "I spent a lot of time lying in bed with my hands on my stomach going, 'This is okay,'" perhaps comforting both the fetus and herself. She didn't stop there in her mission to be mommy-for-a-week. She went to the park and took herself out to eat. Wanda wasn't going to deny the fetus anything. Her attitude was, "Chocolate? Cool! Chocolate coming up! And you want turkey for dinner?" Because she tried to meet the fetus's needs, she says, "I felt a lot better about it." Wanda says this action helped her "feel like I made my peace with it."

Wanda believes the fetus was much too young to be asking her for those things. She comments that it's not like "it had a personality or anything. And not that it could even think." She is unsure about when life actually begins, but still feels that the fetus "knew something was up." Wanda comments, "I didn't want to surprise it." She wanted to say to the fetus, "I'm just telling you what's going on. This is what's going to happen."

Because Wanda tried to fix the painful parts of her first abortion experience, she had a much easier time after the second abortion. She says she did have some pain, "but not as much. I didn't feel as bad. I didn't feel like I'd gone in with my eyes closed." With the second abortion, she says, "I had really thought it out."

A few other things also made her second experience better. It occurred at six weeks, so it was much easier physically, and she felt less guilty. Although Wanda lived for so much less time with the second pregnancy, she appreciated it more and felt "like a creator."

She found pregnancy incredible and now says, "I can't wait to have kids. I'm chomping at the bit. I can't wait to be five hundred pounds pregnant!"

She had a different boyfriend the second time. They had been together for several years. Although he didn't always understand how she felt about her abortion, he tried to be as supportive as he could throughout the experience.

The second procedure occurred in her gynecologist's office. Insurance covered the whole cost and the doctor was kind. Wanda explains, "He was very considerate. Someone not treating me like a complete animal is really, really important." Wanda says of her second abortion, "If a woman has to go through that, I would say that that was probably one of the best-case scenarios for actually having the procedure. Things couldn't have been done any better. I don't have anything to say but to thank the people who helped me."

Ultimately, Wanda's whole experience was easier the second time, during the pregnancy and abortion and after the procedure. Her knowledge of what she would face made all the difference. The operation was not a mystery, nor were her feelings. Armed with experience, she could prepare herself and meet her emotional needs much better.

Patricia: Resolving Childbearing Issues

Forty-three-year-old Patricia, who is white, had two boys in her twenties. Then, when she was 30, her IUD failed and Patricia became pregnant again. She didn't know what to do. Although her family was large enough, she still wanted a daughter. Even if she ended up with another boy, she thought that a new baby would bring her happiness. She had felt "unbelievable emotions in having a baby" twice before and had trouble thinking about "giving up that experience that I had enjoyed so much." Ultimately, though, she felt uncomfortable carrying to term a pregnancy begun with an IUD; she worried that the IUD could have damaged the fetus. "It just seemed too risky," Patricia says. Actually, it would not have been risky. If a pregnancy is to be carried to term, the IUD should be removed, because it can cause infections that could kill the woman. Once the IUD has been taken out, there is no risk of birth defects. Still, it is easy to see how Patricia could feel uneasy. She ended that pregnancy and had a difficult recovery period emotionally. She expected to feel sad, but did not anticipate how strong and intense those feelings would be.

When her diaphragm failed six years later, she thought she would have the same sort of difficulties, both before and after her abortion, but her second experience was much better. She had had a series of X rays before realizing she was pregnant, so it was easier to make a decision, knowing that there was a high likelihood that she damaged the fetus. At 36, Patricia had also come a long way in her feelings about childbearing. In the period between the two abortions, she had resolved not to have another child and says, "I was able to lay to rest the desire for a daughter, too." She derives "a lot of pleasure out of having nonsexist sons," and did not feel that she needed a daughter to make her life complete. Because she felt so much clearer about these issues, she comments, "I had much less ambivalence about not having the child." She didn't feel as sad after this second abortion. In fact, she felt a great sense of relief.

ACCEPTING MULTIPLE ABORTIONS INTO OUR LIVES

Patricia has explained why her decision making was easier the second time. The reasons she felt less sadness or ambivalence with the later abortion are clear. Simply focusing on the first abortion versus the second abortion overlooks an important issue, though: How does Patricia feel about being someone who has had more than one abortion?

Patricia has not found it difficult to accept multiple abortions into her sense of self, because she keeps clear about how she conceived through method failures. She felt quite troubled that her IUD let her down because she trusted it and felt protected. As for the second failure, she says, "I know lots of people have gotten pregnant with diaphragms. They have always seemed riskier to me." In fact, she can't believe she didn't conceive sooner with the diaphragm, given its high failure rate and her high level of fertility.

It is striking that Patricia used the diaphragm at all, knowing that it was risky. Apparently, she could tolerate the thought that she was in danger of another unwanted pregnancy. To her, a second abortion wouldn't be the worst thing in the world. In fact, Patricia framed abortion in an accepting way before she ever faced the issue personally. When she was in college in the 1960s, she knew of several people who had had abortions. This was during the illegal era, but Patricia attended college near New York City, where one could obtain a legal abortion. She notes, "In my closest group of friends, there was one who'd had an abortion. It was not a common experience, but it was something they were very supportive and knowledgeable about." She and her friends seem to have discussed the issue rather openly. Because of this background, when Patricia did have her first abortion, she says, "I didn't feel out of the mainstream at all."

Patricia's mother had two illegal abortions, which made abortion seem even less marginalized in Patricia's eyes. In addition, Patricia discovered how fertile she was when she conceived her two boys very quickly. She figured, "If I'm that fertile, I'm not sure I'm always going to be able to have control" over pregnancy. She knew she might be a candidate for abortion someday. In fact, when *Roe* v. *Wade* passed, she felt relieved both for other women and for herself, because she would never have to face what her mother did with illegal abortions. In addition to these personal experiences with abortion, Patricia worked in women's health care for a while and saw many women involuntarily conceive. Because she views abortion as a common and necessary event that many women experience, she found it painless to accept that she had one, and then two, abortions.

Not every woman feels this way. Our society attaches a stigma to abortion and therefore to those of us who have abortions. The more we have, the more we may feel that we have stepped outside the bounds of acceptability. People might judge us harshly for having several abortions. For this reason, if abortion comes into our life a few times, we may become increasingly silent about these experiences.

This has been the case for 44-year-old Daphne, who has had three abortions. One occurred in her twenties. She cannot remember when the other two happened—somewhere in her thirties or forties. On one level, Daphne is quite forthcoming about her abortions. She says, "I told all my friends. I had no problem with it. It wasn't something that I was ashamed of," and adds, "I'm open about things like that. I really find it very hard to cover up the lies. It's just so much easier to be straight."

On the other hand, Daphne does not like to tell many people about the number of abortions she has had. She comments, "If my mother found out it was three, I'd be just terrified." Daphne worries that even though two of the three pregnancies resulted from IUD failures, people might judge her for the number. They might say, "Come on, don't you learn quick?" or "What is going on, girl, that you can't be more together than that?" Astutely, she notes, "I think I would react the same way." Daphne would be embarrassed for someone to think she hadn't protected herself well and says that rather than telling them how many abortions she has had, she would just say, "I've had experience with abortion." If she ever told a stranger the number, she "would have to clarify right away. Some people might not know IUDs or how they work, but it just sounds flaky." Daphne emphasizes, "I'm not ashamed of the abortions. That was something that had to be done." She does, however, feel embarrassed about "not being in control enough to prevent them." Like Patricia, Daphne frames her experiences as being more about unwanted conceptions than about ended pregnancies.

Thirty-two-year-old Oriana focuses more on how many times she has terminated pregnancies. She has had abortions at ages 18, 19, 25, and 30. Oriana is currently carrying a fifth unplanned pregnancy to term, but does not group that pregnancy with the others; she looks at the outcome more than at the fact of unplanned pregnancy. As for those four earlier outcomes, Oriana says, "I feel very strange about the number. I used to feel very uncomfortable talking about it." She confronts this feeling most often in the medical setting, where she occasionally must write down her reproductive history. Oriana comments, "I used to feel really humiliated whenever I went in for a gynecological exam. It got to the point where I couldn't remember the numbers. I'd write them down and then it'd be like three? It can't be four. How can I put down four abortions?" She adds, "I felt really embarrassed and humiliated that someone of my background and upbringing could have that kind of a history. And that I was really an irresponsible freak for having gone through four of them." She feels as if there are stereotypes about the people who have several abortions and that she does not fit that image at all.

Oriana says, "I just go against all the statistics, because I'm an educated, middle-class woman who knows better and who's used the forms of birth control." Trying to integrate her four abortions into her sense of self, she says, "The image is one of irresponsibility and it's something that I'm still dealing with."

HOW IT FEELS TO KEEP HAVING ABORTIONS

Oriana's discomfort with the number of abortions is the only similarity between her four experiences. Her first two sparked very different feelings from her last two, partly because her life had changed so much between the two sets of pregnancies. If the events surrounding our abortions vary, we might see the experiences as separate occurrences. They may seem to be about distinct times in our lives, raising new concerns and reflecting different levels of maturity. We might have finished with one when another enters our lives.

If, however, our feelings are unresolved, a later abortion can trigger feelings about an earlier one, making the abortions feel interlinked. They may seem to blur together as pieces in an ongoing, exhausting event. This was the case for Toni. She is a 23-year-old African American who had three unplanned pregnancies within sixteen months, with the last one ending four months ago. When she conceived just a few months after the second abortion, Toni remembers thinking, "I can't believe this. I was just in this boat three months ago. And now I'm here again." Toni had not finished sorting out her feelings from one experience when the next pregnancy landed in her life.

Toni felt a range of emotions with all of her abortions. Together, the three abortions made some feelings more intense than they would have been with just one abortion. Each decision has been increasingly difficult to make, prompting more and more guilt. The guilt used to appear as her father's voice in her head, lambasting her for conceiving three times and having abortions. Now her own self-criticism has taken over. She tells herself, "Toni, how could you do this? Toni, look what you're doing."

As Toni surveys the past few years, she feels quite frustrated with the birth control failures that allowed her to conceive. The third time, especially, Toni felt devastated that the birth control let her down. She says, "I was really putting my trust into the fact that this wouldn't happen to me again. Then it happened. And I really felt like I had no control over my life." She now distrusts contraception and worries about pregnancy.

Just as control may seem important after one abortion, it may be essential after several. Toni says, "I've regimented everything. I go to school, go to work, go to the gym three times a week." She does not feel satisfied with having such a regulated life.

The one good thing about these painful experiences is that each has brought Toni closer to her boyfriend. Because she can tell him her feelings, the abortions have "sealed the bond" between them and provided "another building block" of trust. Indeed, Toni's boyfriend is the only one who understands that her emotions are so intense because she has experienced three abortions in a very short period.

WHY WE MIGHT HAVE MULTIPLE ABORTIONS

On an annual basis, doctors perform over 645,000 abortions on women who have had at least one previous abortion. More than 1 percent of women of childbearing age have a second, third, or even sixth abortion each year. One percent may not seem like a lot, but that is roughly the portion of our population that is Jewish. When one reflects on how many Jews one knows, that number may indeed seem large. Why do so many of us have unplanned pregnancies and abortions? We might have repeated birth control failures. Indeed, as was true for Iris, Wanda, Patricia, Daphne, and Toni, contraceptive failures are so common that we may have several abortions during our reproductive years.

There can also be psychological reasons behind multiple unwanted pregnancies and abortions. Some of us try to conceive in order to test our fertility. We may be concerned that a previous abortion has damaged our reproductive abilities. This damage is unlikely; while some women who end pregnancies do suffer from infertility later in life, there is no proof that abortion causes this problem. There could only be a direct connection if an infection develops after an abortion, and symptoms of such an infection are usually apparent right away.

Those of us who feel unhappy about having had an abortion may want to become pregnant again to fix the situation. This impulse may come from denial, an attempt to make it seem as if the abortion never happened. It can result from guilt; we might want a child as a way to right a "wrong" event. Grief can also spark this desire; if we feel a painful void after ending our pregnancy, we may long to become pregnant again so that we can have a child to love and hold. This desire may hit us particularly hard on the pregnancy's projected due date or on the abortion's anniversary.

We may also have several unplanned pregnancies and abortions if we have never taken control of our reproduction. This will be especially true if we suffered sexual abuse in childhood. Just as we were unable to protect ourselves from a molester in our past, we might continue to feel defenseless during sex as an adult. Chapter 11 discusses these and other psychological causes of pregnancy in more depth.

Although any of these psychological responses to an earlier abortion might motivate us to conceive again, we might have another abortion for the same reasons we had the first one. Perhaps we have little money. Maybe the man in our lives doesn't want a child. We might have life plans that do not fit with childbearing. After ending the pregnancy, we may again wish to replace it. A cycle of pregnancy and abortion can develop.

We may need to go through more than one pregnancy and abortion before we understand why we have conceived. Each pregnancy and abortion experience presents an opportunity to look at our feelings and motivations. After a few such experiences, something may click into place for us and make us understand.

PART IV: WHEN RELATIONSHIPS SHIFT

Chapter 13

Breaking Through Silence

Thirty-four-year-old Karen, a Caucasian, has had abortions at age 22, age 28, and just three months ago. With each experience, she has found great solace in discussing her feelings. Karen says, "Talking about it always helps me to feel better. Sometimes it also causes me to cry, which serves to release a lot of the pent-up sadness." Unfortunately, there are few people with whom Karen can speak about her abortions. Her husband is her main confidant. Karen says, "He's always there to listen and to agree with me on the powerfulness of the experience. He also has his own sadness about it. The last abortion was one more tough time to go through together, which reinforces the relationship."

If this sort of sharing brings more intimacy to a relationship and gives Karen the catharsis she needs, wouldn't it be wonderful if she could speak so openly about her abortions with all the people she loves? Karen would like to be able to discuss them, because she has needed support, especially with her most recent experience. She explains, "I felt guilty for getting pregnant, and very alone. I am new to the area and have no local friends. I've never felt I could tell my family about my abortions." Lacking support from those who know her, she decided to speak with a clinic counselor about her birth control failure and her decision. This proved successful. Karen says, "I didn't really know what kind of support I needed, but I got it. It was so nice to be told it wasn't my fault. It happens to a lot of women." This sounds great in theory, but Karen would feel much more reassured if she knew others who had ended pregnancies. She muses, "I sometimes wonder how many other women out there have been through it. I wish I could know that about women I deal with, because then I would know if it's safe to talk about."

Besides not knowing who else has had an abortion, Karen finds that several other obstacles prevent her from discussing her feelings. First, her emotional state has made it difficult to be social. She comments, "It was hard to deal with people when I felt sad and depressed, yet could not share what I was going through. During the pregnancy and soon after the abortion, it was hard for me to leave the house and face the world." Karen refers to the emotional withdrawal that can accompany depression. If sadness depletes our energy and makes us want to retreat from the challenges of socializing, we may isolate ourselves. While this withdrawal may be temporary, it can occur when we most need others' care.

Karen cites another reason for remaining silent about her abortions. She says, "I don't want to risk the judgment and possible disapproval of other people, so it is easier to not tell." Although she fears criticism, Karen emphasizes that she does not remain silent about her abortion because she feels she has done something wrong. She says, "I feel like I have to hide the fact that I had an abortion in order to protect myself from possible scorn, yet I am not ashamed of it, so it seems unfair that I have to hide it."

Even though some might not judge her, she thinks people will not understand her feelings unless they have had an abortion themselves. She feels set apart from those who have not had this experience. In many ways, we have a distinct frame of reference after an abortion. One 23 year old who has had two abortions likens this difference to losing a parent and realizing that others cannot guess what this feels like. She says of abortion, "You won't understand it till you're there. It gives you a different perspective on childbirth, on everything having to do with children. I don't think I'm superior because I've been through it, or lower because I have." She simply feels different.

It is one thing to feel a gap when others lack our frame of reference and therefore cannot understand our experience. An additional problem arises when even we cannot grasp the rationale behind our emotions. For instance, Karen cannot make sense of her grief. She says, "I hated being pregnant. I knew I did not want to have a baby. So why should I feel sad after the abortion?" Karen's abortion experiences seem so far removed from daily life that she cannot communicate her feelings to other people. She comments, "I don't understand the emotions, so I can't very well explain them." Those emotions are from another realm. To describe them would be like returning from war and trying to convey the experience to people who have been sitting in their living rooms, watching the action on television. Even the perfect listener may have trouble grasping such feelings, and when we discuss personal experiences of abortion, we rarely have the perfect listener.

Political beliefs may prevent someone from listening to our feelings in an open-minded way. Ideologies demand that things be black-and-white. On either side of the abortion debate, people have invested so much energy in their beliefs that they may not want to hear anything that opposes those views. Karen has found this to be true on the pro-choice side. She says of her depression and confusion, "I wish it were okay to talk of such feelings in the feminist circles. It seems that for political reasons we cannot." Some abortion advocates might interpret Karen's feelings as a threat to the movement or as a sign of defection, when in reality, Karen's support has not wavered at all. On the pro-life side, people may be unwilling to hear her describe how it felt to have an abortion. They may be appalled that she would do such a thing, and may think that she deserves to feel badly. Even if we have no negative feelings after an abortion, we may find it difficult to speak openly about our experiences. Some people do not want to hear that we are free of pain; that could threaten what they believe to be true of an abortion experience.

No matter how we feel afterward, we may find the subject extremely difficult to broach. There is a stigma placed on abortion in this society. We can discuss the political, legal, and ethical aspects of abortion, but it is not acceptable in many circles to speak about it on a personal level. Often, people would rather deal with the topic in an abstract way, as if only hypothetical women have abortions, not the women they know. If we bring up our abortions, a tension may occur, and some listeners might change the topic. Other listeners may make an authoritative statement about abortion that leaves us no room to say how we feel. Alternatively, they may make an assumption about how we have felt.

Twenty-seven-year-old Willa has concealed her two abortions when people around her have raised the topic. She comments, "If there is a conversation about abortion, you just sit there and pretend you haven't had one, or say things like, 'Gee, I don't know what I would do if I had to have an abortion.'" Willa remains reticent in order to conform to our culture's silence on the topic. She explains, "It is perhaps the most secret of all women's issues. You'll find many more women discussing incest than abortion. You can't really go out anywhere and tell people you've had an abortion without fearing some sort of retaliation from society's values." In Willa's view, the silence about abortion stems not only from people's intolerance of others' choices, but also from a deep-rooted misogyny. She says, "We live in such a female-hating society, and exposing ourselves to talk about abortion is a double-edged sword. But for as long as we don't talk about it, we remain censored, which is what it really means to be a female in a male world."

A Fear of Judgment and a Sense of Privacy

Willa and Karen wish that the reasons they must remain silent would change so that they could receive support. Others of us feel fine about remaining silent and have no desire to break down this wall. For instance, Nora, age 22, has chosen not to tell many people about the abortion she had eight months ago. She is usually outspoken about everything, even to the point of saying things for shock value, but not with this issue. She says, "I'm conscious that I won't tell anyone, because a lot of people think it's bad. They're really grossed out by it." A friend of hers felt that way when he heard Nora's news. She comments, "I just told him I had an abortion and he thought it was disgusting." After that, Nora says she chose not to "tell anyone that my relationship would change with, anyone who would freak out." She has told her mother, but not a sister who also had an abortion. Nora informed a few friends, but not most, including some of her closest pals.

It is not that the abortion has meant nothing to Nora. On the contrary, she has changed many of her views on abortion and feels personally and politically transformed. Why the silence, then? Nora worries that if she tells someone about her pain, it will burden them. She comments, "I don't feel like whining about it." She adds, "I don't like people having to listen to my emotions. I'll be wondering what they're thinking of me, because I'm being so self-centered."

Nora is willing to talk about her abortion with anyone going through one and has done so, but sees no other reason to discuss it.

When she does converse about her abortions, Nora likes to keep her distance. She tells only those who will ask few questions so that she can "answer them and get on with it." It does not appeal to her to be intimate with someone about this topic. The thought of "commiserating" with her sister about their abortions seems "really cheesy" to Nora. For many of us, such sharing would feel wonderful. Nora, though, prefers to be more independent and private.

She is not the only one who feels this way. Randi is a 35 year old who had an abortion ten years ago. She maintains that when you discuss an abortion experience, "You're talking about sexuality. You're talking about something that's very private." For this reason, she would rather keep silent about her abortion. Randi conveys this point by drawing two analogies. First, she says, "I don't discuss my methods of birth control" with other people; to her, it's the same sort of thing. Second, she comments, she is as private about her abortion as about the divorce she had a few years later. Randi explains that she compares the abortion and divorce, "because that was another very large, momentous, intimate, personal thing. I handled the abortion in a similar manner to the way I handled that, in terms of talking to people." The divorce required a bit of explaining, as people noticed she was no longer married or living with her husband. Randi told them only the cursory details, however, and says that, as with her abortion, "It's none of their business. It's not important. It's not going to affect their life. They don't need to know these things."

Randi also remains quiet about her abortion because she worries how others might see her. She explains, "I want people to have this image of me as always in control. Not making mistakes." When Randi and her husband conceived, they used a condom that broke. Even though they took precautions, she blames herself for not using a backup method. She says of the unplanned conception, "I'm not proud of the mistake I made. So I'm not going to tell people that I made a mistake." On top of the way people might view her unplanned pregnancy, Randi worries about how they might judge the pregnancy's outcome. She does not feel ashamed of it, but is "sure" that some would see her as a murderer. As a result, she has told few people about her abortion.

Ricki: Shame and an Order to Keep Quiet

Twenty-year-old Ricki, an African American, has told almost no one about the abortion she had six weeks ago. Much of Ricki's silence comes from her shame about ending her pregnancy. As a Muslim, she believes that abortion is immoral. She had the abortion because her boyfriend, Wayne, who is also a Black Muslim, insisted that a child would interfere with their schooling and career plans. Ricki felt forced into the abortion and never reconciled herself to the decision. Feelings of guilt and shame have plagued her all along, especially at the clinic. Noting, "You don't want nobody to know about it," she explains that she felt ashamed to interact with the clinicians. Ricki says, "They were nice, but I just felt ultimately embarrassed. I didn't want people looking at me and knowing who I was."

Although one wouldn't know it from her silence, Ricki longs to talk about the abortion. She has tried to do this with Wayne, and would like to hear something back from him, but he has been stony. Ricki explains, "I want people to respond to me when I speak. He'll just sit there. He won't say nothing. I'll be talking, talking, talking. I'm talking to myself." She has prodded him, saying, "Are you listening to me? Do you hear what I'm saying? Say something." He refuses. After talking herself "blue in the face," Ricki has become frustrated and has stopped trying to elicit his feelings. She says, "The more I ask him questions, the more he won't tell me. So I just sit back and hope one day he'll tell me."

Ricki figures that it would solve a lot of her problems if she knew how he felt. She says, "I would feel like finally somebody feels the same way. Like, I'm not the only one who's suffering. You feel like you're losing your mind and you shouldn't be tripping, because he's not tripping." Ricki reasons that because they played equal roles in conceiving the pregnancy, they should have the same amount of feeling about the abortion. Since she seems to have so much more emotion than Wayne, she feels like something is wrong with her and feels very alone. She says, "You feel like you're the only one" who has had an abortion, "especially if you can't talk about it."

Wayne not only refuses to discuss his feelings, but has also ordered her to remain silent about the abortion. Ricki has decided to ignore his wishes and to share her feelings in an interview for this book, although she will not tell him this until after the interview. Laughing, she anticipates how he will react to the news: "Oh, he'll be mad! He'll be like, 'I thought you weren't going to tell nobody about this. I hope you didn't say my name.'"

Just because Ricki has come forward with her story does not mean that she feels less ashamed about her abortion. She says, "If I had a choice, I would walk in here with a bag over my head, just so I wouldn't see you. I don't want nobody to see my face." Why has she subjected herself to such embarrassment by coming for an interview? She says she rejoiced at the opportunity to speak, thinking, "Oh, finally, someone wants to hear what I have to say!" Ricki explains, "I wanted to talk about it, but not with someone I knew." According to Ricki, the interview provided the "outlet" she needed. She believes in going through an abortion experience with as much support as possible and advises other women, "Try to have someone there for you who will really talk to you about it." Ricki adds, "I can't see going through it and not talking about it and coming out healthy. I don't think I came out all right, because I didn't talk about the stuff I would like to have."

Marilyn: "I Was Now Speaking a Different Language"

Marilyn also has not spoken about her abortion to her satisfaction, but for very different reasons. She is a 28-year-old white woman who had an abortion eleven months ago. During her pregnancy, all her preconceptions about abortion fell by the wayside. Whereas she had once viewed it as a way to stop being pregnant, she now feels that the experience is about deciding whether or not to have a child. For Marilyn, that decision was agonizing. She spent a few weeks feeling muddled, strung out, and highly emotional. She and her boyfriend planned to marry and have children soon anyway, but there were a few conflicts. The pregnancy brought those problems to the forefront, forcing Marilyn to make several life decisions all at once. Should she and her boyfriend marry? If so, where should they live? He was from Italy; choosing a country would mean that one of them would make several adjustments. Did she want to give up her work and be a full-time mother?

She and her boyfriend spent a lot of time mulling over these questions. They tried to visualize the life that all three of them might have in a few years and invested a great deal of emotion in these fantasies. A very real child began to inhabit their minds. Although they decided not to carry to term and chose to split up, Marilyn and her boyfriend came a long way from thinking of a fetus as it might have been in the first trimester. She now speaks of "the baby" or "the child" at the center of her abortion decision, rather than "the fetus."

Because of her new vocabulary, Marilyn finds it difficult to communicate with most people about her experience. She explains, "I have a tendency to keep silent about the abortion, because what I have to say about the abortion is not understood by a certain kind of politically correct person." For example, her therapist reacted badly when Marilyn used the words "baby" and "child" and expressed ambivalence about her abortion. The therapist said, "Before we go on, I think you should know that I'm very feminist and I'm very pro-abortion." Marilyn responded, "So I'm not?" Still astounded, she laughs, "I have always been a rabid feminist, bordering on man-hating. And that was the first time anybody ever accused me of not being a feminist!" The problem was, as Marilyn puts it, "I was now speaking a different language." Marilyn cannot go back to the way she used to discuss the issue. She comments "I feel like I can't use that vocabulary anymore." Her new language isolates her from anyone who does not share her perspective.

Marilyn has faced "real incomprehension" from people other than the therapist. After she split up with her boyfriend, she began to date someone new. She found him incapable of understanding her feelings. His attitude was, "So, what's the problem? You had an abortion and that's what you do when you get pregnant and you don't want to have the baby." He could not see why she still might be upset some months later, why she might grieve the loss of the child she imagined. In his mind, the abortion was a solution and should have put an end to the problem, not created other problems.

Marilyn cannot make him understand her experience, because she does not fully grasp it herself. She says, "I still can't understand how I feel and why I did it and if I should have done it and I try to avoid thinking that way. It's a feeling of incomprehension and of somehow not having made a free choice, of not having been able to think about it very clearly." So much occurred during that time and little of it felt logical to Marilyn. How can she communicate that experience to others? She does not feel she can. Consequently, she says, "I don't talk about it anymore. I have not actually told that many people."

Brittany: "No One Else Is Going Through What I'm Going Through"

Since her abortions at ages 19 and 20, 22-year-old Brittany, a Caucasian, has found it difficult to speak about these experiences. She agrees with Marilyn's assessment of the atmosphere around abortion, saying, "It's such a charged topic that it's hard for people to sit still and not have an opinion." Because abortion is so loaded, Brittany hesitates to broach the subject. She says, "I don't usually like to bring up things that are controversial. Like, I wouldn't want to talk about someone's religion with them in a way that was offensive, unless I felt like there was already some bond between us." If that bond existed, Brittany says, nobody would feel attacked within the discussion. Because Brittany does not want to risk being pounced on for her abortions, she says, "I don't talk about it very much."

Brittany knows several people who have had abortions, including her mother, but has not had an easy time communicating with them. She comments, "The people that I knew who'd had abortions were pretty shut down about it." Perhaps they have unresolved pain about their abortions and find it difficult to discuss those feelings. Maybe they have grown so accustomed to being silent about their abortions that they cannot open up easily.

Although Brittany has had bad experiences speaking with both those who have and haven't had abortions, she does not feel that her listeners need to have had abortions. Instead, she wants others to approach the topic with more openness. Brittany has heard people talk about abortion "in a surface way," saying, "I could never do that." That rigid approach can "push some buttons" for her, making her take their statements personally. She feels that people ought to think "more creatively about the issue."

Brittany has tried to build bridges with women who have shared her experience. When she went for her second abortion, she saw how many women were in the waiting room and how alone they seemed to feel, herself included. Brittany comments, "I think that it was really hard not being able to talk to other women. It's really hard that we were each" going through the experience "individually." She approached one patient and introduced herself. The other woman said, "This is a really bad time," implying that she wanted to be left alone. When more people filed into the waiting room, Brittany "didn't keep taking the initiative." It wasn't working. She regrets, though, that all the women seemed to be thinking, "No one else is going through what I'm going through."

Brittany feels dissatisfied with this situation. She thinks that we should support each other as we experience abortions, that "there should be a lot more help and a lot more people offering themselves, saying, 'I'm here for you.'" Brittany encourages other women to "Go after people who will be there and who are devoted to listening to you, not to giving you advice." That ideal, of course, may be a far cry from our individual realities. But her idea makes a lot of sense. If we feel isolated during an abortion experience, we do not need to accept this as inevitable. Instead, we can speak to other patients in the abortion facility. We can consider who might listen in an unbiased way to our feelings. At the very least, we can try not to cut ourselves off from support, as the patient at Brittany's clinic did.

IS HAVING AN ABORTION MAINSTREAM?

One 39 year old gives a compelling reason for remaining silent about the abortion she had a year ago. It is hard for her to find the right tone when she shares such a bit of news. This issue arose when she had to excuse herself from work on the day of the procedure. "What do you say to people?" she wonders. "Excuse me, I'm going out for an abortion?" Politically, she feels, "You should be able to say that." She believes in the right to have an abortion; why should she have to skulk around as if she were committing a crime? On a personal level, however, she finds that information too private to divulge. Abortion does not seem to her as if it is entirely in the mainstream. It is somewhat shadowy, dragging behind it the weight of its old illegal status.

She touches on a major reason for the silence, shame, and isolation many of us feel after an abortion. We may see abortion as somehow illicit, taboo, off-limits. It might seem shady to us, lurking on the unmentionable edges of society, much like venereal disease or prostitution. Feeling this way, we might not be inclined to tell people about our experience. We might fear that if others know about our abortion, we will seem unacceptable to them. Even if we remain silent about our experience, we may already feel that our lives have become somewhat tainted because we have had contact with this stigmatized activity. The silence surrounding abortion certainly reinforces this sense that abortion is improper or unfit for polite conversation. When few women feel free to speak openly about their abortions, it seems as though abortion is not an okay experience to have had, and that we are not fully okay if we have had one. As one 42 year old puts it, two decades after her two abortions, "Society treats women who make a sensible choice like pariahs." If we have more than one abortion, we may feel pushed even further to society's margins.

No matter how many abortions we have, the pervasive silence about abortion experiences would make each of us believe that we are the only one ever to have ended a pregnancy. One 23 year old felt this way three years ago during her pregnancy. She recalls, "I felt so lonely and exceptional in my dilemma." As she lay in the recovery room after her abortion, she asked the nurse how many abortions the clinic performed. The answer was 500 a month. Learning that this many people have abortions reassured her that she was not alone. Still, she feels, "Abortion seems to be a closeted experience, an experience with no voice. To me, this gives the antiabortion side more power. If those of us who want to talk are given a forum–look out. We'd be loud."

Beth: "There Was a Certain Shame and Stigma Around It"

Beth, a Caucasian, also feels that silence surrounds the abortion experience. She had an abortion in 1973, when she was 27 and about to be married. She didn't want to give birth because, as she says, "I was supposed to be a bride, not a mother!" Plus, an unwanted child had strained her brother's life and marriage; she vowed that this would not happen to her. Her younger sister helped her locate an abortion clinic. This sister was the only person who knew about the abortion. Beth did not talk about it and says this was how abortion was handled back then. She recalls that abortion was "shrouded in shame and silence," even though she lived in the liberal city of New York and even though abortion had become legal nationally. People felt that "nice girls don't do it." They also thought that if you do have an abortion, you shouldn't "go around broadcasting it." Beth adhered to that social more and remained silent. She explains, "Within my family and setting, there was a certain shame and stigma around it. I felt I didn't have the freedom to tell my parents."

In her thirties, Beth had a miscarriage and two stillbirths. These experiences were so painful that when she accidentally conceived again at forty, she ended the pregnancy. She wanted a child badly, but could not risk more heartbreak. Beth has told few people about her abortions. She comments, "I don't know if others can understand my decisions–they were very complicated for me." Beth adds, "I feel like with the second abortion, a lot of people who went through all those pregnancies with me wouldn't understand. They'd say, 'How could she do that when she wanted a baby so much?'"

Beth laments having gone through an abortion without support from loved ones. She believes that being silent "makes you feel like you've done something wrong, that you're a bad person." Silence and guilt enhance each other.

Beth is now in her forties. In some ways, she doesn't feel it is any easier today for women to speak about their abortions. She has taken many Women's Studies courses and has learned that silence permeates women's lives, not just in the realm of abortion. Indeed, women have been silenced throughout history. Their concerns have been devalued as irrational or unimportant. For a long time, women did not realize that their dissatisfactions and experiences were similar. That is where some of us still are with abortion–suffering in silence.

Feeling That the Stigma Ended with Legalization

If, like Beth, we came of age before abortion was legal, we may have felt a stigma around it at that time. Unlike Beth, we may have thought it disappeared after *Roe* v. *Wade* passed. That was the case for Olivia, a 46-year-old African American who had an abortion in California in 1970. It was legal in that state then, but because abortion was illegal nationally, she sensed a large taboo on the subject. Olivia says, "I remember a sense of doing something that society didn't approve of and feeling guilty about that. There seemed to be whispers and shadows." She recalls feeling ashamed and "a little dirty," after her abortion. Olivia attributes these feelings to the "taboos of society." She explains, "It was not something that you talked about at work. Or something that you told your family about. It seemed that people always whispered when they said the 'A' word."

Then, when abortion became legal, the experience seemed much more legitimate to Olivia. Legalization pulled abortion out of the shadows and made it discussable, at least in a general way. Olivia felt better about her abortion and opened up about it. She says, "In the long run, I probably told everybody. It's not something that I keep secret and I think that that is a direct result of the reproductive rights movement. I don't think it's a medal of honor, but it certainly is okay to have had an abortion at some time." It seemed so "okay" to Olivia that she became a pro-choice activist a few years later.

Sensing Little Stigma

If we live in a liberal area and if our friends or relatives have had abortions, we may see abortion as the norm. While we may not tell everyone about our experiences, we might feel free to discuss them with intimates. Most of the women in our lives may have had abortions. In certain circles, abortion is a fact of life, not an aberration. A 25 year old who had an abortion seven years ago feels this way. She says, "I've been surprised to find out just how many people I know have had abortions. That makes me feel less of an anomaly. I laughed the other day when a friend said she hadn't had an abortion–I thought she was the anomaly!"

Forty-two-year-old Heidi, a Caucasian, has always seen abortion as fairly mainstream. She came of age when abortion was legal in New York, but not in the whole country. When she attended high school in Massachusetts, she and her peers knew they could go to New York for an abortion, and some of them did. Heidi shrugs,

"That was the next state, so it wasn't that big a deal." She adds, "I went to college in New York, so that seemed like not a big problem." Access was the main issue that arose for her crowd with regard to abortion. After college, Heidi lived on a commune. It was the 1970s, and she says, "It was really a different time. People were just jumping into bed with someone that they'd met two seconds ago and would never see again. And if you got pregnant, you just took care of it and went on. So within the context of the community that I was in, it was absolutely no big deal. It was just like having your teeth cleaned." When Heidi became pregnant at 24 and had an abortion, she had very little trouble emotionally. It helped that abortion wasn't nearly as hot a topic back then. She recalls, "Unlike now, there wasn't this huge public debate about it. There were no protesters, there were no bombings of clinics. Plenty of doctors just did it in their offices." Although times have changed, Heidi still feels in the mainstream in terms of her abortion and mentions it whenever it is appropriate. Many of her friends have had abortions, but some have not. That does not seem to be the issue so much as that when Heidi had an abortion, it was quite acceptable.

PUNCTURING THE SILENCE

Whatever level of stigma each of us feels in terms of our abortions, it seems undeniable that we cannot speak of it as freely as other topics. Many of us cannot speak of our abortions at all. While that silence might be fine for some, it creates problems for others. There can be a sense of isolation. Some of us carry around a weighty shame about the unmentioned and seemingly unmentionable. We might feel that others do not fully know us, that this hidden part of ourselves is vital and needs to be revealed. We may even believe, as gay rights activists do, that silence equals death, that remaining quiet about a central part of one's identity or a transformative event in one's life is akin to not being fully alive.

At some point after an abortion, we may try to break through this restricting silence. We might talk about our abortions with the people in our lives so that they can know us better. We may try to obtain their support for our decision. Some of us speak out in an attempt to shake off shame and find out if others have been through the same thing. We may speak to strangers or to those who think they know us best. Both are ways of "coming out," of reconciling our private and public selves.

Paige has had this experience recently. She is a 22-year-old Palestinian American who had an abortion four years ago. During her pregnancy, she shared her news with her boyfriend and a few friends. They all supported her decision, but not to the degree Paige needed. Her family did not know about her plight. They are Orthodox Christian and regard both premarital sex and abortion as sins; she could not share her news with most of them. Paige did tell a cousin who was also a co-worker. Paige recalls, "She listened, but I felt a distance between her and me." Overall, Paige says, "I felt totally alone with my decision." The whole experience, she notes, "triggered feelings of loss for myself. A sense of loneliness in my life."

Eventually, she shared the experience with her mom and brother. Paige recalls, "My mother could not believe that I had gone through it by myself and felt very sad for me. My brother said he was sorry, but seemed very uncomfortable with the whole topic." Telling her family members seems to have helped somewhat, but not greatly.

Then, a few months ago, Paige attended a seminar on personal growth. There, she told 150 people about her abortion. Paige recalls, "I felt very relieved after I shared this. It was like I came out of hiding. Many women came up to me and told me that they had had the same experience and the same feelings. Many women go through it and never talk about it, like it never happened. This was very reassuring for me to hear. It also felt good to feel safe enough to share it with such a large group of people. It was like a huge burden was lifted off my shoulders." Paige finally felt surrounded by people who understood her feelings and who wanted to listen to her experience. Having so many people offer support must have felt confirming, giving Paige the sense that others approve of her feelings and decision. She says that "sharing it with people outside of the shame and guilt of the whole thing" helped her feel better about herself.

Paige has "done a lot of work" on her feelings about her abortion. Her speech at the seminar proves how far she has come, and helped her feel even more resolved. Paige could not have predicted this transformation, just as many of us cannot anticipate that pain about an abortion can give way to peaceful acceptance. Abigail, who is white and 24, had a similar experience, never imagining the day she would speak out about her abortion.

Abigail: "I Thought I Would Want to Keep Silent Forever"

When Abigail conceived at age 19, she told two friends and her boyfriend, all of whom supported her through an abortion. This support helped her accept the abortion somewhat. When she became pregnant again at 20, however, she had no such bedrock. She spoke to her new boyfriend, mother, and the two friends who had been helpful before. In terms of support, Abigail says, "I feel I only got half of what I wanted." Her boyfriend was not terribly enthusiastic about her having an abortion, which was tough for her. The whole decision was excruciating. Abigail knew no one who had had two abortions, and did not want that to be part of her identity. She questioned the morality of a second abortion. Immobilized by indecision, Abigail did not end the pregnancy until the sixteenth week.

After both abortions, Abigail retreated into silence. She notes, "Every time I heard discussions about abortion, I wanted to jump in and give my two cents," but she dared to do nothing of the sort. She explains, "I feared judgment and accusations of 'baby killer.'" Feeling "bound up in shame and fear of being found out," she wondered what would happen if others discovered her secrets. This intense concern "gnawed" at her. After the second abortion, Abigail had especially low self-esteem, because she blamed herself for conceiving again and ending another pregnancy; her feelings of worthlessness account for her paranoia, in her opinion. Silence and shame reinforced each other.

Over time, though, all of this has changed for Abigail. She comments, "My self-esteem increased when I realized that the whole world was not out to get me, but that I was out to get me, and I was my own judgment and support in the long run." Abigail started listening to other people's abortion experiences and pro-choice convictions. She began to see that "life moves on" and that no one intended to hurt her. When some people did find out about her abortion and "mildly confronted" her, Abigail discovered that she could maintain herself and handle other people's knowledge of her abortions just fine.

Now, Abigail occasionally discusses her abortions. She comments, "I didn't expect to be as willing to speak about my experiences. I thought I would want to keep silent forever." The topic arises when she explains to new partners why contraception is so important to her. She has tried to redress people's ignorance about abortion and defends abortion politically and socially. Abigail is willing to talk about her abortion, if asked. She notes that "telling even an edited version of my story" helps her understand herself better.

Chapter 14

Family: When We Confront Our Biggest Fans and Harshest Judges

As Mindy, who is white and 22, grew up, her mother ingrained a message in her: "You're not having a baby as a teenager." She said that if Mindy ever conceived, she would insist that Mindy have a abortion. When Mindy's mom, Beryl, discovered that her daughter was regularly having sex, she reiterated her point, saying, "If you ever get pregnant, I'm dragging you, whether you like it or not, to have an abortion done."

Some women might feel relieved to know that their mothers are pro-choice. Mindy did feel a little bit of that. She comments, "I knew that I wouldn't have to worry about ridicule from them" if she were pregnant and her parents ever found out. At the same time, she felt angry at her mom's warnings and thought, "Screw you, Mom." More conservative about abortion than her mother, Mindy is critical that her mom ended two pregnancies. Beryl had those abortions because she was unhappily married to an unfaithful husband. When she conceived a couple of times, she felt it necessary to end the pregnancies, so as not to compound the family misery. Eventually, she divorced, remarried, and had Mindy. Beryl made it her mission not to see her daughter repeat any of her mistakes.

When Mindy conceived at age 21 and had an abortion, she did not share this with Beryl. Mindy explains, "There was no way I was going to tell her, because I didn't know how she would react and I didn't feel like listening to 'tsk tsk, I told you so.'" Mindy did hint at the situation during her pregnancy, calling her mom to ask about the symptoms of pregnancy. On some level, she may have wanted her mother to know. Beryl asked the reason for the question. Mindy said, "I was just curious," but Beryl didn't buy it. "Are you pregnant?" she asked. Mindy retorted, "If I were pregnant, would I be calling you?"

Still, Beryl probably saw through this lie. A year later, she revealed that she knew about the pregnancy, and said, "I can't understand why you wouldn't come to me." Mindy said, "I had no idea how you would react." Beryl ended up reacting fine. She remained consistent with her earlier teachings. In fact, she is so accepting of Mindy's abortion that she answered an ad seeking volunteers for this book and gave Mindy's name.

Even though Beryl reacted well, Mindy may have been wise to refrain from telling her the news. Parents might voice one belief in the abstract, but have very different standards when it comes to their own child. They might approve of premarital sex for others but not for their daughters. Some families are tinderboxes waiting to explode over matters much less volatile than sex, pregnancy, and abortion. It is hard to know how anyone will react to these topics; family members with already charged feelings are a special case. We may need to think carefully before telling our families our news.

In some cases, we know that our families outright disapprove of abortion, so telling them is out of the question. Even if we tell them nothing, we may have unresolved feelings where they are concerned. Many of us carry around images of our parents in our minds. If we keep hearing our parents' disapproving voices in our heads, we may feel guilty or angry at ourselves about the abortion. In this way, family members can play a large part in our abortion experiences, even if they don't know a thing about the pregnancy.

That was the case for 21-year-old Veronica. Her family emigrated from Central America when she was 11. Although the family does not practice Catholicism anymore, the mother has given her children conservative values, advising them against premarital sex and instilling in Veronica a reverence for motherhood. Much like Mindy's mother, Veronica's mom often said, "I don't want you to make the same mistakes I did." Her own mistakes? She had two children out of wedlock, as was common in her country.

When Veronica moved to the United States, she met peers with liberal opinions. Veronica decided that premarital sex is fine, as long as one is mature. She was comfortable with this choice, until she became pregnant. She recalls that when she had a positive pregnancy test a year ago, "I felt really guilty, and the first thing that came to my mind was my mom." She knew her mother would have her "six feet under" if she knew. Her mom would dislike several aspects of the situation. Veronica was her golden child, "her miracle baby." Veronica's mom had four stillbirths, then bore Veronica prematurely. Because Veronica survived the odds and was the only daughter, her mom put her on a pedestal and bragged about her virtues. If her mother learned that Veronica had an abortion, it would tarnish this image. Veronica did not want "to step off the pedestal."

Veronica's mom would also have been enraged about her daughter's sexual activity and the conception. Veronica imagines that her mom would scream, "How could you do this to me? Look what I had to go through because I didn't have a husband! How could you be selfish and stupid enough to let that happen?" She seems to have commanded Veronica to lead the perfect life that she did not lead. Veronica has to get right what her mother feels she got wrong. This legacy only adds to Veronica's guilt. She explains, "When I felt guilty, it wasn't because I felt like God's going to punish me. It was more like I've disappointed myself and I would be disappointing my family if they knew." A final issue that would have troubled Veronica's mom was the choice to end the pregnancy. She feels, "You got pregnant. Have a child. Tough. You take care of it however you manage to take care of it."

Because Veronica went against so many of her mom's beliefs, she felt troubled. She explains, "It was hard, because all along she had been telling me those things," telling Veronica she was perfect, "and I had incorporated some of that into my image of myself." Her mother does not know about the abortion, and if Veronica can help it, she never will. Still, her mom has played a role in her experience, living in her head, dictating values, and dispensing judgments. Veronica has somewhat separated from her mother, making her own life choices and carving out her own identity. If, however, her mom's criticism remains in her mind, Veronica may need to detach herself even more, discarding those views and paying more attention to her own values and beliefs.

TELLING OUR PARENTS AND SEEKING THEIR SUPPORT

Whether or not our families approve of abortion, we may feel a need to let them know about this event in our lives. It might feel as if we are hiding something from them and that this prevents us from being as close as we would like to be. We may think that they could support us. Alternatively, we might want to confront those voices in our minds and see what they would really say. Their responses may surprise us, or may be eerily predictable.

Meeting with a Parent's Judgment

Cassie, who is 25 and white, knew that her fundamentalist mother viewed premarital sex as a sin, and abortion as murder. Still, Cassie felt guilty for not telling her about the abortion she had at age 22. She finally told her mom that she conceived and had to have an abortion, because the fetus wouldn't have survived. Cassie comments, "The only way I could tell her was to lie. And that was fine with her and she accepted that."

Then, Cassie conceived again at age 24. She and her boyfriend decided to carry to term and had a quickie wedding. Cassie told her family about the marriage and impending birth. She recalls, "My sister was pregnant at the same time. So everyone was excited." Then, Cassie and her husband decided that they could not cope with a baby, and she had an abortion. Telling the family was tricky. Cassie notes, "I knew I couldn't just not say anything. So I called them and told them I had a miscarriage."

That abortion occurred ten months ago. Since then, Cassie and other family members have began to break a long silence about how their stepfather molested them during childhood. In this spirit of truth-telling, Cassie told her mom the real story about the second abortion. She explains, "When we'd been discussing the abuse in the family and I started feeling close to her, I felt like I had to tell her the truth, because I hated the lie. I hated that I was out there in marches and working in clinics and yet I couldn't even tell my own mother the truth. I told her. And I just got complete silence at the other end of the phone." She observes that this is how her mother deals with anger, rather than by raising her voice. Cassie found this response unacceptable and would not drop the subject. Finally her mother said, "Well, I know why you lied." Cassie knew that her mother had jumped to the wrong conclusion; she thinks Cassie could not admit to such an immoral act. Cassie corrected this assumption, saying, "No, I lied because I didn't want to hurt you."

A short time after they hung up, Cassie wrote her mother a detailed letter. Cassie told the truth about the first abortion. She also criticized her mother's attempt to raise her children as fundamentalists, which Cassie sees as detrimental. Cassie notes, "I wrote about why I hated her church and what she did to us and what she's still doing to my younger brother." That was five months ago. Cassie has heard nothing more from her mother or siblings.

Twenty-three-year-old Toni also met with disapproving silence when she told her mother about her first abortion, but she was not completely shut off. Toni explains her parents' values: "My parents are from the South. And some of their beliefs come from their upbringing, in terms of the church. Black people are very church-oriented." Her parents object to abortion and premarital sex. Moreover, she says, "My mom is sixty-five and my father will be seventy-four in June. So they're very old school." Therefore, she did not want them to know that she ended pregnancies at ages 21, 22, and 23, the last abortion occurring just four months ago.

Still, Toni found it difficult to say nothing about these experiences, especially after her first one. She explains, "My mom and I are close, but I didn't feel that I was sharing something with her." Telling her mother could remove that barrier to intimacy, she reasoned. First, Toni told her she had had sex, and believes her mom was thinking, "Why is she telling me that she's sexually active? She knows that's not something her father and I approve of." Wanting to space out the hard-to-handle news, Toni waited a few days before telling her mom about the abortion. Toni thought her mother would be sympathetic. Her mom did understand why Toni had mentioned her sex life. But she had none of the empathy Toni had hoped to find. She simply commented, "Your father doesn't need to know."

Toni did not expect this reaction. Instead of hearing, "I'm sorry that you had to go through this," she was made to feel, "I've really screwed up that there's this big secret that we just won't talk about." She felt guilty and ashamed to think that she had done something that disappointed one parent so much that she wouldn't share it with the other one.

It was hard for Toni to feel that she had failed them. She was the favorite kid, born ten years after their sixth child. Toni notes, "Everything they wanted to do with their other kids, they did with me. All the mistakes they learned from having their kids, they tried to perfect. I was their last chance. But I ended up disappointing them anyway."

She let them down further, she feels, when she temporarily withdrew from school several months after she told her mother about the abortion. By then, Toni had ended two more pregnancies. Distraught by these traumas, she decided to spend some time away from school pressures. Unfortunately, because Toni's mom had taken the news of the first abortion so badly, Toni could not tell her parents that there had been two more and that she was quite depressed now. Toni adds, "I wanted to spare them that." Toni simply told her mom, "I can't be in school right now." She explained that there was too much stress, which her mother accepted, especially when she observed how tired and preoccupied Toni was. Toni met her needs by going home and having a mental rest. She notes, "Without their knowing it, I got them to nurture me and give me all the things that I missed from being away. I missed the reassurance. I just needed my mom and dad and their support in every way."

Vivian: Wanting to Tell Her Parents

Twenty-two-year-old Vivian, who is Caucasian, has much more liberal parents. They are Catholic, but pro-choice. Vivian is very close to them and feels she could have told them about the pregnancy she ended a year ago. During the crisis, she did not tell them, however, because she wanted to be self-reliant. Vivian explains, "This was an area in which I had to assert my independence. I felt like this was something I had to get through without telling my parents." She wanted to prove her strength both to herself and to them.

Since that time, however, she has wanted to let her family know about her abortion. She had a chance to tell them once, when her mother called, needing to vent anger at a pro-life advertising campaign. Vivian's mother said, "I just had to talk to you about this. It's just so infuriating for them to take choice away from us." Vivian recognized that this was her opportunity to tell her mother. At the same time, she "just didn't want to get into it." She has a strong sense of privacy, and the need to keep a boundary between her mother and herself seemed keen at that moment. Plus, Vivian thought, it would be almost too opportunistic to say, "Well, speaking of abortion, let me tell you. . . ."

Vivian continues to weigh the pros and cons of telling her parents about the abortion. She comments, "One of the cons is it'll be bringing this thing up that is very much in the past now." On the other hand, she notes, "I'm keeping a secret that I don't think I should have to keep." She says that being so hush-hush about the abortion "makes me feel guilty about what I've done, which I shouldn't." Telling them will end all of that. Plus, she points out, "There's no reason they shouldn't know." Finally, Vivian feels that there are benefits to letting them see how strong she is. She explains, "Part of it is a certain, 'Look what happened to me.' I want them to know I got through this thing without them."

Timing continues to be a problem. Whenever Vivian intends to tell her parents, they reveal that their marital problems have reached new heights. The summer after Vivian's March abortion, she went home for a weekend. She recalls, "They were having all these problems and thought they might split up. I just couldn't give them another thing to worry about." That fall, she again contemplated talking to them about the abortion. Another of their problems interfered and Vivian felt less inclined to tell them. Now, a year later, her mom is going to stay with Vivian for a time. Vivian's parents have decided to divorce. Vivian says, "When I found out she was coming, I thought, 'That'll be a good time to tell her.' And now, they're having a crisis again! And I'm like, 'Tough shit, I'm telling her. I don't care if this is going to add to everything else! That's just the way it is!'" Vivian laughs hard. Then she adds thoughtfully, "But maybe I won't tell her."

When Parents' Needs Prevent Them from Giving Full Support

Vivian seems to have a good relationship with her parents. Apparently, they listen to her when she speaks. Others of us may find that our parents always seem to have more important things to think about. We may feel as if our news pales in comparison to their worries. They may not hear what we say, or might interpret the news as being about themselves. For this reason, one 19 year old chose not to tell her mother that she was pregnant two months ago. She explains, "Her tendency would be to make it like something bad has happened to her. She'd be like, 'Oh, poor me. My daughter's pregnant.'" Our parents may fail to see that we are communicating something about ourselves, not them.

Yvette, who is 28 and white, found out just how narcissistic her parents were when she told them about her abortions. She didn't mention the abortion she had at age 16 until six years after the fact. When she let them know, she says, "I don't remember them having a reaction. It was an 'oh' thing." They were "too busy" to pay attention to her news.

Three months ago, Yvette ended another pregnancy. This time, she told her mom before the procedure occurred. Yvette wanted her to react with warmth and love. She explains, "I had hoped that with something like this, she would have come through. If my daughter got pregnant, I think I immediately would have been there with Chinese food, some flowers. Even a couple times. But she didn't do that." Instead, after her mom heard the news, "Within five minutes, she managed to change the topic to something about herself."

Right after the procedure, as Yvette's boyfriend Rod drove her home, they had to stop by Yvette's mom's house to pick up something. Rod went into the house to retrieve the item. Yvette instructed him, "Tell her not to keep you hostage. I want to go home." Rod relayed this message to Yvette's mother, who responded cavalierly, "She'll be fine. Just let me show you the rest of the house." Even at that sensitive time, Yvette's mother overlooked her daughter's needs and made herself the center of attention.

In reaction to her mother's lack of support, Yvette notes, "I felt lonely and uncared for. I think if my mother had been there for me. . . ." She trails off, unable to articulate how much better the experience would have been. Trying again, she says, "It's not just a broken wrist, where you have a cast on your wrist and then it heals. It's much, much more." Her mother failed to understand how important the experience was to Yvette.

Narcissistic parents simply cannot see their children for who they are. Instead, the children appear to be their appendages, cogs in their own wheels. A pregnancy signals that a daughter is a sexually active adult. An abortion reflects that she can make her own decisions and act on them. These facts may threaten a parent who would rather see a daughter as a dependent youngster. If we have parents like this, we may try to break through their self-absorption by telling them about an abortion, saying in effect, "Look at me and my life, for once!" If the parent cannot or will not do this, it may feel devastating.

At the same time, it can help us to realize our parents' limitations. The way Yvette's mom reacted to her abortion illuminated something that Yvette feels she needed to see. She comments, "It really brought my relationship with my mother into focus. In a crisis, you find out who your real friends are." Yvette adds, "I feel differently about her. I don't feel like I can depend on her. I feel like the grown-up. She's a child still." Now, Yvette recognizes that her mom has never really been there for her. This is a painful but valuable lesson. Knowing her mother's limits, Yvette will probably expect less from her mom and suffer fewer disappointments. Realizing similar things about our parents can help us separate from them emotionally and define ourselves without their interference. We may begin to tell them less about our lives, taking more risks after freeing ourselves from their criticism. Although it can be depressing to realize that they cannot provide a safety net when we fall, it can be exhilarating for us to see that we can take charge of our own lives. Yvette has certainly found this to be true. She says that many events have caused her to separate from her mother, but that the abortion "pushed it a little faster." Now, she says, "I feel like I can live without my mother." She adds that "independencing" herself from her mother has helped her feel stronger and more mature.

When Families Receive the News Well

Sometimes, parents are able to provide exactly what daughters need after an abortion. There may be no conflict, only love, warmth, and understanding. That was what Randi, who is Caucasian, found ten years ago when she ended a pregnancy at age 25. After the procedure, Randi drove thirteen hours to her parents' house. She planned to tell them about the abortion when she arrived, but began bleeding on the way. Feeling "absolutely terrified," she called her mother and told her what was happening. The mother immediately called a knowledgeable friend, and then relayed the friend's advice to get some rest.

It turned out to be a good decision for Randi to tell her mother. At first, Randi was not sure it would be, even though her mom and dad have always been beyond reproach as parents. She recalls feeling "mortified" when she told her mother the news over the phone, and reassured her mom, "It's nobody's fault. We weren't as careful as we could have been, but we weren't careless." Her mom first reacted as an ardent abortion rights activist. She said, "Oh, I'm so glad. I'm sorry you had to go through it, but I'm glad that all my fighting had a personal effect." Randi's mother was also sad because she wanted a grandchild. But, says Randi, "She knew it wasn't the right time, and she knew she'd be a grandmother sometime." The mother dealt with the situation by joking, "My daughter has decided this wasn't the right time to make me a grandmother." This experience brought Randi and her mom much closer. Randi explains, "We had another basis for intimacy. And it was something we agreed–that I had the right to have the pregnancy terminated." In fact, Randi's mother feels so comfortable with this decision that, just as Mindy's mother did, she answered an ad for this book on her daughter's behalf.

Thirty-one-year-old Annika found her parents equally supportive. She ended her pregnancy at age 26, but waited four years to tell her parents about it. She delayed partly because they live abroad and she wanted to tell them in person, and partly because it took her a long time to reconcile herself to her abortion. She explains, "I wanted to be at a certain point with it myself, to be ready for whatever reaction" they had. It was still important after all that time for her to tell them. She says, "It seemed that they didn't really know me if they didn't know about this. So I wanted to share that part of myself with them." It turned out that they were very understanding. Annika told her mother that she had been pregnant and hadn't carried to term. Her mom empathized with how hard that decision must have been, which Annika found comforting. Annika explains, "She knows me and she knows how much I love children." She recalls, "My mom was crying with me!"

WHEN AN ABORTION SPARKS FEELINGS ABOUT CERTAIN FAMILY MEMBERS

Even though Annika's parents took the news so well, the matter wasn't as simple as it appeared. Before Annika ever told them, she had to work through "tremendous guilt feelings" where her mom was concerned. Annika explains, "I had this huge issue around my mother, because I was the age my mother was when she was pregnant with me. And she has always been a really wonderful mother. My mom was always there for us when we were little. And she was really loving and warm. So I felt like my mom had been the ultimate good mother and I was the ultimate bad mother, killing my child." Annika felt inadequate for being unable to live up to her mom's example. Plus, she could not stop thinking about the "eerie" age coincidence. Before the abortion, this similarity made her think, "Oh my God, what if she had done what I'm about to do?" Feeling grateful to be alive, Annika didn't know how she could justify denying life to the fetus she carried. Eventually, Annika's guilt ran its course. She says the comparison she kept drawing between herself and her mother "just stopped all by itself."

Our Mothers

When we become pregnant, it is natural to think more about our own mothers. How did they feel to be pregnant? How did they put up with the challenges a pregnancy can present? Like Annika, we may compare ourselves with our mothers. One 18 year old named Evelyn has done this a lot lately, because she and her mom were pregnant practically at the same time. Her mom gave birth three months ago, and Evelyn ended a pregnancy ten days ago. The concurrence has been hard for her. She notes, "I see my mother with my baby sister all the time. I'm jealous but excited about my future. Someday that will be me with my perfect, healthy little baby." Evelyn has also struggled because in having an abortion, she violated her pro-life beliefs. She explains, "I was raised in a Catholic family where abortion was unheard of. In addition, my mom has been pregnant eight times and has lost four children, so I was taught how precious and special life is." Evelyn adds, "Not only did I have tremendous guilt from my upbringing, but I also felt sick that I was voluntarily killing my baby when my mom went through so much pain unintentionally losing hers."

Through our pregnancies, we may gain a new appreciation for our moms. After her abortion, one 23 year old felt a wave of empathy for her mother, who had once experienced a stillbirth; suddenly, the daughter knew how much grief her mom must have felt. She comments, "I knew a little bit more what my mother thought as a mother and as a woman. I felt like I was more in touch with what she'd been in touch with all these years."

We might feel more of a bond. If we tell them about the pregnancy, we may hope that our moms will feel more bonded as well, and will intuitively know how to treat us. Sharing knowledge about the joys and troubles of living in a woman's body can draw us together.

It can be hard if we feel a new link to our mothers, but are unable to tell them about our abortions. We may regret having to hide these events from them. Six years after her abortion, one 30 year old feels this way, especially because her mom has worked in many abortion clinics. The daughter says, "The only difficult thing has been not telling my mother. I'm too embarrassed—plus now it's been so long, she'll be hurt I did not tell her sooner." A year after her abortion, a 25 year old feels the same way. She comments, "I wanted to tell my mother, but somehow couldn't. I didn't want to hurt her, although she would have dealt. My mother had helped one of my friends years earlier deal with her abortion. I still haven't told her. Sadly enough, I don't know why."

If we feel more connected to our moms during pregnancy, we may be especially grateful if they can support us through the abortion. Filling out a questionnaire about the abortion she had eleven years ago reignited one 29 year old's gratitude for the support her mother and sister gave her. She writes, "I'm thinking now that I should thank them again. Perhaps I'll call them tonight." She recalls, "My mother held my hand throughout the procedure. I've always felt so grateful to her for that, but also sad that she witnessed the abortion, rather than the birth of a grandchild."

We may feel guilty or sad about denying our parents grandchildren by having an abortion. If they have no grandchildren and mention this frequently in wistful tones, or if we are the only one of their offspring who has not yet reproduced, the unplanned pregnancy can seem particularly ironic. This issue has arisen for 44-year-old Daphne, who has never wanted children. She comments, "My mother keeps talking about grandchildren from my brother. And they're trying to have more. In fact, it's really ironic that they're trying so hard to have another one," when Daphne has conceived against her will and ended three pregnancies over the last two decades. This issue can take on new dimensions if our parents are ill and face death. That was true for one 25 year old who had an abortion two years ago. In a letter about her experience, she notes, "My mother died recently and one of my first thoughts was I could have given her a grandchild."

If our mothers have had abortions themselves, they may be especially empathic. Before abortion became legal, many of them saw unwanted pregnancies burden people's lives and marriages. They may feel strongly that their own abortions saved them in this regard and that their daughters should have the same chance at avoiding misery. Then again, if our moms have unresolved feelings about their abortions, they may act strangely about ours, growing tense during conversations about them, or having outbursts of rage or sadness.

Whether or not our moms have ended pregnancies, our abortions can stir up uncomfortable feelings for them. They may experience our decision to end a pregnancy as a rejection of the way they lived their lives. Our choice may make them face any ambivalence they have about being a mother. Maybe they would have liked more of a say about when they gave birth. Fifteen years ago, when one 36 year old had the first of her four abortions, she learned that her mother had tried to abort her, and had failed. Perhaps to distance herself from the pain, this woman describes that conversation by referring to herself as "you": "Imagine after your first abortion, all the guilt, etcetera, and your own mother turns to you and says, 'You're so lucky to be able to have done this so safely.' She went on to explain that she and my father had traveled far to find and pay for abortive medicines for the termination of her pregnancy with me." While this story may be unusual, it highlights the ambivalence that our mothers may have had about their own pregnancy histories, an ambivalence that our abortions can trigger for them.

Our Fathers

It can be awkward to discuss our sexuality with male family members. As we turned from girls into women, this issue may have become more charged. Our fathers, in particular, may have become like guard dogs, warding off predatory men, making sure we dressed in Victorian fashions, or issuing occasional threats. One 17 year old who ended a pregnancy a year ago recalls such warnings vividly. She explains, "I was raised to think that premarital sex was bad. Abortion was never mentioned because premarital sex should not be a part of my thoughts. My father once said, 'If you make a mistake, I will never forgive you.' We were having a discussion on my attendance at a party. He said I would probably drink and that would lead to the inevitable." If our dads have said such things, they may have little faith in our judgment and may not be supportive if we conceive.

In other cases, our fathers may have sent mixed messages. For instance, a 27 year old who ended a pregnancy two years ago notes, "My dad was really strict and would say, 'If I catch you sleeping around, I'm going to kill you.'" However, she adds, "My parents told me that if I ever got pregnant, I could come to them and talk to them." Apparently, neither she nor they saw the contradiction in those two messages. How could she have felt safe telling them about a pregnancy, not knowing whether they would help her or kill her?

Some dads may surprise us when we tell them about our pregnancies. For example, one 20 year old heard threats from her father during her adolescence. She recalls, "He didn't seem to care about anything when I was thirteen to eighteen, except that I mustn't get pregnant, because he would be financially responsible." She did conceive at age 18 and told her father and sister. Referring in particular to these two family members, she notes, "I was surprised that when I told people about it, they said they were sorry. I expected them to be disappointed or even disapproving because I had let it happen." If we tell our fathers that we have conceived, they might feel angry only at the man who impregnated us, not at us.

Our fathers may have imparted early messages about sex and pregnancy with good intentions. They might think back to their own youth and realize how easily unplanned pregnancies occur. They may put energy into warning us about sex and pregnancy, not because they feel that sex is sinful, but because of their own pasts. When we do conceive unintentionally, some fathers rise to the occasion and provide as much support as they can.

Twenty-one-year-old Fritzi found that this was true when she conceived two years ago. She points out that her dad is "the most liberal man in the world." Before she conceived, he knew she was sexually active and was comfortable with this. After Fritzi discovered her pregnancy, she told both parents right away. Both were accepting. They told her that they had conceived her before marriage and had married for that reason. This was in no way a punitive story. They merely wanted to tell her that the same thing had happened to them when they were young. Plus, they let her know that when Fritzi was in high school, they had ended a pregnancy for fear that the fetus would be disabled.

Many of us believe that our fathers will be hurt or disappointed, so we refrain from telling them about our pregnancy or abortion. We may want to spare our dads the pain that our information could cause. One 23 year old feels that way. She explains, "My father does not know. Nor will he ever, hopefully. I don't think he'd be angry. I just think it would really hurt him that I had an abortion." Not only does abortion conflict with his religious beliefs, but he would probably also think, "I really didn't want that to happen to my daughter." She does not want him to know about all the pain she experienced, because he would think, "What a shame." She adds, "That's not the kind of life he wants for me."

Our Siblings

Just as our fathers may be uncomfortable with the idea of our sexuality, our brothers may not be at ease with the news of our pregnancy or abortion. Some of our brothers have driven us to abortion clinics or filled prescriptions for medicine. Brothers may have been through it themselves after impregnating women. However, they may not know what to say to us about our abortion, and might prefer performing practical actions to talking with us about our feelings. Some brothers are not helpful at all. That was what one 28 year old found when she ended a pregnancy five months ago. Gina deliberated over her decision, thoroughly investigating single parenthood, but taking into account that her mother had been a single parent, which had been difficult for the whole family. When Gina told her brother about her pregnancy, she received "instant misunderstanding and shock" that she was even considering single parenthood. She was dismayed at his reaction.

Sisters may not be much more empathic. Seventeen-year-old Blair, who is both Asian and Caucasian, has an older sister who went through Blair's calendar and found out about her abortion. Blair says, "I got *hell* for it." A year later, the sister still says things such as, "You don't want to go around acting like a whore and getting pregnant. Again!" Blair calls such snide comments the "one challenge I haven't been able to overcome" in her abortion experience. The jabs are "nerve-wracking" and disillusion Blair about her sister's character.

Our sisters' pregnancy histories may matter to us when we go through abortions. Dana, who is now 27, has long been concerned with her sister Loretta's reproduction. When Dana was 20 and Loretta was 18, Dana showed her pictures of chopped-up fetuses. Dana said, "Loretta, you've got to be very careful with your boyfriend so you don't get pregnant." Loretta began to cry. Unbeknownst to Dana, Loretta had recently had an abortion. Four years later, Loretta wrote to Dana about the abortion. Dana read the letter before going to a class. She recalls, "All of a sudden, I burst out crying in class for my sister." She recalled the pictures she had shown Loretta and felt badly.

A year after Loretta sent that letter, both sisters conceived. Dana had an abortion, and Loretta announced her plans to carry to term. Dana recalls, "I was upset that my situation wasn't different. I thought it would have been neat if we could both have a baby at the same time." Now, seeing Loretta's baby triggers Dana's feelings about her abortion. In addition, because Loretta carried to term, Dana feels that she cannot tell her father about her own abortion. She explains, "I would never hear the end of it. I think my dad would say, 'Look at Loretta. Look at her baby. Why can't you do something like that?'"

Since many of us feel competitive with our sisters, their pregnancy histories may prevent us from bonding with them as we go through abortions. Their plans may be out of sync with ours, as Loretta's were with Dana's. Their beliefs may also be different, causing them to judge us for our choice. This need not be the case, however. For instance, one 22 year old has only good things to say about how her three teenaged sisters responded to her abortions at ages 19 and 20. She comments, "They're terrific. And they have more insights than a lot of people about what has gone into my decisions. They can tell that I'm a very loving person, that I would love to be a mom as many times over as I could. And they also are able to see where the limitations are in my life. I think they trust my thinking a lot more than older adults or some of my contemporaries." She adds that the two youngest were just preteens during her first abortion, but still responded well. She notes, "Young people really allow people to live their lives. I think a lot of adults try to get in there and control things." While several adults critiqued her decisions, her sisters ignored all of this and told her, "It really doesn't matter to us. We love you." She does not know what they think about abortion, but observes that they managed to overlook any personal feelings they may have had about the issue and to give her the support she needed.

Our Children

If we already have kids at the time of our abortions, we may find that being with them keeps bringing the abortion to mind, making guilt or grief more acute. One 42 year old had some trouble with this on the night of her abortion two years ago. Her 5 year old wanted to play "the game of being born and being a magical baby." Usually, this game gives them both pleasure, but that night, she says, it was "too close to my feelings about giving un-birth. I was writhing with discomfort, but he didn't really notice." If we have a child at some point after an abortion, it may also set off some feelings about the decision we made. For instance, one 37 year old had an abortion at age 18. She later adopted a girl, whose biological parents were also 18 years old. To realize that her adopted daughter could have been aborted made her quite sad. Our children exist because we (or a biological mother) chose birth over abortion; because they represent the "yea" in contrast to the "nay" of the abortion, reflecting on their existence may make us doubt our choice.

Alternatively, being with our children may make us feel good about both the birth and the abortion decisions. Each choice may reinforce the other. That is how one 38 year old feels. She had an abortion at age 24 and had babies at ages 29 and 33. She comments, "The miracle of pregnancy, birth, and watching a child grow is no less a miracle to me because I chose not to live it the first time I was pregnant. My birth experiences were wonderful. Birth when we choose it is a cherished, powerful miracle." She did not approach abortion and birth in opposite ways, but with the continuous philosophy that children deserve mothers who are ready for parenthood. With this attitude, we may have an abortion for the sake of children we already have, children to whom we want to give all our resources. One 30 year old had an abortion at age 25 for this reason; she already had two children, but felt that they "needed more than they were getting." She says her abortion gave her "more appreciation for the children I have. They are so precious. Their quality of life helped me to decide it was not the best idea to have more children just then."

If, like this woman, we end a pregnancy for the sake of the children we already have, we may have ambivalence about denying them a sibling. That was the case for 49-year-old Sylvia two decades ago. Her son was only seven months old when she conceived. She had an abortion for his sake, and explains, "I believe if I'd had the child, I would have been devastated and not capable of being a very good mother to him. It was hard enough being a single parent to one baby. I didn't feel I could manage two and maintain any kind of quality of life." At the time of her abortion, she was clear about what she needed to do on a practical level. Still, Sylvia says, "I needed to cope with the guilt of knowing my wonderful son could have had a sibling." She has been able to accept her decision rather easily, commenting, "I don't feel guilty. I did what I had to do for my son." Twenty years after the fact, she says, "I've been a really good mother and I have a fabulous son. Once in a while, I think about what it would have been like raising two children instead of one (private schools, clothes, 'Would I have been able to buy a house?') and what it would be like in my later years to have two children to 'take care of me' instead of one."

Our desire to provide our children with siblings may be straightforward, as in Sylvia's case. Alternatively, feelings of loss or guilt about the abortion may masquerade as concerns about providing our kids with a sibling. That is the case for one 27 year old. She had a daughter at age 22, and then ended pregnancies at ages 24 and 26. She comments, "I definitely feel a loss. I feel like I'm missing a child. I find myself asking Carina if she would like any brothers or sisters. She always says 'No.'"

We may want to tell our kids about our abortions, but may need to wait until they are older so that they can understand. Twenty-two-year-old Brittany had already told her 2 year old, Courtney, that she was going to be a big sister before Brittany changed her mind about the pregnancy. After the abortion, Brittany told Courtney, "We're not having a baby," explaining, "The baby isn't in there anymore. It's not alive anymore." That seemed to satisfy Courtney, who hasn't raised the topic since. Brittany comments, "Someday, I'd like to talk to her about it. But I haven't dealt with enough of my own feelings that I feel like I can effectively communicate with her." In the meantime, Brittany worries that Courtney could confuse the abortion with vengeance. She may believe that Brittany became angry with the baby and killed it. Brittany has not figured out how to broach this subject.

We might wonder how to discuss our abortions with any children we have in the future. One 32 year old feels that her kids should know about the four siblings they could have had. Currently midway through a pregnancy, she wonders whether her child will ask, "How come you didn't abort me?" She muses, "Will I be honest and say, 'I considered'?" She had initially intended to end this pregnancy as well. She does not know how to explain to her child why he or she is different from the other four. Another woman, age 42, has had two kids since her abortion. Although her boys are young and would not understand what she was talking about if she mentioned her abortion, she doesn't think it will be hard to tell them when they are older. If they mention abortion, she will say, "Before you guys were born, I did have an abortion. I was already with your dad and our relationship was pretty new and shaky." She shrugs, "I'm really honest with my kids. I think if you address these things very openly and without a lot of baggage, then it's fine."

Beyond discussing abortion with our kids, we may end up helping them through their own abortions. This was true for 75-year-old Irma, who had an abortion fifty years ago. Her daughters have done the same thing. She held one daughter's hand during the procedure. Irma observes, "I was disturbed when my daughters had to go through abortions, because it's a tough experience, but I knew they wouldn't be happy marrying the men and they didn't want to become single mothers. I helped as much as I could."

Chapter 15

Friends: When Pregnancy and Abortion Test Platonic Ties

When Simone, who is age 39 and Caucasian, ended a pregnancy a year ago, she did not intend to burden her friends with her problems. They dragged the secret out of her, though. As she puts it, "I told people in circumstances in which I couldn't hold it back any longer. I was telling people because it was forced out of me." Her friends could sense that she was unhappy, and when they didn't buy any of the reasons she offered, she had to explain why she was so depressed.

Telling her friends turned out to be quite helpful. First of all, she found out that "everybody has their own story," that she was not alone. Her women friends told her the worst and the best parts about their abortion experiences.

She received support for her decision from her friends. They thought that, given the pressures in Simone's life, "to have the baby was just lunatic." Simone says, however, that she did not necessarily want her friends to support her decision. She explains, "I didn't want people to say, 'I think you're doing the right thing.' I didn't want to convince people." Simone means that she did not want to bully her friends into seeing the situation her way. Instead, she just wanted them to listen. After that, Simone wished to know, "Where do you think I am leaning, given all the things I've said to you?" She says she wanted "a reflection from my friends of where I was." She spoke only to her very close friends in this way, which was a good choice; she could trust them to be her mirror.

Simone also needed their empathy. She spoke primarily to people who had had abortions, and notes, "I really wanted somebody to say, 'Yes, I understand what this dilemma is about.'" If they could feel what she felt, or understand the depth of her pain, she would feel less isolated in her troubles. She seems to have received this empathy. When her friends gave advice, shared their experiences, listened to her talk, agreed with her decision, and tried to understand her feelings, they met her needs. It is fortunate that Simone was conscious enough of what she needed to direct her friends in how they could best help her. It is also quite lucky that her friends were able to provide all of this.

Sometimes, things are not so clearcut. When we experience an abortion, or any crisis, we may expect support from the people in our lives. But "support" is a vague word, one that means different things to different people. If Simone's friends had insisted that her decision was right, even before they heard her feelings, she might have felt frustrated or disappointed. Another woman going through an abortion might have felt annoyed if people did *not* automatically say that her decision was good. It partly depends on how honest we need our friends to be. If we ask them whether an outfit makes us look heavy, do we really want to hear the truth? When we go through an abortion, we may want friends' truthful opinions. On the other hand, their respectful silence may fill us with gratitude.

For example, when 23-year-old Wanda had abortions at ages 19 and 22, she had different needs from Simone. In the first situation, Wanda's boyfriend had abandoned her. She was a physical wreck after fifteen weeks of pregnancy. Her car wasn't working and her town had no public transportation. It was raining. And she had little food at home.

Wanda's friend did the best she could to fill in the gaps. She took Wanda to the clinic. In a few days, she visited Wanda, bringing flowers and food. Wanda felt tremendously grateful for this help and care. When Wanda ended her second pregnancy three years later, her friend was quite considerate again. Even though the friend was traveling, she made a point to check on Wanda right after the procedure. She called from a diner somewhere in Texas, which really cheered Wanda up.

Wanda's friend met her physical needs, such as transportation, and her emotional needs, by showing affection. This friend also tried to empathize, saying, "I feel bad for you," and "Everything's going to be okay." These responses were warm and appropriate, but fell a little bit short of what Wanda needed. She laments, "Nobody could say, 'I know what you're going through.'" Wanda adds, "Nobody really knew what to say." Her friend tried hard to give Wanda what she needed, and Wanda's needs were not unreasonable, but she did not get exactly what she wanted. She appreciated her friend's efforts and their relationship survived the abortions, but Wanda felt the keen absence of a few essential things: validation, understanding, and guidance in making it through her experience.

When Friends Don't Meet Our Needs

If we want friends to help us through an abortion experience, we may find our friendships tested. Sometimes our needs match our friends' ability to give. At other times, there is a mismatch. When our friends don't live up to our expectations during this crisis, we may feel quite disappointed. We may have believed that our friends were so close that we could rely on them completely. Suddenly, we see that the relationship was not quite what we thought, that our friend could not deal with heavy events in our life, or that she or he was not able to listen to our feelings. The friendship may reveal itself as rather superficial, based more on having fun than on true caring. We may be shocked to find the bond so weak. If we have always tried to be there for our friend, we might resent the lack of reciprocity and the friends' seemingly conditional love. After the abortion reveals the flaws in the relationship, the friendship may not seem to have much of a future. The abortion may become off-limits in conversation and any related subjects might feel risky to discuss. We may decide that we have no time for people who cannot understand what the abortion means to us, especially if it has altered our sense of self or life direction.

We may feel inadequate if an abortion shows us that we lack a circle of dependable buddies, that we don't possess the popularity so vaunted in our culture. Having friends often gives us a sense of self-worth; when our friendships fall apart, we may experience a loss of self-esteem and feel a need to find new friends quickly. We may begin talking about the abortion with people who are not close to us, both to elicit supportive comments, and to see if they react better than our friends did. We might talk about the abortion with acquaintances to screen them as friends on the basis of their reactions and even to accelerate the process of letting them know us. They may respond well, and we may feel close, or the heavy topic and our neediness may scare them off.

Preferring to Be Independent of Friends During a Crisis

Some of us would rather circumvent the problems that can arise when we discuss our abortions and would prefer to be self-reliant. For instance, we might go to the abortion facility without any friends present. As one 25 year old puts it, seven years after her abortion, "My friend dropped me off and picked me up, but I didn't want people to make a big deal out of it (holding my hand and whatnot), because I never like to impose or 'need' emotional support. I didn't want anyone else involved—not even my boyfriend. It was my issue to deal with, I thought." Another woman also went through the abortion procedure solo, because she does not like to depend on others. Nineteen years after her abortion, this 43 year old notes, "I think it would have been hard for me to have anyone I knew that close to me (i.e., to stay through the procedure)—not because it was a 'bad abortion,' but because of problems I had about borders, boundaries, and intimacy."

Irene, age 19, has handled her whole abortion experience in a similar way. Since she ended her pregnancy two months ago, she has tried to be self-reliant, even though her friends have offered support. One of her friends said, "I'm going to be here for you to come and talk to me." Irene says, however, "If someone starts showing me support and holding me, that's when I break." She feels she can hold herself together better without such kindness. Irene has mixed results in concealing her unhappiness about her abortion from her friends. She comments, "I do a very good job of convincing them it doesn't bother me. But sometimes I just get quiet." Her friends sometimes ask, "What was wrong through that lunch?" and Irene responds happily, "Oh, you noticed?" It sounds as if Irene appreciates such attention, despite her attempts to hide her feelings. She feels torn between letting herself be cared for and maintaining the autonomy she values.

We may find ourselves without friends' help during an abortion experience, especially if we have conceived at a time of great change, a period when we are growing away from our friends. For instance, one 28 year old had no friends to support her when she had an abortion three months ago, because she was recovering from a drug addiction, and found it necessary to stop associating with addicts. She explains, "I had to drop all my friends. And it's really hard to make new friends when you're an adult and you're working and you're not going to school anymore. So I don't really have anybody." Another woman, age 45, was also in the middle of overhauling her life when she ended an unplanned pregnancy thirteen years ago. She comments, "I had only one close friend at the time who had transitioned with me from my old life to my new life. And I shared the situation with her. But aside from that, I hardly talked to anybody about it."

CONFLICTS THAT ABORTION CAN CREATE IN FRIENDSHIPS

Since Becky, a 25-year-old Caucasian, ended her pregnancy two months ago, she feels pleased that only one person was critical of her news. Becky comments, "I was really lucky, because you don't know what people's views are." Still, Becky feels that it wasn't enough that people didn't criticize her; she wanted their support. As Becky went through the most traumatic experience of her life, she felt that everyone minimized her pain.

For instance, Becky's roommate from college seemed to gloss over the news. She sent a present for Becky's birthday, which occurred four weeks after the abortion. When Becky called to say thanks for the gift, she told her friend about the abortion. Becky expected her to say, "Oh my God! I can't believe this happened to you!" Instead, she was "more laid-back about it" and "didn't get overexcited about it." Her casual response saddens Becky, because her friend does not seem to understand what a big event this is in Becky's life. Plus, Becky notes, "Two years ago, she would have been the first person I told." The friend's cool response emphasizes how they seem to have lost that intimacy.

Becky's current roommate was even less responsive. Madeline gave her a card, but had law school finals and couldn't handle Becky's problems at that time. Becky recalls, "We made a deal that I wasn't going to listen to her problems about her law school finals and she wasn't going to listen to mine. That was the way we said we'd get along. I felt like hers were nothing compared to mine, but I had to be sympathetic to her, too." This arrangement didn't feel very satisfactory. Becky explains, "By the time she got done with her law school finals, it was two weeks after my abortion, so I didn't really feel like I needed to talk about it with her anymore." Plus, Madeline had been less than sensitive the day after the abortion. Becky explains, "I got the abortion on Saturday. And we do the cleaning on Sunday. I was staying out of the house so that I wouldn't think about it. She left me this note that said, 'I'm stressed out and I managed to do all my cleaning. How come you didn't?'" Becky was astonished at this attack. She exclaims, "She's my friend! This is a girl that I had been friends with since high school!" Recently, Madeline said to Becky, "I can't believe my roommate had an abortion," as if this thought disturbs her. Perhaps it is just as well that Becky and she never spoke in depth about the abortion.

Becky has had conflicts with two other friends in regard to her abortion. Her co-worker, Daisy, conceived a month before Becky did, and decided to carry to term. Daisy speaks about her pregnancy all the time, which has been hard for Becky to hear. This situation may also present problems for Becky because many of us feel uncomfortable speaking about abortion with a pregnant woman. It is as if her fetus is sacred and any mention of ending a pregnancy is sacrilegious. If Becky feels this way, she may see Daisy's pregnancy as one more reason she cannot discuss her abortion.

Becky's friend Nelson, who is Mormon, certainly views abortion as sacrilegious, or worse, and would not hesitate to tell Becky this if he learned of her abortion. Unfortunately, he came into town during her pregnancy and came to see her right away. When Becky greeted him, she was thinking self-consciously, "I'm pregnant, I'm pregnant, I'm pregnant!" Nelson looked her over and said, "Oh, you look really skinny!" Two weeks after her pregnancy ended, they saw a movie that had a scene about abortion. Becky sat frozen in her seat, afraid to react. She comments, "I felt weird going out with him after the abortion. If he ever found out, he would hate me. He feels really strongly." If, like Becky, we cannot tell a friend about our abortion, we may feel less close, as if the friend does not really know us now. Unfortunately, our friend will not even know we feel this way.

For several reasons that Becky has named, a pregnancy and abortion can challenge friendships. We now explore other ways abortion can cause conflict between friends.

When Friends Don't Know How to React to Our Situation

Our friends may have no idea how to respond to our pregnancy and abortion. This is especially true if they are young and have not experienced abortion, pregnancy, or even sex. One 18 year old found this to be the case when she ended a pregnancy two years ago. She recalls, "Two of my friends didn't know how to handle it, so they just pretended like it didn't happen." A 22 year old faced a similar situation when she had an abortion last year. "My friends helped, but they were as much in awe as I was," she says, adding, "They had never dealt with that before. They didn't know what the hell to do. They didn't know how to act." We may understand that our friends are as scared as we are about our unplanned pregnancy, and forgive them. Or we may feel let down that just when we rely on them, they fall to pieces. We might expect that once they overcome the initial shock, they will rally around us. Unfortunately, this might never happen. Our friends may hope that the whole issue blows over and feel relieved when things seem to return to normal.

When Friends Have Babies or Baby Issues

If our choice is out of sync with our friends' pregnancy plans, it can create conflict in the relationship. Jealousy, judgments, or awkwardness can supplant acceptance and openness. For instance, when 46-year-old Olivia ended a pregnancy twenty years ago, her close friend was carrying to term. Olivia's abortion took place in December. A month later, her friend gave birth to twins. Olivia told her friend about the abortion, but found it awkward. Moreover, Olivia had a hard time adjusting to her friend's delivery, because she was "longing for a baby" herself. Olivia acknowledges that it was strange to want a baby when her pregnancy was unintentional, the result of a fluke birth control failure. She felt, however, that she deserved to have a baby as much as her friend did. Seeing her friend's babies only increased her desire to have children. The irony was just too great–here were two women who wanted babies, and there were two children, but they both belonged to the same woman. Eventually, this painful situation actually helped Olivia resolve her feelings about her abortion. She recalls, "I spent time with them, and that got out whatever it was I had inside that I wanted to take care of screaming, smelly, little things."

When we have abortions, we may also find ourselves out of sync with friends who are struggling to conceive or to carry a healthy fetus to term. Our accidental conception and decision to end the pregnancy may cause them great distress. Thirty-two-year-old Oriana has had abortions at ages 18, 19, 25, and 30, and notes, "I have a very close friend who's been having trouble conceiving and desperately wants a baby. She's seen me go through two abortions and it's put a strain on our friendship." To make matters worse, Oriana is now five months into another pregnancy. She didn't plan this one either, but decided to carry to term. Even though her friend, Dinah, had trouble seeing Oriana end two pregnancies, she also had a hard time when Oriana decided to have this baby. Dinah told Oriana, "Your life is in shambles right now. You can have a baby whenever you want one. I can't. Why are you choosing to have this baby now?" Oriana explains, "This friend was advocating abortion for me because I wasn't in a relationship, I wasn't married, I wasn't sure about my partner, financially I was up a creek, I had no health insurance. And since she knows my history as a baby-making machine, of all times, why choose now to have a baby?" Dinah has tried to support Oriana's last choice, but it has been hard. Oriana muses that the best scenario might have been "if I could have done a handoff, giving the baby to Dinah."

When Friends' Views of Abortion Conflict with Our Own

Dinah is pro-choice and did not criticize Oriana's abortions. This, unfortunately, is not always the case. Just as abortion divides our country, this gulf can easily separate friends. Before either friend faces an unplanned pregnancy, it may not seem relevant. When the issue arises, however, it can imperil the friendship, as we will now see from several examples.

Hallie: Feeling Set Apart from Pro-Life Friends

Hallie, age 22, conceived two years ago at the end of "a five-year born-again Christian phase." Hallie had become religious when she lived with her pro-choice, religious family. She explains, "I became a born-again Christian to rebel against them." Because of her new religious practice, she says, "I was pro-life. But I never thought abortion should be illegal. I just never saw myself getting one."

When she conceived, however, everything changed. She was in her third year of college, three thousand miles from her family and her born-again friends. Hallie recalls, "As soon as I found out for certain that I was pregnant, I did not hesitate in my decision to get an abortion. I was only twenty and wanted to get my college degree. I knew that I would not be a good mother at the time, because I would have so many regrets and would resent the child for taking up my time." Hallie told many people in her life about her decision–the guy who impregnated her, her parents, aunt, cousins, and her college friends. Since her abortion, she has continued to speak about it without reservation. Hallie comments, "I talk about it openly with people who want to know about it, and if they really seem to want to understand what the experience was like, I will tell them about it in great detail. It is good for me to talk about it and it is good for them to know." It is also important to discuss abortion experiences, Hallie figures, so other women "know that they are not alone."

Despite this philosophy, Hallie remains silent about it with her friends from home. She remarks, "I knew that I could never talk to my born-again Christian friends again, because I could not explain to them why I chose to have an abortion." She feels set apart from those who are pro-life and says, "When I hear pro-lifers talk, I get very angry because of my newfound wisdom–you never know until it happens to you." She now prefers to be with "people who are open-minded and accepting." Hallie notes, "I felt fortunate to have gotten a new perspective on the whole issue, although it meant that there was a group of people who would never be able to understand my experience."

Vera: Friends Pressured Her to Carry to Term

Vera also hung out with a pro-life crowd before her first pregnancy. Vera is a Latina 26 year old who ended pregnancies at ages 16, 21, and 22. The first abortion remains the most vivid for her, because of the way her friends pressured her to have the child. Vera recalls, "One friend told me she'd get a job to help support 'us.'" Several months after Vera's abortion, another friend disparaged her choice. Vera's sister had conceived at the same time as she, but had given birth. When Vera showed this baby to a friend, the friend said, "See, you could have had an adorable baby like that if you hadn't had an abortion."

These comments felt quite hurtful. To make matters worse, Vera relied on her friends to help her. She was unsure of her decision and needed people to ease the situation. Her boyfriend was unsupportive. Her family was Catholic and pro-life. Although they did not really discuss abortion during her childhood, Vera says, "I do have a vague memory of right-to-life stickers–my dad's." She could not let her parents know about her pregnancy.

As Vera looks back on that first pregnancy and abortion experience, she comments, "I wish more people had encouraged me to discuss my feelings, instead of giving me theirs." Fortunately, Vera notes that with her second and third abortions, "The people I was involved with were more mature and supportive."

May: It Was a Personal Issue, Not a Political One

Sometimes, our friends may be so used to viewing abortion as a political issue that they find it difficult to see it any other way. If they are entrenched in abortion rights ideology, they might be unable or unwilling to understand that abortion can cause personal conflicts. When 25-year-old May had an abortion twelve months ago, she found that her close friend Stacy treated the issue as political, not personal. Stacy has worked extensively defending clinics against protesters. She has never had an abortion, but her sister had one and experienced no emotional difficulties. This reinforces Stacy's belief that women do not have problems with abortion, that this is only pro-life propaganda.

Stacy was very helpful to May on one level. May recalls, "Stacy was actually really supportive through the whole thing. She lent me money, she came with me, and just was there for me." In other ways, however, Stacy did not understand May's needs. When May discovered that she was pregnant, she talked her decision over with Stacy. May felt that abortion was probably the best option, as she was still in graduate school, had no money, and had become pregnant from a one-night stand. Still, she did not feel entirely sure. Stacy urged her to have an abortion. May says that after their conversation, she felt "bothered" by Stacy's insistence. She muses, "You have to let people make their own decision. It's just as bad to say, 'Of course you'll have an abortion,' as it is to say, 'Of course you'll have a kid when you're nineteen.'" May acknowledges, however, that she expected this response from Stacy, and figures she spoke to Stacy because that was what she "really needed" to hear. If she wanted encouragement to carry to term, she could have talked to someone else.

Their communication problems did not stop there. May anticipated that there might be protesters at the clinic. She told Stacy, "I need some help. I can't go through the protesters alone." Hearing this, Stacy felt even more motivated than usual to stand up to the picketers. May was frustrated by this response and dropped the issue. She remembers thinking, "I'm not doing this to prove that abortion is a woman's right. I'm doing this because I have this crisis in my life that I have to deal with. This isn't a political thing for me at all. There's a big difference to me between the whole political movement for abortion, which I'm committed to, and this whole personal thing. This is my life. This is what's happening to me. And if there were protesters and they hit me, that would hurt me. And if they called me evil, I wouldn't agree with them, but I would still feel evil." May feels that this distinction between the politics of abortion and the personal experience of abortion is crucial for people to understand, especially the people who are her friends.

BONDING WITH FRIENDS BECAUSE OF AN ABORTION

Despite all the possible reasons for being unable to connect with friends when we end pregnancies, it is certainly possible to maintain or even improve friendships during abortion experiences. Our friends often provide the bulk of the support we receive, which can confirm for us that they love us and that the relationship is solid.

During the illegal era, female friends were often the key players in a woman's abortion, helping her locate someone who would perform the procedure. That was true for Irma fifty years ago when she conceived at age 25. It was World War II and she was in the Women's Army Corps. She recalls how her friend, Delores, helped her: "I felt terribly alone, until I got enough courage to confess to Delores that I was pregnant. She made me feel better, telling me that when she was a naive virgin before joining the Army, a boy had gotten her pregnant–she hadn't been sure quite how. Her mother had arranged for an abortion." Delores helped Irma find some pills, which were supposed to "bring you 'round." They went together to a motel room, where Irma inserted the pills into her vagina. Nothing happened. Another friend came to the rescue. Irma says, "Mona, my friend in New York, told me about a doctor who would do an abortion for three hundred dollars." Irma ended her pregnancy in New York. She felt very grateful for the help these two friends gave her. In fact, Irma is still so close to Delores that she sent her a questionnaire so that she could contribute her abortion experience to this book!

Even though abortion is usually easier to obtain these days, there are still plenty of ways our friends can support us. We may feel grateful if they agree wholeheartedly with our decision. To one 25 year old who had an abortion a year ago, such support meant everything, especially because she and her boyfriend split up at that time. She says that after she confirmed her pregnancy at a clinic, "I drove home with Adele, whom I've known for fifteen years. We smoked cigarettes. I spoke with all of my friends, and one of their mothers, whom I have also known forever. She said that whatever decision I made she would support." Her friends gave her similar assurances.

Many of us appreciate having our friends come to the abortion with us, especially if the man who impregnated us is not present at the procedure. One 37 year old had a friend hold her hand at her abortion sixteen years ago. She recalls, "I felt good about her involvement. I usually do stressful, traumatic things alone, so this was good for me." Her friend also supported her in a disagreement with the doctors about receiving a sedative.

Sometimes, having a friend to discuss our experience with makes all the difference. Talking about something so intimate can make us feel bonded. Twenty-one-year-old Fritzi, who ended a pregnancy two years ago, was able to speak openly about the abortion with her best friend from high school. Fritzi didn't tell her for a while, because they were at different colleges and hadn't caught up on each other's lives in about a year. When Fritzi did share her experience, she says, "I felt like it brought us closer, because I was sharing something private with her." Another woman, 30-year-old Faith, also found that talking about her abortion with an estranged friend had a conciliatory effect. Although they had lost contact for a year because of a conflict over a man, they got back in touch soon after the abortion she had at age 24. Faith comments, "She told me then she had experienced the same thing. Discussing our experiences helped re-form an old, long-lasting friendship. She is my closest friend." Not only did they grow close, but Faith felt less alone in her experience. She realized "that this happens a lot, to anyone, anywhere."

It can be especially meaningful if a friend overcomes ambivalence about abortion and can support us. That was the case for 27-year-old Tanya, who ended a pregnancy at age 19. Although her best friend had always said she would not have an abortion, she had no objections to helping Tanya. As soon as Tanya discovered the pregnancy, she called her friend in a panic. Tanya explains, "I didn't have any money to pay for it. I thought my friend could help me find a way to come up with the money. She did. She cashed a few of her savings bonds to pay for it. I ended up paying her back about six to eight months later. I felt like she was saving my life." Not only did the friend finance the abortion, but she drove Tanya to and from the clinic and stayed with her during the procedure. All this from a person who thinks on some level that abortion is wrong!

Thirty-five-year-old Randi also found great understanding from her best friend, Kendall, even though Kendall is Catholic. Randi knew Kendall had reservations about abortion, so when Randi ended a pregnancy ten years ago, she deliberately hid it from her. Randi explains, "I was afraid of her reaction and afraid that it would change our relationship." Soon after that, Kendall conceived and decided to carry to term. She complained to Randi about her nausea, and Randi responded, "Oh, yeah, I know what you mean." Kendall thought Randi was currently pregnant, so Randi clarified what she meant and told her about her experience. She recalls that in response to this news, Kendall "was not upset that I had done it, but more upset that I had trouble telling her. She has the guts to say that until you're in that situation, how can you really be sure what you would do?" Because Randi saw how open-minded Kendall could be, she had even greater respect for her than before.

The more our friends help us through an abortion experience and understand our feelings, the more indebted to them we may feel. One 22 year old felt this way when she ended a pregnancy two years ago. Her male friend helped her by coming with her to the clinic and giving her emotional support. She comments, "He really carried me through it all. I felt an overwhelming debt to him for at least a year afterward." This, unfortunately, had a negative effect. She says, "Jordan was right there the whole time offering his shoulder, and after a while I did end up leaning on it quite a bit. I got dependent on him and ended up falling in love with him, which was bad, since his girlfriend was my good friend." Jordan did not happen to be available, so that was perhaps not the best turn of events. Still, the strength of her feelings attests to the way in which trust and understanding may unite us with a friend who helps us through an abortion. Knowing how a friend has met our needs so well, we may find that we are quite prepared and willing to assist friends if they, in turn, face unplanned pregnancies and abortions.

Chapter 16

Partners: When the Crisis Highlights a Relationship's Strengths and Weaknesses

A few months ago, when 25-year-old Becky told her boyfriend she was pregnant, he panicked. Becky recalls, "He just didn't know what to do. He didn't know how to react. He would hike in the hills by himself." Twenty-seven-year-old Riana faced a similar situation with her boyfriend six months ago. She says, "The whole thing was freaking him out far more than me. He waffled between extremes, from frightened but solid support, to getting drunk and high to try to make it go away." These women found that they had to fend for themselves as they sought abortions. Not surprisingly, both of those relationships fell apart around the time of the abortions. Neither the men nor the relationships could withstand a force as strong as a pregnancy, or an event as powerful as an abortion.

Twenty-one-year-old Fritzi did not have to prop up her boyfriend during her pregnancy two years ago, but she did have to clarify that her body belonged to her, not him. She says, "It made him feel good to think there was something inside me that was part of him. It was possessive. It just made me feel like a flowerpot!" Their relationship did not last long after the abortion, mostly because it was undefined and "based on having fun."

Unlike these women's partners, some men react to unplanned pregnancies in helpful, caring ways. While the conception is likely to be a shock, a man will not necessarily evade this challenging situation. Sally, age 52, found that her partner had a trustworthy response to her pregnancy. Twelve years ago, they had been involved for only six months when they conceived while using the rhythm method. The pregnancy distressed Sally's boyfriend. He had impregnated his previous partner, who claimed to have been using contraception; she gave birth around the time Sally conceived. Because of these accidental pregnancies, Sally recalls, "My partner was totally traumatized and wanted to rush out to have a vasectomy. I worried that if our relationship did not survive, he might find himself in a relationship where he desired to have children. He was certain about his feelings and went ahead with the vasectomy." His reaction was quite responsible, if also a bit frantic. Sally was equally intent on being responsible; she ended the pregnancy. Neither blamed the other, or had overly high expectations of the other's support. Their relationship continues to this day. In fact, they have been married for five years.

Our partner's immediate reaction to the news of our pregnancy is not the only thing that affects whether the romance will survive. His role in the decision making, his level of support, and his attitude toward the abortion can make a big difference.

HOW INVOLVED WE WANT OUR PARTNERS TO BE

We expect different things of the men in our lives during pregnancies and abortions. One woman may want her partner to help her make a decision. Another woman may want him to leave it entirely up to her. Those varied expectations can make this a confusing time for both men and women. We now look at what individual women have wanted from their partners during this crisis and how this has affected their relationships.

Simone: "His Opinion Was Really Important and Formative to Me"

When Simone, who is 39 and Caucasian, found herself pregnant a year ago, she had no idea what to do. She and her husband, Vic, had had a baby seventeen months before. They both were in the middle of career transitions and planned to conceive in the next year when their lives had stabilized a bit. It seemed overwhelming to them to have another child this soon. Simone recalls that her first response was, "I can't possibly have this child." Her second response was, "How can I not have it?" Then she entered a "third, nebulous stage" in which she realized that she could not make this decision on her own. "I really had to make it in concert with Vic," she muses. "His attitude toward it was very, very important to me."

Until then, Vic had given Simone the space she needed to make a decision. She says, "He was very sensitive about not telling me what he thought until I had somehow worked it out." More than sensitive, Simone thinks Vic was strong and clear in his approach to the problem. He told her, "I am willing to be convinced by you and I'm willing to go through it all" if she felt it were essential to give birth. Vic cautioned her, however, that he saw "the future of this child as bleakness and darkness." When Simone heard that, the picture swung into focus. She thought, "I just cannot do it alone." Ultimately, she says, "The fact that he wasn't happy about the pregnancy really swayed me."

Simone realized that she could not have this child, but could not reconcile herself to having an abortion. She deliberated and agonized. Finally, she chose abortion, but without much conviction. Simone's muddled approach to the situation irked Vic, especially since they had already reasoned their way to the most logical choice. Simone notes, "He was angry at me for not being able to make the decision in a more commonsensical fashion."

Vic stayed with her throughout the procedure and was positive about their choice. Afterward, though, they began to fight about it. Vic insists that Simone pins responsibility for the abortion on him, because she says he was "one of the convincing factors" in her decision and that "his opinion was really important and formative" to her. He wants Simone to own up to the choice. Simone believes she has, but acknowledges, "Maybe it's an easy escape for me. It's easier to say, 'Because he wasn't supporting this pregnancy, I did it,' than for me to say, 'I didn't want to have the baby.'"

Their conflict may revolve around the role each believes Vic should have taken in the decision. Vic apparently thinks he should have had a hands-off approach, at least until she needed his input. When that time came, he gave her the "answer." He seems to have felt that this should have cleared things up, that there was no need for lollygagging. It might have felt confusing to voice his opinion and then to have his good advice ignored.

Simone has a more mixed idea about his role. She resented his attitude in the beginning, "because he didn't have to go through the procedure" and "because it wasn't happening in his body." It was easy for him to be so clear about the decision when he did not have to face the moral qualms that Simone confronted in the operation's physical realities. She notes, "Men can have opinions and we really need to take counsel with them, but they don't have to go through it." Then she rethinks this opinion, saying, "On the other hand, he was there for the whole thing. So it was as if he did go through a lot of it."

Simone seems to have valued his help with the decision, but needed him to understand that a decision that is logical to the brain may not be so obvious to the heart. She also appears torn between seeing the decision as one they should have shared and one over which she should have had autonomy. She may have seen the choice as something to discuss, but the emotional part as something she would have to experience solo.

Their marriage is certainly intact. They are currently five months into a new, planned pregnancy. Still, because they had different expectations of what the abortion required of them, that topic remains a hot spot in their relationship a year later.

Wanda: "I Wanted Him to Read My Mind"

Like Simone, 23-year-old Wanda, who is Caucasian, had mixed ideas about the support she wanted from her live-in boyfriend, Colin, when she conceived six months ago. Her first abortion at age 19 had been a disaster, mainly because her boyfriend at the time abandoned her. Wanda concluded that this is how men react when women conceive, so she felt "terrified" when she discovered her second pregnancy. She dreaded telling Colin the news, and thought, "He's going to walk. I really love this person and I've been so happy with him. I'm pregnant and now he's going to leave." Wanda did tell him she was pregnant and issued a threat at the same time: "If you're going to leave, leave now. If you make me one promise you can't keep, then I'm not responsible for my actions." Colin reassured Wanda, "Whatever you want to do, I'll be there." Colin was true to his word. He and Wanda talked at length about their situation, and eventually chose abortion.

In the days after the procedure, Colin cared for Wanda, giving her hugs, seeing that she took medication, and shopping with her for sanitary pads. He took two days off work to be with her. "I think he was as supportive as he could be," Wanda notes. She adds, however, "I don't think he wanted to pretend like he understood when he didn't."

Although he was so responsive to her physical needs, her emotional ones eluded him. This issue actually arose before her second pregnancy. Because her first abortion had been so traumatic, she had unresolved feelings about it that returned occasionally. One night, she and Colin drank wine and Wanda began to think about how much she missed the fetus. She recalls, "The more I thought about it, the more hysterical I became. I was crying." Colin did not comprehend her feelings. In fact, he belittled them, saying, "Honey, you're just drunk." This was, Wanda says, absolutely the wrong answer. She grew outraged and yelled, "I'm not drunk. I can't make you understand." Wanda laughs now as she thinks about his reaction. She says, "I'm wanting to kill him. And the poor guy's cowering in the corner." The next day, Colin asked, "What was that about?" Wanda shrugged it off, saying, "I don't know. You're probably right. I was just probably upset because of the wine." She does not actually think her emotions were so inconsequential.

Her second abortion brought up less intense feelings, but there was still significant grief and moodiness, which confused Colin. His lack of comprehension angered Wanda. She explains, "I would get frustrated with him because I wanted him to read my mind." She wished he would check in with her about how she felt. When he failed to notice her moods, she became even more upset. Moreover, she hated that he didn't share her feelings.

The matter of how Colin felt about the pregnancy and abortion weighed on Wanda's mind more and more. Once, during an argument about something unrelated to the abortion, she brought it up. Wanda said, "You never told me how you felt about that." She recalls that Colin "looked at me like I'd just stabbed him." Indignant, Colin spat out, "I didn't want to influence your decision. I didn't want to impose my opinion on you one way or another. This was your choice." He was outraged. Not only had his valorous gesture been overlooked, but it had actually become a source of criticism. Wanda responded, "I appreciate that. But that doesn't mean that you don't have feelings." Colin couldn't believe his ears. Wanda recalls, "Oh, he was not pleased. And honestly, I didn't realize that it was such a sore spot with him until I actually said it. The look on his face—he was just stunned. He wasn't expecting that and he didn't want to talk about it anymore."

Later, however, when Colin was less enraged, he shared his feelings with Wanda. He told her, "If you had decided to have that child, I would have been a father for the rest of my life." That idea seemed both good and bad. On the negative side, says Wanda, "It would have changed his identity." At the same time, Colin was thrilled about the pregnancy. He said, "There was this part of me that was so happy. But I didn't want to tell you that." He didn't want to make her decision any tougher than it had to be.

Six months after the abortion, Wanda can see things more from his point of view. She comments, "He doesn't know what to say. He doesn't have the feelings that I have about it. I'm not saying that this was of no consequence to him. I believe that it did affect him. But he didn't have as much at stake in it as I did. And I've got to respect that, too."

Despite her compassion for his feelings, their relationship is languishing and may end soon. Wanda says the abortion plays only a small part in that. The larger issue is that their communication has deteriorated. This lapse in communication probably accounts for most of the ways in which Wanda and Colin could not connect after her abortion. He tried hard to do what he thought was right and to give her the proper space; he cannot understand why his efforts went unappreciated. She did her best to communicate her feelings to him, and had trouble accepting that he neither comprehended nor shared those emotions. She wanted the intimacy that comes with discussing feelings, particularly after the abortion. He saw the importance of talking before the abortion. The tragedy here is that Colin and Wanda had the best intentions and acted as lovingly as they could.

How Women and Men Approach the Decision Differently

Simone's and Wanda's stories show how men and women tend to have different needs when they make an abortion decision. Women generally wish to talk about their feelings, because they want to explore and vent their emotions and because such sharing feels intimate. They may feel indecisive and truly want men's perspective, particularly if they have always made decisions in tandem. A woman may include her partner in the decision in an attempt to consider his feelings. Some women also feel that their partners ought to give the matter some attention and that women should not bear the burden of the decision alone. Beyond discussing the decision with their partners before the abortion, women may want men to come to the procedure and to offer support there. Women may hope that their partners will talk about feelings for as long as they persist after the abortion.

Men tend to approach the matter quite differently. For many, the first priority is to resolve the problem that the pregnancy presents. They may feel that they must take charge. They concern themselves with the practical issues, especially the decision. If they attend to emotional matters, they might prefer to focus on the woman's feelings. Expressing their own feelings may seem to burden her or add to the confusion. They may want to appear strong and invulnerable, believing that this will reassure the woman. Individual men have different ideas about when they should step in and give their opinion, but they often feel that once they have voted for or against the pregnancy, they have done their duty. Some men may feel upset that even though they have expressed a well-thought-out opinion, the decision-making process lingers, seemingly without structure or discipline. They may also be enraged that they are so powerless over the final outcome. Some men are bewildered if a woman feels quite emotional after the abortion, which should have solved the problem.

Adding to this melee are issues of gender politics. For a long time, women have insisted that because pregnancy affects their bodies, the decision must be theirs. Many men have respected this perspective. It has become fashionable, however, for men to explore their sensitivity, voicing their feelings and asserting their responsibilities. The issue of how involved men should be in the decision seems to change with the times.

Given the vast differences between the way men and women approach this issue, it is no wonder that communication can fall apart. If partners want different things from each other, one may fail to meet the other's needs and may seem to have the wrong priorities.

Sharing Power in Abortion Decisions

Two partners may have a great deal of tension whenever they make decisions. They may struggle for power. As a couple decides the fate of a pregnancy, it is crucial for them to be able to communicate. Each must have room to express feelings. If one dominates, the other will not have this space. The subordinate partner may feel hurt, angry, and powerless.

For example, when 20-year-old Ricki told her boyfriend, Wayne, that she was pregnant a few months ago, his response was, "You have to get an abortion." To Ricki, this was unthinkable. Both she and Wayne are Black Muslims and don't believe in abortion. Wayne felt willing to overlook his principles, as he and Ricki are in college and have no money. As Ricki considered the pros and cons, she felt "split in two." For several weeks, Wayne pressured her to end the pregnancy. She waited for him to change his mind, and explains, "I wanted him to say, 'Don't have it,' so I would have an excuse not to have" the abortion. When his last-minute change of heart did not occur, she went ahead with the abortion. She never reconciled herself to this decision, but only followed his orders. For this reason, she has found the abortion difficult to accept. Their relationship has continued, and they plan to marry sometime. It is possible, though, that Ricki will not always carry out Wayne's commands. She may listen more closely to her own feelings in the future.

Like Ricki, 22-year-old Brittany wanted to keep the baby when she conceived two years ago. Like Wayne, Brittany's boyfriend Dean wanted her to have an abortion. Brittany, however, was the one with power when she and Dean made the decision. They had already had one baby and one abortion together, and Dean had supported those decisions. With this new pregnancy, though, he expressed "doubt about the whole thing," as he was depressed about his career and did not want to be saddled with another child. Plus, he and Brittany weren't even dating; they only shared parenting responsibilities. He showed Brittany his resistance by sleeping with other women.

Brittany was unable to hear his point at first. She wanted to have her baby, no matter what, and figured he would eventually overcome his resistance to the pregnancy. Then, after receiving a friend's advice, Brittany began to see that Dean's reluctance about the pregnancy "wasn't going to go away" and that he would be angry if she carried to term. As she observes, "He felt like it was being done against his will." Brittany looked at their relationship honestly. She notes, "I have this pattern of wanting to control everything, and he has a pattern of letting other people control him." She saw how that was true in this situation, and decided she didn't want things to be that way. She realized that being in control was not the same as being powerful. Exercising true power would mean listening "to what someone was saying about their concerns." Brittany ended her pregnancy and began to talk with Dean about the relationship. In six weeks, they reunited.

A pregnancy decision can highlight a power imbalance in a relationship, one that may have gone unnoticed before. It may not seem like such a big deal to let one's partner have his or her way from day to day. With a pregnancy, however, it may suddenly feel intolerable to have one's needs and wishes overlooked. The pregnancy prompted Dean to assert himself at last, which was quite necessary. Brittany began to see that power wasn't about winning, but about being flexible and unselfish. Because both of them shifted the balance of power, they were able to move toward equality in their relationship.

Wanting to Deal with the Pregnancy Alone

Some couples handle an unexpected pregnancy by having each person make a decision separately and then sharing their conclusions. Others of us insist on doing everything ourselves once we realize we are pregnant. We think this should be very much our own experience and want little help or interference from our partners. Sharing this decision with a man may violate our political beliefs. Many of us insist on total sovereignty over our bodies and feel that asking a man his opinion is unsavory or even dangerous.

We may not tell our partner about the pregnancy at all. This is especially likely if we have had a noncommittal relationship with him and do not want to burden him with the news. Some women feel fine about this decision. Others are slightly unresolved about it. That has been Tanya's experience. A 27 year old who had a fling at age 19 with a friend of a friend, she comments, "I barely knew him and certainly didn't feel like I could ask for money from him. I really felt like it was all my fault and that he was not to blame." Later, she changed her mind. Tanya explains, "I felt a bit guilty about not telling the man I was with. He may have benefited from knowing what I went through and maybe would have taken better precautions in the future." She has seen him a few times since the abortion and notes, "He has no idea that I became pregnant by our encounter." It can feel very strange if the man who impregnated us is oblivious to his significance in our life.

HOW THE EXPERIENCE TESTS THE RELATIONSHIP

Any crisis can reveal the worst and best in a relationship. A pregnancy and abortion highlight the conflicts or bonds that always existed in the romance, but were never so sharply apparent. Problems may have reared their heads before, but the couple may have tried to ignore them. A pregnancy can make problems unavoidable, both in the short term as the couple clashes over making a decision, or in the long term as incompatible desires for the future emerge. A relationship that might have lingered in a flawed state for years may suddenly seem unviable. The end can come more quickly, partly because an unexpected conception forces two people to look at their future in a way they may not have done before. As one 32 year old puts it, a pregnancy "speeds up the whole process of a relationship. People may end up breaking up more quickly after that, because you've already looked down the rosy path and said, 'Ah, no! I like you, you're good in bed, you make great lasagna, but I'm not ready to have a baby with you.'" She also notes that a pregnancy and abortion "actually can make the relationship a little closer, because you touch upon some core issues." The pregnancy and abortion experience may signal to a couple that they love each other more than they even knew and that they always want to stay together.

They may feel that conceiving together is so noteworthy that the pregnancy alone has forged a special bond between them. The crisis can heighten emotions and strengthen convictions, providing a wonderful chance for intimacy. Each may feel as if the other person has revealed a true self and that they can trust who that other person is. Two people may come out of an abortion experience saying, "If we could make it through that, we can survive anything." They may feel that the romance has passed a test with flying colors. We now explore the ways in which a pregnancy and abortion can affect a relationship, from devastating it to ensuring its survival.

When There's More of a Tryst Than a Relationship

When many of us conceive, we are not in a monogamous, set-in-stone relationship. We may have an on-and-off romance, or a one-night fling. It can be confusing to find ourselves pregnant but not to know quite where we stand with the guy or what to expect from him. That happened to Elissa, who is Caucasian and 24. She met Miguel nine months ago, when she began to work at her father's company. Miguel, a South American who drove a company truck, was off-limits; Elissa's dad forbade her to date anyone in the company. Elissa and Miguel developed a "passion" so strong that they became involved anyway. She explains, "It was very obvious that this was dangerous for both of us." Not only were their jobs at stake, but Miguel also lived with a woman, who knew about his relationship with Elissa. He was married to a third woman, as well.

Elissa had trouble sharing him. She says, "I had him one night a week. Nothing about that feels whole." Her relationship with Miguel also felt unsatisfying because he was sometimes distant. She knew that the relationship was not "healthy," but could not stay away from this "caring, consuming, dangerous affair." Making things even more difficult, Elissa and Miguel conceived after two months. Elissa soon suspected that she was pregnant and recalls, "The idea of carrying his baby seemed absolutely wonderful. I told him that I hoped, to a certain degree, that I was. He held my stomach. We made love that night."

The next day, they planned to go to a clinic for a pregnancy test. He didn't show. Furious, Elissa took a test at home, which was positive. She let him have it for not meeting her, but told him about the pregnancy. He smiled and said he wanted her to have the baby. Elissa recalls, "For a moment, I considered having it. And I was a woman who didn't want children, who knew he was already involved, who knew this was crazy. I understood the sad stories of women having a baby to keep a man. I felt pathetic." Despite her urge to carry to term, she knew this was unrealistic. She eventually opted for abortion. She explains, "It was my decision mostly–and he agreed to respect me," even though he wanted the baby so much that he told his family and girlfriend that Elissa was pregnant.

His enthusiasm about the pregnancy prevented him from supporting Elissa at the abortion. The night before the procedure, she recalls, "He was cold and horrible. Miguel did not hold me all night." His coldness persisted the next day. At the clinic, Elissa sobbed for an hour after the abortion, which had felt violating and lonely. Miguel responded by saying that every woman there was smiling, except her. He also said he had heard from the doctor that Elissa complained during the procedure. When Elissa and Miguel left the clinic, she began to scream at him and told him "what a bastard he was." She says, "I was totally out of control. At the same time, I wanted his comfort more than anything on this planet, and I had never felt so far from him." Elissa goes on, "The next morning, he apologized. And said he had wanted that baby." That week, he was hot and cold.

Now, five months have passed since her abortion. Elissa feels confused about him, but continues to see him. She says she is angry about his "inability to cope, to give me what I needed and deserved." She also resents that she has loved him well and has not received much love back. It helps that Miguel has "admitted how horrible he was."

The pregnancy and abortion have exacerbated the problems in their liaison. Miguel was not fully committed to her before they conceived. When Elissa most needed him during the experience, he acted as if his participation and caring were not essential. Part of his ambivalence may have come from his excitement about the pregnancy. But before she ever made a decision about the pregnancy, he showed his feeble commitment by not meeting her for the pregnancy test. This affair doesn't seem to have much of a future, but it might have gone on longer if a pregnancy had not interfered and made Elissa need more.

When Pregnancy and Abortion Destroy the Relationship

A pregnancy also disrupted Clarissa's relationship with Russ. Clarissa, who is 30 and Caucasian, had 3-year-old twin girls when she and Russ conceived five years ago. They had been dating for a year and felt very close. When Clarissa discovered the pregnancy, she was thrilled, but Russ was adamant that having a child would ruin his life. Clarissa explains, "He had plans that he would have to forget about." Clarissa planned to have the child anyway. She recalls, "I explained to him that he wouldn't have any obligation to us, that we wouldn't ask anything of him." But, she says, Russ could not "bear the thought of knowing he fathered a child and was not involved in his life."

Clarissa suddenly understood Russ's position. She muses, "I never considered how much of an impact it would have on his life, whether I did or did not have the child. I realized how selfish this was. I was thinking of myself and the baby, but not of him and not completely of the baby." She figured Russ might come to love the child in time, but decided she could not gamble with such a vital matter. Clarissa explains, "It was important that I came to that serious realization about the child's relationship with the father. I had a poor relationship with mine and I wouldn't wish that on anyone. (I was also unwanted.)" Clarissa feels pleased that she took Russ's feelings into account. She notes, "My final decision to have the abortion was probably the most selfless thing I ever did."

Russ came with her to the abortion. Clarissa notes, "I made sure he came. I didn't have to coax him, but I would have done anything necessary to make sure that he was there through it all. I can't imagine not having him there just to completely understand the experience. What we were both doing and what it was going to mean to both of us. He saw the entire procedure." He cried during the surgery. Clarissa recalls, "I looked at him and saw tears rolling down his face. When I saw his tears, I lost it and broke into a deep sob."

Clarissa and Russ shared the decision making and felt connected during the procedure, but that was not enough to preserve the relationship. "It deteriorated from that point on," she notes. The pregnancy had exposed irreconcilable differences, mainly in their reproductive plans. Russ said he never wanted kids, which didn't sit well with Clarissa. This conflict became even more pronounced after the abortion. Clarissa recalls, "He couldn't stand to be around my kids after that. Perhaps they were too much of a reminder." A few months after the abortion, when he actually told Clarissa that he did not want to see her girls anymore, she said, "See ya," and ended the relationship promptly. "That same day, done, over, no more," she says emotionlessly. She says that breaking up was not difficult "after all we'd been through. I ended it and for the most part didn't look back."

When the Relationship Suffers, but Survives

Sometimes, relationships take a hit during a pregnancy and abortion crisis, but recover and become stronger than ever. That was the case for 22-year-old Mindy and her boyfriend Kurt. They had dated for five years before the pregnancy and had problems off and on during that period. After she had an abortion seventeen months ago, they broke up. Now, they are back together and feel as though they will marry someday. At their interview for this book, they both discuss how the abortion temporarily ended their romance.

Kurt explains, "I don't think it was because of the abortion we broke up. It was more the fact that there was a total breakdown in communication. And the abortion, that "was probably the last straw that broke the camel's back." Mindy comments, "It's not really that the communication was bad." Kurt cuts in, saying, "You expect for me to communicate to you in one way, but you never told me that. You would expect me to do something, but it would never come back to me as, 'Why don't we do this?' And since I had no idea how to act . . ." He trails off and Mindy concurs, "It was a mess."

Mindy later elaborates on the problem. After the abortion, she and Kurt returned to their separate colleges. She wanted him to keep calling her to find out how she was doing. Instead, she says, "I didn't really give him a chance to call me, because I called him ten times a day. I just felt like he wasn't acting the way I wanted him to act." He wasn't as "concerned" as he might have been, which made her angry and depressed. They broke up in the March after the November abortion, and Kurt immediately began dating someone else. Both he and Mindy felt relieved to stop arguing and to stop facing their problems. Mindy muses, "We both needed to get away from each other, because that had caused so much pain for each of us separately and between us. We each needed to be by ourselves to get over everything." They did sort out their feelings on their own. By the end of that summer, they reunited. The relationship improved immensely. Mindy explains, "When we started going out again, we could talk about it." That was about nine months ago.

If a pregnancy and abortion stir up a relationship as it did for Mindy and Kurt, it may not take a breakup and reconciliation to improve matters. For instance, 28-year-old Yvette and Rod, her boyfriend of three years, felt turbulence around the time of her abortion three months ago, but readjusted and now plan to marry. Yvette believes that a desire to settle down with Rod contributed to her pregnancy in the first place. She explains, "It was the second time I screwed up on birth control pills in a year. I've been taking it for five years. Suddenly we're very happy and I screwed up twice." Yvette continues, "It was obvious to me after the second time why it was happening. I wanted to invest in this little nest and make it more of a home. I unconsciously wanted to get pregnant."

As much as Yvette may have wanted to conceive on an unconscious level, she was devastated when she took a home pregnancy test and it "turned the wrong color." She came out of the bathroom sobbing and told Rod the test was positive. He didn't handle it very well. Yvette explains, "He's a great guy. He just has that typical male attribute of not knowing what to do if I'm too emotional. After about an hour, he was comforting me."

Rod rose to the occasion that day, but didn't know how to respond to Yvette's mood swings. She attributes the problem to a few things. First, she says, "He's not a good talker." Second, she usually expresses so many feelings to him that he doesn't know which ones to take seriously. Third, he seemed to lack empathy. Yvette comments, "I feel like he didn't try to really understand how horrible it was emotionally." Rod came with her to the abortion and held her hand. After the procedure, more problems arose, however. Yvette explains, "He had imagined that once I had the abortion, I would just be back to normal. But I was much worse than I had been before. And he wasn't very supportive. He went and played his bass." Yvette laments, "It was the time I needed him most."

Since then, one more problem has come to the surface. Yvette says she is "totally afraid of getting pregnant again," which affects their sex life. She does not feel that she can be terribly open about this fear with Rod, however, because as she explains, "I don't want to discourage him. I don't want him to become less sexual." There is a context for her fear. Yvette explains, "He's the first one I've been with who didn't get disinterested in sex with me after three months, like all the other guys I've been with. They want to go have sex with somebody else. And we've been together for years, and he just wants to have sex with me. It's great. I feel like there's a delicate balance and I don't want to disturb it."

Aside from this problem, their relationship has improved since the abortion. Rod proposed soon after the procedure. She's been proposing for two years, and he has refused, but now he likes the idea. Yvette comments, "Ever since the abortion, he sure does hold my hand a lot. And he's a lot warmer." The reason? Yvette believes both she and Rod have changed. She explains, "I have been more loving. Less jealous. I don't know if that's because of the abortion. It might have helped me grow up." Rod concurs that she has changed. Also, he now sees her as "somebody who's capable of having a baby." Yvette muses, "I think he realized that he really did want us to have kids some day." The pregnancy caused some problems in their romance, but has ultimately brought them closer.

When the Crisis Strengthens the Relationship

A pregnancy and abortion can make a couple closer without causing any problems. The partners can speak openly about their most serious feelings and may realize the depth of their love and commitment. This was true for Carrie and Olin seven years ago, when Carrie was age 35. They had met in September and had begun dating right away. In January, they moved in together. The same month, Carrie conceived. She recalls how that affected their romance: "We had to talk seriously very quickly, because this was a very important issue–a life and death matter. We had to have our communication be very clear." He already had two children from a previous marriage. Carrie had none, but wanted some badly. Before she met Olin, she figured that if she reached her mid-thirties and had no partner, she would become a single parent. When she conceived, some of these ideas lingered. Olin dismantled her "fantasies" and "ideals" about parenting and was, as Carrie says, "very clear about how difficult it would be for us to start that way." She explains, "It was really his input and our working it through that led us to decide to terminate." Without his intervention, she says, "I would have just gone along with it. If left to my own devices, I wouldn't have thought it through clearly. I would have just let the pregnancy happen and crossed my fingers."

They talked about their feelings for a long time, which not only helped them make the best decision, but also created intimacy. Carrie recalls, "I felt incredibly positive about the communication" that they had. She adds, "We met the challenge to talk about it."

Carrie observes that the pregnancy "cemented our relationship. It gave us a crisis to work through." She adds, "It caused us to define ourselves in a way we wouldn't have had to before then. We had made that commitment to each other" and "going through something like this" really "reaffirmed" that commitment. Shortly after the abortion, they married. They now have two sons, whom Carrie and Olin conceived when they were ready.

HOW THE ABORTION AFFECTS SUBSEQUENT RELATIONSHIPS

If our relationship does not survive an abortion, we may become involved with a new partner at some point, and might want to tell that person about the abortion. Maybe we have asserted the importance of birth control and want to explain the reason for our concerns. Or we may see sharing this experience as a path to intimacy, a way to share ourselves.

Telling New Partners About Our Experiences

Nineteen-year-old Irene faced this situation soon after the abortion she had two months ago. Two weeks after her abortion, she had a one-night stand with a guy she met at a party. Both had drunk a lot, but Irene was lucid enough to think about safe sex. She was on the pill, but didn't tell this guy about that. Instead, she said, "I would prefer we use a condom." Laughing in amazement, Irene recalls how he said, "Don't worry about it. What are you afraid of?" She answered scornfully, "Ooh, I'm afraid of maybe getting pregnant." He did not see her point. "I won't get you pregnant," he said. Irene responded, "Oh my God! What are you talking about?" Still, he maintained his original stance–that contraception was not necessary. Irene recalls, "He seemed to find it very amusing that I was actually concerned about this. He took the whole subject extremely lightly." She then told him about her recent pregnancy, figuring that would change his attitude. Instead, he shrugged, "That's not a big deal." He is the only new partner she has told about her abortion. She explains, "The reaction was so negative that I haven't told any other men yet." While his response was not very encouraging, he may not be the best litmus test.

We may not anticipate just how hard it will be to discuss the abortion with a new partner. It may seem so far in the past that we may not expect the large amount of emotion we still feel about it. "I thought it would be easier to talk about," says a 27 year old who had an abortion at age 19. She adds, "It was difficult talking about it with my boyfriend (now my husband), but once I got it out, I was very relieved." We may see telling a new partner about it as an uncomfortable task that we must accomplish.

In contrast, we may find it pretty simple to tell new partners about an abortion. A 38 year old notes that telling her lover about the abortion she had at age 24 went smoothly. She says, "Before we married, I told my husband that I had been pregnant and had an abortion. It was not an issue between us." If we have resolved our feelings about the abortion and need little support for the way we felt, we may find it painless to discuss. In fact, when we tell new partners about our abortion, we may focus less on our emotions and more on how they respond. If they are not shocked, the conversation may not seem that significant.

If we tell new partners about our abortion, we may learn that they have previous experience with this matter and harbor strong feelings about it. That was true for 23-year-old Wanda, who found herself in a "truly twisted" relationship with Al right after her abortion four years ago. Al treated Wanda as a substitute for his ex-girlfriend, whom he had mistreated during their abortion experience. Wanda explains, "He felt badly about his girlfriend. I was a proxy person to whom he could go, 'There, there sweetheart.'" Wanda also treated Al as a substitute for her boyfriend, who had abandoned her after her pregnancy. She jumped at the chance to talk to a man about the abortion. Al and Wanda forged an immediate intimacy. After two months, though, they had worked through their feelings about the abortions and had nothing further to say. Wanda feels amazed that they ever engaged in this arrangement, but feels grateful that Al helped her understand her feelings.

Even if our new partners have had no experience with abortion, we may feel more bonded with them after sharing our experience. For instance, an 18 year old told her boyfriend about the abortion she had at age 16. She notes that this conversation "brought us closer. He was upset, but very supportive, and glad I had told him." Another woman, age 29, feared telling her boyfriend about the abortion she had at age 18. She explains, "I was worried about my boyfriend's reaction–if he would have a conflict with it or think less of me for it. But he took it in stride. He's a reasonable, understanding, and open-minded guy. He understands my position and loves me for me." We may have such a positive reaction from our new partner that it confirms how solid our relationship is. One 31 year old found this when she told her partner about the abortion she had five years ago. She notes that he "really understands it to an extent that has surprised me." He understands her so well in general that they plan to marry next year; the abortion may be just one more area where he intuitively grasps how she feels.

Unlike these women, we may choose never to tell new partners. Just as we may remain silent about the abortion with family members and friends, we might think that our partners would judge us, or that our relationship would not benefit from such a disclosure. One 56 year old had this point of view when she married many years ago. She never told her husband about the pregnancy she ended at age 25, because she did not know whether he would approve. Besides, she doesn't feel that telling a spouse everything about oneself strengthens a marriage. She didn't feel strange about her silence; the abortion had no relevance to her marriage. Aside from the reasons she named, she may have hesitated to tell him about the abortion because in any relationship, it can be tricky to decide how much to talk about an ex-lover. Such talk can be healing and bring us closer to our new partner, or it can seem intrusive. If we do speak of the pregnancy to a new partner, we may want to act as if we conceived by ourselves. It might not feel safe to mention the other man.

Criteria for a New Partner

Whether or not we tell our new partner, we may take the abortion into account when we select the next love of our lives. It may seem essential to date someone pro-choice. As one 25 year old who has had two abortions notes, "I would never sleep with anyone who wasn't pro-choice. That was true before also, but I wasn't as stringent. Now, I would never sleep with anybody who would try to force me to carry a child that I didn't want." We may figure that a pro-choice man won't condemn us for our abortion and will be open to abortion if we conceive again. Plus, if we feel more pro-choice than ever, we may find it inconceivable to sleep with a political "enemy." We may require a new partner to have the same views as we do, not only on abortion, but also on pregnancy, sex, and birth control.

If we realize during our abortion experience that our partner feels differently than we do about having kids, we may try to find a man of like mind on this issue. This criterion can seem more urgent if our ex revealed a resistance to having children, or if the pregnancy made us realize just how much we want to have kids. We may begin to screen out people who don't have the same urge to parent. As 30-year-old Clarissa puts it, five years after her abortion, "If I couldn't see myself having a child with that person, I would not start a real relationship. I'd usually find out how they felt about children very quickly."

No matter what our specific criteria are for a new partner, we may long for a more solid relationship, treating romances more seriously and becoming pickier about our partners. Sheila, a 26-year-old Asian American, feels this way two years after her abortion. During that crisis, her partner shattered every belief she had about their relationship. Before they conceived, they planned to marry. Then, he delayed that plan, suggesting that they keep living together to see if the relationship improved. When they conceived after a method failure, the situation worsened. Sheila was unsure what to do about the pregnancy. While he did not force her to have an abortion, she felt she had no alternative. Sheila notes that his reaction "confirmed my worst fear–that I was essentially alone in this specific crisis and the relationship as a whole." She comments that after the abortion, "The already deteriorating relationship buckled under the pressure of living together without a clear idea of what we wanted."

Sheila says she now treats their romance as a "learning experience" and a "reminder to me that I should be very selective about my lovers." She explains how her method failure reinforced this belief: "No birth control method is completely reliable. With that in mind, the men I choose to be in a relationship with are all potential fathers. Ideally, I would only choose to be with a man who could be an enthusiastic partner and father. I want to be with someone who could rise to the occasion." Unlike some women who quickly screen out men who have no interest in fatherhood, Sheila believes she can only learn about a man slowly. She comments, "I know that it takes time to develop a relationship and really get to know someone's true character. Although I am a very physical and passionate woman, I can and will wait for physical intimacy with my next partner. I want to be sure of him."

Chapter 17

Gender Awareness: When Feelings About Women and Men Change

Three years ago, when Nicola was 22 years old, she had her first abortion at a feminist health center. Nicola, who is Caucasian, calls it an "amazing, great place" for several reasons, starting with the procedure. A woman from the clinic held Nicola's hand throughout the surgery and told her what to expect. Nicola recalls, "She explained every touch. 'Now you will feel a hand on your buttock. Fingers opening your labia.' She told me when the speculum was going to be inserted, when I was going to feel pain, how long it would last, and how to make it easier. 'Imagine a weight on your abdomen. Breathe deeply. Now you will feel some cramping. Now you will again.'" Nicola also appreciated the female doctor, and comments, "She was friendly and nice and explained the whole procedure to me." The abortion hurt, but because these women supplied Nicola with so much knowledge, she says she found the procedure "less traumatic than a lot of regular gynecological exams I've been to, with impersonal male doctors who don't tell you what they're doing." She found the clinic atmosphere reassuring, too, and says, "There was a blackboard in the bathroom where women had drawn pictures and written their thanks and relief. There were all kinds of women in the waiting room–teenagers and college students and a mother with her three-year-old son." The patients also recovered together from their abortions. Nicola recalls, "There was such a supportive feeling in that room, even though we didn't talk to each other. All of us were going through the aftermath together, rather than alone in some small, sterile room. It seemed impossible to feel shame in that situation, surrounded by women who had just been through the same thing. Recovering with other women took away all feelings of loneliness and made me feel strong and hopeful."

What Nicola has described is more than just relief. At her abortion, Nicola had a heightened awareness of gender. She felt close to the female clinicians, to the women who had left messages on the bathroom blackboard, and to the other patients. Pregnancy and abortion are such female experiences that they can easily make one feel closer to other women, and perhaps more distant from men. This chapter will explore how an abortion can spark strong feelings about both genders.

FEELING CLOSER TO WOMEN

An abortion may make us gain a new appreciation for women. We might have a higher regard for those who preceded us in fighting for abortion rights. As one 23 year old says six months after her second abortion, her experiences with ending pregnancies "helped me see women as fiercely strong. I felt a part of a long history of struggle, and I am so happy to be here today behind all of those who earned these rights I enjoy." In ending pregnancies, she has become part of a certain community, whose members she respects and with whom she has much in common. Another 23 year old has a similar sense after two abortions. She feels "more in touch with every single woman in the world" because her unplanned pregnancy opened her eyes to the challenges women share. She now has "tons more female friends," whereas she used to befriend mainly men.

Solidarity with the Other Patients

We may leave an abortion facility feeling more bonded with women, not because the clinicians were warm, as in Nicola's case, but because of how we have interacted with the other clients. In fact, if the clinicians are cold, the patients may offer each other extra support. That was the case when Vivian, who is age 22 and Caucasian, had an abortion a year ago. The clinic was, as Vivian describes it, "a real assembly line. It had probably a hundred women on Saturday and it was really impersonal. I was told that you get some counseling. None at all." Vivian found the clinic staff quite abrasive. The male doctor used the instruments quickly and "shoved the speculum up really hard," which made Vivian scared and tense. She adds that one nasty woman barked, "Get up! Put your legs up!"

In this cold environment, where no one provided counseling, Vivian found herself providing this service to a distraught 18 year old who moved with her through the clinic. Vivian recalls that this young woman began saying, "I don't believe I'm doing this. This is horrible." Vivian tried to address her fears, asking about her feelings. The irony of the situation did not escape Vivian. She comments, "I was counseling her! And here I am sitting in this paper gown myself, thinking, 'I shouldn't be the one having to do this!'"

Vivian experienced more female solidarity as she recovered from the general anesthesia. She woke up, realizing that she was in a room with other women who were also awakening. At first, Vivian found it weird that people watched her come out of unconsciousness. Then, she appreciated the chance to share this moment with other women. She comments, "It was actually neat, because we all were sitting around. And this girl who'd been upset was now cracking jokes. It was a real bonding. All these women who'd just been through the same thing." She feels that the women supported each other through this experience. Vivian also liked that "a real variety of people" with different ages and faces had come together like this. She found that unity "really powerful."

Wanda, age 23, had a similar experience. At age 19, she went through a physically difficult second-trimester abortion, as did the other clinic patients that day. She remembers that another woman was in so much pain afterward that it "sounded like she was going to die." Wanda put her hand out to the other woman, murmuring, "It's going to be okay. You're going to be okay." They lay on stretchers, holding hands. The other woman asked for her phone number at the end, so that they could talk about their feelings. She did call Wanda once, but they never actually spoke again. Wanda wishes they could. As she puts it, "It was like someone you'd been through a war with."

Virginia: "My Female Friends and My Mom Offered the Best Support"

We may bond with women in realms beyond the abortion facility. For instance, 19-year-old Virginia, who is white, black, and Native

American, felt closer to her mother and female friends when she ended her pregnancy a year and a half ago.

At first, Virginia's friends did not play a central role in her experience. She turned for support to her mother and the guy she had dated for five months. Virginia gives her mom and boyfriend a lot of credit for the way they responded. She observes, "They were both wonderful (especially Mom), but nothing they said or did was quite what I wanted." That dissonance between their warmth and her dissatisfaction continued at the abortion. Virginia's mom and boyfriend sat in the waiting room during the procedure and visited Virginia in the recovery room. She notes, however, "I didn't really want them there. I didn't want to talk to anyone. I think I would rather have been alone for a while."

In the period after the abortion, her boyfriend seemed ill at ease and ashamed of the abortion. Their relationship ended seven months later. In contrast, Virginia's mom kept telling her daughter how proud she was of her "for making a mature decision and handling it well." Virginia calls this support "most important" and says it "did so much for me."

Virginia did not expect much support from her close female friends, and told them about the abortion only after it happened. She may have had low hopes where they were concerned because she feels "a little withdrawn" when friends who haven't had an abortion discuss that topic. She doesn't feel that they can understand her experience. Her friends surprised her, though. She says they were able to "just be honest, talk to me, hug me," which was exactly what Virginia needed. Plus, since she ended her pregnancy, three of her friends have also had abortions. Virginia notes that those three friends "have an unspoken understanding about some things that I could never have explained."

Virginia explains that when she dealt with her mother and female friends, "I never once felt judged, only loved. They helped me deal with my emotions and cared for me, but never seemed to pity me." Because her girlfriends and mother were so wonderful, Virginia comments, "It made me feel closer to women. My female friends and my mom offered the best support, while my boyfriend just couldn't talk about it. It made me realize that there are some things a man will never be able to do that a female friend can. I really wanted him to put his arm around me and love me and listen to me. He was so uncomfortable that he couldn't, but my girlfriends could." Because the women in her life seem to have so much empathy, Virginia found the closeness she needed from members of her own gender.

Opal: "Compassion for Womanhood on a Global Level"

Virginia felt closer to women because they were empathic toward her. After an abortion, we may experience a variation on this; we might feel a rush of empathy for other women. We may see ourselves as having the same elements of power or powerlessness in our lives. Thirty-seven-year-old Opal now feels "compassion for womanhood on a global level." In this spirit of solidarity, she wants to blur the distinctions between people. Instead of indicating her race on her questionnaire, she writes, "I don't believe in color." She did say in an earlier phone call, however, that her last name is Native American. Opal states that her abortion at age 22 supplied only part of her global compassion. The rest came from her "varied female experiences." One way she expresses this compassion is by noting that twentieth-century women have unprecedented opportunities, and therefore challenges. She comments, "We are the first women to enjoy choice, especially in regard to reproductive rights. We have no role models and it's difficult." This lack of foremothers to guide the way may be what motivates Opal to be there for other women.

FEELING DISILLUSIONED WITH MEN

What also drives Opal in that direction is that her abortion experience awakened her to large inequities in gender relations. Henry, the man who impregnated her, was 31, nine years older than she, and had a great deal of influence over her decisions. She recalls, "He totally refused to take any birth control responsibility." Opal, who was engaged in substance abuse at the time, had little control over her own behavior, much less his. When they conceived, Henry pressured her to end the pregnancy. His relationship with Opal was "nonbinding," as he had other commitments. Opal notes, "He had a child from a previous marriage and couldn't handle even that responsibility." His pressures swayed her. She explains, "I got caught up in the trap of feeling that I had to be fair to the sperm donor's request that I get an abortion. The guy really objected: it was going to screw up his life, he had another kid, it would hurt the other kid, etc." Opal's ex-lover, a woman, also felt that Opal was too young to become a parent, so she encouraged Opal to end the pregnancy. Opal says, "She had had an abortion before, so she was understanding." Opal's abortion turned out to be incomplete. When Henry discovered this, "He flipped and began to apply more pressure."

All at once, Opal understood a few things. She explains, "This guy was a huge asshole, and I suddenly realized I wasn't making the *choice*, and reproductive freedom was supposed to be about a woman's right to choose." She went ahead with a second procedure, which did end the pregnancy, but she never saw the situation in the same way again. Opal now says: "I was under the illusion that I was a free person and that I wasn't taking any of that sexist crap. Right. There I was, giving up my freedom of choice, because I felt sorry for some lying guy. That guy who I later found out had a history of beating up women and never paid a dime of child support for the kid he claimed to love so much. He wanted control and power over my choice and, like a stupid idiot, I fell for it. I think even without his pressure, I would have still decided to abort. I was unprepared for motherhood. But it would have been my choice. Now I feel that I gave away my power."

She feels that surrendering her choice to an older, dominant man was "just the tip of the sexist iceberg" for her, the start of "one, long chain of events." Henry went on to beat her. She left him. At age 23, Opal conceived again. She "adamantly refused an abortion" because she was so angry about having been pressured into one before. She gave birth and delivered once more at age 26. She does not indicate whether those children were Henry's. When one of her kids was 2 years old, Henry kidnapped him. Opal had Henry arrested, but the court only "slapped his wrist with, 'Bad boy, stop that,'" and insisted that her son had to continue seeing Henry, even though he feared being taken again.

Opal fumes that this society "lets men basically own women and children, but lets them take no responsibility for any of their rearing." She feels enraged that men think they have a right to control her body through laws, violence, and social conditioning. To redress this injustice, Opal insists that women should exclude men from female reproduction issues. She says, "If an individual woman feels the need to be 'fair' and include the sperm donor in her decision, that's her decision. For me, I think it's very dangerous to let men have any say over any part of our lives." She notes that while there are individual exceptions, collectively, men "do not have our best interest in mind." While she might have remained angry just at Henry after her abortion, Opal has taken a broader view and has extended these personal experiences into a wide political framework.

Like Opal, we may feel disillusioned on a personal level in our relationships with men, and then generalize from those personal experiences to form a worldview about gender relations. As we realize that what has happened to us also occurs elsewhere, we may not feel as isolated or as focused on the particulars. Instead, we might think in terms of patterns and trends. It may feel as if we have risen to a higher level, with a grander perspective on the way the world works, the way people relate to each other, the way things should be. We may feel convinced that we know the truth and feel an urgent need to spread our knowledge and to counter ignorance. Feelings of anger and power may go hand in hand as we seek to correct problems in whatever ways we can.

Sabine: "I Don't Believe in Love or Marriage Anymore"

Twenty-three-year-old Sabine, who is African American and who ended a pregnancy two years ago, has gone through such a process. Drawing on her abortion experience, she feels outraged that some men threaten women's autonomy in reproductive decisions. Sabine found her abortion so wrenching that she swears she will never have another and considers herself pro-life in that way. She sees this as entirely different from having people who are incapable of becoming pregnant step in and tell her what to do. When men presume to be experts on something that has never happened to them, it trivializes her pain and her intelligence.

Aside from her anger about male attempts to restrict abortion, Sabine feels greatly disillusioned about men and their capacity to commit to women. This rage also comes directly out of her experience. Sabine recalls, "I got pregnant with my second boyfriend in college. This is when I was crazy in love with him." She says their relationship was like a "fairytale." They both wanted to keep the baby, and Sabine felt "really pleased" about the pregnancy. She and Frank lived together and planned to marry before the baby arrived. Then, Sabine's mother intervened, saying that having kids would ruin Sabine's life as much as childrearing had ruined her own life. Without her mom's support at this crucial time, Sabine fell apart. She figured she wasn't ready to parent if she could not handle her mother's criticism, so Sabine decided on abortion. This choice was excruciating. She notes, "I would get hysterical if I thought about it." In response, Frank would just laugh.

He continued to be just as insensitive in the year and a half in which they stayed together after the abortion. Sabine felt ongoing pain about the abortion, but he couldn't understand her emotions or handle the heaviness that had settled into their relationship. Sabine remembers, "I tried to talk to him about it sometimes, but he avoided it." Sabine noticed that he was "backing off" from her in general, but did not understand why. She also realized that she was losing her sense of self. Sabine comments, "It started to dawn on me that I didn't have my own life anymore. I moved out, but we were still going out."

Frank began to see other women, but lied to Sabine about this. Sabine left town for Christmas break and called Frank every day. Once, a woman answered the phone. When Sabine questioned Frank about this event, he said that this woman was now his wife. Sabine was so distraught that when she returned from vacation, she went over to his house to speak with him. She recalls, "He let me in. And all of my stuff was packed in garbage bags next to the door. She had already moved in with all her things." Later, Sabine discovered that Frank had lied about being married. He had met this woman three weeks before telling Sabine this fib, and they had become engaged, but had not yet married.

Frank may have found it easy to exchange one woman for another in a matter of weeks, but Sabine does not think it is so easy to go on loving men. Believing that they don't hang around, she figures that if she ever gives birth, she had better count on being a single parent. She says, "I don't necessarily believe in being in love with someone. I don't believe in marriage anymore. I used to think it was a celebration that two people have because they've decided that they want to spend their lives together. And now I just think it's garbage that people make up to get what they want."

Sabine sees a new guy on a regular basis, but notes, "I've never really been in love with him. I think of him like a friend, and if we got married, just a long-term companion." She has not even told the bulk of her disillusioning abortion experience to this new partner. Sabine mentioned that she had an abortion and left it at that. She explains, "I have little faith that men can understand what it's like." He told her that his former girlfriend and several friends have had abortions. Sabine is not impressed. She shrugs, "It's just not the same. Men can be there and I think men can be really sensitive. But they will never, ever know what that's like. They can feel like they ought to know, but they won't. Just like I'll never know what it's like to be a man, to experience the things that men experience."

Melinda: "The General Insensitivity of Men"

Like Sabine, 42-year-old Melinda has had a wholesale disillusionment with men. She had so many infuriating experiences with them during her second abortion and was so stunned by "the general insensitivity of men" that she says, "I've never gotten over it." With her first abortion at age 20, she felt some of this. Her partner thought they should have the child and did not support her decision or help pay for the abortion. It was her abortion at age 25, however, that showed her certain truths about gender relations.

At that time, she led a mostly lesbian life, so she had no birth control. When she slept with an old lover one night, she asked him to wear a condom. Rudy said he would put one on before getting too excited, but continued with sex. Melinda tried to stop him and says he virtually raped her. She fumes, "I still feel he was cowardly, disrespectful, and misogynist never to acknowledge his responsibility in the event."

By the time Melinda discovered the pregnancy, Rudy had gone abroad. She sent a letter and a telegram, asking him to help finance an abortion. He did not acknowledge either missive. Meanwhile, Melinda's father, Bart, learned that she had tried to extract money from Rudy. Bart "chastised" Melinda for taking this action, saying that she had "exposed" him. He may have meant that Melinda made him look like he wasn't providing well for his daughter, which seems a peculiar and self-centered reaction. To make matters worse, even though he knew Melinda needed money, he offered no help. Melinda sought financial aid from a social service agency. There, she says, the woman told her that "white girls didn't have problems getting money and that I'd better just go to my rich daddy and get the money." Finally, Melinda appealed to her female friend's mother, who lent her the money. Another friend, Oliver, helped Melinda obtain an abortion at the hospital where he worked.

The day of her abortion, Melinda called her workplace and said she was sick. Her supervisor did not receive the message, and called Bart to find out where she was. Bart said that Melinda "was busy having an abortion" and would be out for a few days. The supervisor tried to tell her own boss that Melinda had "female trouble." When the boss didn't buy this line, he forced her to tell the truth. The day Melinda returned, there was a holiday luncheon. She recalls that her supervisor's boss, "the pig of pigs," announced to the assembled staff, "The new medical plan won't cover things like abortions, as Melinda can tell you." Melinda laments, "The whole table knew why I'd been gone for a week."

This was the final blow. She felt enraged that, as she says, "All the men in my life (except my gay friend, Oliver) were totally unsupportive." She notes that Rudy and her first partner "were not supportive, caring, or particularly understanding of my decisions." Melinda adds, "I stopped feeling like I could tell my dad things after my second abortion." Finally, "being publicly humiliated" by her supervisor's boss was hard to take. Taken together, these experiences with men made her feel illegitimate. As Melinda puts it, "I was viewed as a slut." Because these men treated her with so little respect and acted as though her actions were unacceptable, she notes, "It took a while to fully feel I'd been 'a good girl' in spite of it all."

After these betrayals and disappointments, Melinda became even more politicized than she had already been. She comments, "I was so angry at being considered unworthy, unneedy, a bad girl, etcetera, by male society that I just got more militant as a feminist." Melinda adds that she could see from both abortions that "women were seen as inferior" and "treated as pariahs." These realizations, she says, "were significant in developing my feminism." She certainly saw a sharp contrast between the way men had acted toward her and the way women helped her. Melinda felt quite grateful that her friend's mom had lent her money and didn't pressure her to pay it back immediately. This experience must be partly why Melinda says, "My relationships with women changed. I am able to get support from my sisters, friends, and black men, but not from others."

FEELING WARMLY TOWARD MEN AND ALIENATED FROM WOMEN

Melinda feels angrier at men and closer to women since her abortion. This is a common pattern. It is possible, though more unusual, to feel the other way after an abortion. Men may seem more supportive. Their distance from the issue can help them be more objective and less presumptuous about how we feel. Women may disappoint us if we expect them all to be warm and caring. For some women, the abortion issue may push a few buttons, particularly if they have had abortions or if they have carried to term unhappily. They may have too many feelings about their own pregnancies to give us the love we need.

Toni's abortion experiences have made her feel that women can be quite cold and unsympathetic. She is a 23-year-old African American who has conceived and ended three pregnancies in the last two years. Once, she lay in the recovery room cramping after the procedure and crying in her discomfort. A nurse told her, "Crying's not going to take away the pain." Her comment provided no solace to Toni. Instead, Toni says, "It just intensified all the feelings inside me, because there was no one to say, 'It's okay.'"

As Toni proceeded through her abortion experience, her disappointing encounters with women continued. Her female friends tried to be responsive, but they haven't provided what Toni needs. Toni comments, "I feel like they're pitying me." Because of this, she has become more close-mouthed with them about her problems. When they are not overly solicitous of her feelings, they swing to the other extreme, minimizing her pain. They have murmured apologies that she feels unhappy, but Toni says, "I don't think it's affected them that it's their friend" who is experiencing such dramatic events. She says that while "they feel sympathetic that a woman has to go through that," they don't say anything like, "I feel badly for you personally, Toni. I understand you." Perhaps they don't want to pretend that they understand. Alternatively, Toni thinks that they may have picked up on how ashamed she feels about her abortions, and they might think it best not to make too big a deal about the subject. She has only told her two closest female friends, who are her roommates, so maybe her sample is rather limited. But Toni feels that she has noticed this trend in many women's behavior, especially with pregnancy issues. She notes, "In cases of abortion or childbirth, I don't think women are as sympathetic with one another."

In contrast, Toni has felt a great deal of warmth and understanding from the men who know about her abortions. This trend began in the abortion facility. She recalls, "The doctor I had the second and third times, he introduced himself to me both times. He had a button that said 'Doctors for Choice.'" This button reassured Toni of his good intentions. He seemed to value his work, rather than just having been stuck with that job. The doctor didn't let the button do all the talking. He addressed Toni's concerns and spoke to her with respect. Toni notes that her male anesthesiologist was also very kind. She comments, "Maybe I'm picking up patterns, or maybe I'm making up patterns. My male doctor and my male anesthesiologist were all very supportive. But this nurse I had was just so cold."

This pattern of male supportiveness continued outside the hospital. She comments, "I talked to my boyfriend and my brother about it. They seem to be very compassionate and sympathetic." She feels astonished that although "they don't know what it's like," these men seem to "have ideas of the experience." Toni's boyfriend, who has conceived with her all three times, was especially loving and kind during her second and third pregnancies. He, himself, had so much pain about the abortions that he confided in his best friend. This friend and Toni were not close, so she was afraid that he might judge her. But, says Toni, "He was very supportive. He'd be like, 'How are you doing?' And I could tell he was asking indirectly how I was doing with that issue, because he didn't know how to talk about it. I could tell he was really concerned." After seeing so many men respond to her feelings with warmth, Toni comments, "Men seem to be more compassionate and more caring or sensitive about issues that are very women-specific." She figures that they are more feeling precisely because they can never go through the experience themselves. Toni's speculation may well be right. Some men might feel respectful of territory that is not their own, and may approach such matters with curiosity, sensitivity, and compassion.

IMPROVING GENDER RELATIONS

As we go through abortions, many of us want supportive, sensitive women and men by our sides. In order to have this, some changes need to occur, and not just concerning abortion. We will now explore suggestions about how to achieve this revolution.

Women Supporting Women

We have met Sabine earlier in this chapter. A 23-year-old African American who ended her pregnancy two years ago, Sabine felt entirely alone as she went through her abortion experience. It wasn't just that her boyfriend treated her badly, putting her belongings in garbage bags and lying about his marital status. Sabine feels that throughout her experience, there was no mentor to guide her, no one to help her chart this unknown territory. In Sabine's abortion facility, none of the patients even talked to each other.

Sabine sees room for improvement. She comments, "Women should be in every place of abortion to support the women who are going through it." She feels that the doctor's gender is not important, but that women's presence is essential to provide a warm, affirming atmosphere. Sabine explains, "I think that women are women's biggest asset when it comes to things like this." Ultimately, Sabine says, "I think you need women's experiences to know what it's like." She feels strongly that she would have benefited from knowing about other women's experiences before she had her abortion. Sabine muses that with this information, "I think I would have done things differently. I would have known what to expect. I probably would have gone to a place that offered more support. And I probably would have gotten counseling, both before and after it happened."

Sabine does not think women's support of other women should exist only with abortion. She feels that as girls grow older, they should have an older woman who can guide them through life. Sabine notes, "I had some people who did that for me. That was great." She now tries to help troubled young women by volunteering as a mentor. This work has served as a great outlet for her. Sabine observes, "Studies show that the relationships that prolong men's lives are relationships with women. And the relationships that prolong women's lives are also relationships with other women. I think that's really important, women's relationships with each other. Helping each other through all kinds of things is going to get us where we need to be." In Sabine's view, if women support women in all ways, the help women give each other during abortions will merely be an extension of that support, not an anomaly.

Valuing Women's Roles and Choices

Twenty-eight-year-old Marilyn, who is Caucasian, has begun to support other women more, but mostly in her attitude toward them, rather than with any actions. A PhD candidate who has thrown all of her energy into her studies, Marilyn has long seen it as "anti-feminist to have a baby and to get married" and has scorned traditional female roles, both for herself and others. When Marilyn conceived a year ago with her Italian boyfriend Stefano, she relaxed these ideas to the extent that she and Stefano planned to marry and spoke often of having a child. At the same time, Marilyn couldn't imagine being a mom. She comments, "I had banished all thought of traditional female roles and functions from my mind to the point where I could not accept the possibility of motherhood."

An unplanned pregnancy brought these values to the foreground. Marilyn felt strongly that she could not pursue intellectual work if she had children. The pregnancy made Stefano articulate his beliefs, ones Marilyn had not heard in the two years of their relationship. He saw motherhood as "organic," a process that could flow with the rest of daily life. Stefano felt that "the female role is one of power" and that motherhood only adds to this power. At the same time, he saw a woman as "an automatic unit that fulfilled certain functions and would be happy doing that." Even though he approved of abortion, he didn't see pregnancy as a matter of choice–more as an event one does not question. Marilyn was shocked to discover that he harbored such ideas. She says adamantly, "I did not want to have a relationship with a man who thought that. I did not want a child with a man who thought that." For several reasons, they ended the pregnancy and the relationship.

Marilyn notes that although they split up, they both came closer to the other person's way of seeing the issue. She comments, "It was driven home to him that it was a matter of choice." For her part, Marilyn has begun to value motherhood in a way she never did before. She sees that many people in American society treat motherhood as dismissively as she once did, and views that as a problem. She feels much more supportive of mothers and child-care providers, and concerned about a society that doesn't value children or motherhood. If people supported motherhood, Marilyn believes that more women who face unplanned pregnancies could carry to term, knowing that they could have help. Motherhood need not stay as traditional as it has been, she realizes. Men and women should share parenting responsibilities in "some more equitable way." At the same time, she feels that we need to hold onto "traditional female qualities" and "not dismiss those qualities from the face of the earth." She thinks that the ability to nurture others has been undervalued for too long. Marilyn argues for more compassion for all of women's roles and choices, which ultimately gives women more freedom to be whoever they want to be.

In addition to supporting mothers and motherhood, some of us feel strongly that this society should stand behind those of us who do not want to become mothers. There is so much pressure to reproduce that some people don't take us seriously if we say we don't want children. One 22 year old who has a 3 year old notes, "I hear people talking to my daughter right now as if, of course she's going to be a mother. And I think that's a mistake. That pressure contributes to a lot of women getting pregnant without deciding that that's really what they want to do." She feels that women need examples of other women who plan their reproduction, so that having children becomes a conscious choice, not a cultural inevitability, or a biological inevitability resulting from unplanned pregnancies. If our culture made these changes, she thinks, abortion would no longer be as necessary.

Improving the Way Men Treat Women During Abortion

Many of these suggestions hinge on what women can do to improve the situation for other women. As we try to alter our culture, it is good to begin by changing ourselves. But we are only half of the story. What about the men involved in pregnancies and in our lives? Many of us feel frustrated by their attitudes and wish they would respond to issues of sex, birth control, pregnancy, and abortion differently.

Some women want men to respond better in specific ways, such as being more willing to put on a condom, or accompanying them to an abortion clinic. Others want men to be more sensitive in general. Natasha is a 33-year-old Russian immigrant who feels this way. She ended pregnancies at ages 20 and 28. In both cases, she was engaged to the men with whom she conceived. Each time, she found them "unprepared, weak, and immature" and pronounces their lack of care appalling. She feels enraged that neither man wanted to carry the pregnancies to term. Natasha comments of her second fiancé, "There was nothing pleasant about letting my body and soul be scarred again for no better reason than my man's being irresponsible and selfish."

Neither man knew how to handle the crisis. Natasha recalls, "They were always confused and in my first case, even denying the fact that it was possible (for he always claimed to be impotent). My men would never show me their respect in the way of going with me to the clinic, or openly admitting their part in that rather tragic experience." Her second fiancé was particularly helpless about the situation. She recalls that when he came to see her after the abortion, "His eyes were wet, but his face was more of a stranger than an involved supporter. He did not know what to do next, and I hate him for his inability to be strong and in charge. We could never gain back the respect and intimacy we had shared prior to the abortion." Natasha resented these men throughout her pregnancies and explains poetically, "Carrying a pregnancy after you decide in favor of abortion is the hardest and most depressing period, for each day reminds you of what has been betrayed and ruined, and the breakup with a man to whom you committed your feelings, body, and dreams." She adds, "After my second abortion, my innate trust in the power of the man has diminished. Not that I could not trust or was not willing to start a new relationship, but rather I did not expect from them enough affection, stability, and character for a while."

She feels closer to women now, saying, "I can relate more to many of them, and can empathize with a higher level of understanding, and may be able to help." Natasha does not want to be separatist, however. She recognizes that the relations between the genders "are profoundly complex, evolving, and always a two-way agreement" and would like to improve the way men and women relate to one another. Her bad relationships with men have signaled to her that the changes must occur throughout society, both in men and women who are already grown, and in the generations we produce and educate. She says we should rear responsible males, whose strength is mental, not just physical.

Making Abortion More of a Joint Endeavor

Many of us say that we want men to be involved in our abortion experiences, offering support, taking equal responsibility for the conception, paying for half of the procedure's cost, and coming with us to the abortion facility. At the same time, others of us state that men should stay out of our way when we make abortion decisions. We let men know in no uncertain terms that they have no say over what goes on in our bodies. Hearing two contradictory messages may feel confusing to men. When exactly do we need men's support, and when should they give us space? How can they get it right?

If the man in our lives is domineering and orders us to carry out his wishes with the pregnancy, we are certainly right to keep him out of the decision making. This is just the sort of man who should not be given a say, as he is acting in his own interests, not ours. In contrast, if a man is sensitive to us and respectful of our needs, he will likely stand back and let us make our own decision. Because he is sensitive and respectful of us, he can probably be trusted with full partnership in making the choice.

In many cases, then, it would not be detrimental to involve the man in the decision, at least to some degree. This might help both men and women. We would not feel as alone in the situation, and men could begin to explain how they feel. As a 31 year old who had an abortion five years ago notes, "I think society isn't acknowledging the issues that men have around this. And they're probably almost equally intense." She began to wonder how her abortion affected her partner. She thought, "Oh my God. What did I do to you by doing this? What does this mean to you?" She wondered whether he felt that she had rejected him by ending the pregnancy, and says, "This was part of him. Literally part of him that I didn't want to have. And it must feel very rejecting on some level, no matter how conscious that may be to a man." She also sees that a man might feel "completely helpless" if he wants to have the child and if he "can't do anything about it."

Out of love for a man with whom we conceive and end pregnancy, we may indeed want to hear how difficult the experience has been for him. We may need to wait before listening to his feelings, so that we don't feel overburdened. It may also be better to talk when we do not need him to mirror our emotions; otherwise, if his feelings don't have the depth or intensity that ours do, we may feel even more alone in the experience.

Making the abortion a joint endeavor might bring a new level of intimacy to the relationship and help both partners resolve their feelings. As a Caucasian 24 year old named Ingrid observes one month after her abortion, men and women must deal with an abortion together and grieve together for their losses, so they can "stay connected." Ingrid explains the source of her grief: "I feel very close to my boyfriend and I may marry him, so to think it was best to abort with a man I love is sad and painful." They had dated for a year and lived together when they conceived. After Ingrid learned she was pregnant, she "wanted to feel angry" at her boyfriend and "wanted to run away from him," but says she was "nervous he'd be mad at me." Ingrid also feared that he would be angry that she didn't want to have a child with him just then. They "talked through all this," however. He supported her decision and stayed by her side during the procedure, for which Ingrid felt thankful. She says that out of her entire experience, "What remains vivid was just before surgery began, my boyfriend was looking at me and holding my hand while I was crying." After the abortion, they went to a therapist to discuss how the experience affected them. Ingrid says, "I question if he and I still need to deal with it more."

She did not exactly make her decision with her boyfriend; it sounds like she made it on her own and then consulted with him. From that point on, however, they have shared all parts of the experience, at least as much as is possible. Ingrid says that lately, she has been thinking about the "delicacy of emotions and two people in love losing a possible child." She seems to have approached the situation with full awareness of that "delicacy"; not wanting to rip the fine lace of their relationship, she has proceeded cautiously, trying to preserve a balance between their feelings. This joint endeavor seems to have worked. Moreover, it seemed like the only option, given how close the two of them are.

PART V: MOVING ON

Epilogue: Feeling Better After Abortion

Many of the women in this book answered the questions, "What advice would you give someone going through an abortion? What advice do you wish someone had offered you?" They have offered their thoughts on a wide range of topics. Some of the advice is meant for those who have experienced the procedure, while other words encourage those making a decision. Some of the advice is contradictory. Take from it whatever seems useful.

Be Logical, Calm, and Thorough When Making the Decision

When we receive a positive pregnancy test, many of us want to resolve this issue quickly, even scheduling an abortion for the next day. However, panicking won't help. Several people offer advice about adopting the proper mindset when deciding a pregnancy's fate.

Some believe that it is best to be pragmatic in making the decision. One 38-year-old Latina says, "Take off the rose-colored glasses society would glue to your head, and view the situation coldly, dispassionately, and objectively. Are you really ready, willing, and able to bear a child, rear it, and provide for it? Or are you only ripping yourself up because that's how you've been told people are supposed to behave?" Another woman, age 29, is of like mind when she says, "Make the decision based on what you want for yourself and for your children when you are ready to have them. Don't let society dictate what you do. Don't let emotions such as guilt or fear cloud your judgment. Think logically instead of emotionally, if possible." These women base such statements on their own experience–it worked well for them to focus on practical realities when they went through their own abortions, so they recommend that others do the same. As one 42 year old says, "Since I'm so matter-of-fact about this issue for myself, my only advice is: Do it! Don't hesitate if you don't want the child. Why bring a life into this crazy place if you are not sure about it? It's not something to be taken lightly. Parenthood is a job for life."

Although these women did not have many conflicts in their decision making, other women do not find it so easy to make a choice about a pregnancy. They believe it is important to give the matter ample consideration. One 23 year old recalls that when she found herself pregnant three years ago, she decided that becoming fully informed would help reduce her stress. Darian and her boyfriend went to Planned Parenthood to talk to someone. She comments, "I am not usually one to talk excessively about a decision I have to make–I rely on myself heavily, especially in times like this. But this was a big unknown, and Reid and I needed to know what we were in for. I did not go there for advice concerning my decision. I knew what I wanted. I just needed to know where to go, what to expect." Gaining information may help us slow down and think, rather than panick and take immediate action. The information we gather before an abortion can also help stave off regrets afterward. One 23 year old emphasizes the importance of entering an abortion with full knowledge. She says, "Think about it. Think long; think hard. Consider everything that you're doing. Get the facts. Talk to people. Don't let anyone force your hand in the decision. Get a copy of *Our Bodies, Ourselves*. And know exactly what the procedure is going to be. Know exactly what it is that you're doing."

Many women emphasize, as this woman has, that there should be no coercion in the decision. As one 46 year old advises, "Don't let anyone (even him) decide what you should do. It's good to consider his feelings in your decision, but follow what's right for you." Going through an abortion because others have pressured us in this direction makes the abortion hard to accept. The decision must come from within.

How can we block out other voices and determine what we really want? The key is listening to ourselves. One 29 year old says that with her three abortions, "I have followed my intuition and I am at peace with myself. Follow your instinct," she instructs others. Another woman, age 58, agrees and says, "I have great faith in the basic wisdom of human beings, if only they can wade through the morass of 'shoulds' and 'oughts' that interfere with clear choosing." She believes that the answer lies within, ready to be discovered. The challenge is to find the courage to do what we feel is necessary.

Looking inside for answers can certainly help, but that is not the only way to make this decision. Sometimes things seem more muddled in our solitude. Talking to other people is a good way to break through cyclical thinking and to see the situation in a new way. We might choose to talk to a counselor to attain some clarity. We may prefer to speak with those directly involved in the situation, especially our partner. Some of us talk the decision over with the fetus. We either imagine what the fetus might say, or actually try to communicate with the fetus's spirit. Even if the conversation is one-sided, it can help us articulate our feelings. One 42 year old recommends saying the following things: "Thank the child for coming into your life, but remind it you are not ready, and wish it well on its journey. Forgive the child, yourself, your partner, and the life cycle."

Talking about our feelings with the people in our life can cut through any denial that hampers us during an unplanned pregnancy. That's what 21-year-old Veronica believes. She realizes how easy it is to think, "This can't be happening to me," and to have an abortion without much reflection. Remaining silent only bolsters such denial; if we don't discuss our feelings and decisions, we may not examine them closely. After the abortion, we may begin to think more about what we have done and may doubt our decision. We will probably find ourselves on firmer ground if we think about our decision clearly and honestly beforehand. For this reason, Veronica says, "It's really important to talk about it as you're going through it. Find somebody who's going to listen to you and who's going to be open-minded." In her view, talking is a way of thinking out loud and being truthful with oneself; it is hard to deceive oneself with someone else listening.

Twenty-two-year-old Brittany has a similar idea, but would like the listener to intervene when he or she hears denial. Brittany advises the listener not to reassure the woman making the decision. She explains, "It's not a time for comfort. Women in this position need people to be realistic and tough with them." She feels that if a listener helps a woman see the situation clearly, the woman won't look back after the abortion and say, "Why didn't someone push me harder to think about why I was doing this?" Peeling away layers of denial before the procedure helps to prevent regrets. If we do a lot of the thinking and feeling before the abortion, there will probably be less to sort through afterward.

Consider the Essentials When Making a Decision

Thus far, we have heard good advice on what mindset to assume while choosing the fate of a pregnancy. But what should one take into consideration? One 40 year old suggests that a woman should think about "the practical realities–how each path could affect her future relationships, job training, economic stability, community opinion of her and the child." Sometimes, people making an abortion decision do not think about what they want, but about which option seems socially acceptable. The stigma surrounding abortion may deter them from ending a pregnancy, although that may be the best choice.

Several women offer reassurance that abortion is a good decision that brings relief. One 43 year old observes, "Though the abortion experience may be somewhat unpleasant, it's short, and it's over. Motherhood lasts forever. Abortion is not a sin; let's hope it doesn't become a crime!" Another woman, age 23, points out, "When it is over, they will not only have removed the fetus, but also the pressure on your life."

Abortion can be physically and emotionally painful, but fearing such pain is no reason to choose birth. So says Brittany, who recently tried to communicate this to a pregnant friend who was unsure of her decision. She leaned toward abortion, but said that thinking about abortion was heartwrenching. Brittany comments, "I didn't think there was any reason for her to become a parent before she had decided that it was the right time." She adds, "I was encouraging her to have an abortion, because I really didn't want her to" choose birth "out of fear of the feelings" that abortion might bring. Her friend chose to carry to term. Brittany is pleased, but says, "I feel like she's going to struggle with knowing that she wouldn't have had a child" if she hadn't had an accidental conception.

Brittany told her friend to make each option a reality. Brittany explains, "I gave her the perspective of spending a couple of days having decided that she was going to have a baby. And to tell people she trusted that decision. People she would feel comfortable with if she changed her mind. But also to tell them not to pass it on. And to spend a few days with the decision *not* to have a baby." Brittany explains that this method can help us feel that we have made a particular decision, instead of living as if either option is possible and as if we always have an "out." Telling others about a decision and seeing how we feel about their reaction can help us see if we feel committed to that choice.

There is another way to explore what each option might be like. One 27 year old says, "Talk to people who have experienced unplanned pregnancies and ask them about their feelings and decisions." She did this when she conceived at age 21. She recalls, "I spent half a day with a single mother (this is when I thought I was going to have the child). We talked very openly about the pros and cons, and although she was really happy about her decision, she helped me see that I was just not ready to have a child." Our culture often glosses over parenting's challenges, romanticizing it and even treating it as inevitable. Observing a parent and child might awaken us to the realities of parenthood.

If we cannot find another person to talk to about birth or abortion, we might seek written accounts of others' feelings. There is a growing literature about abortion experiences, and much has been written about parenthood. Understanding how birth and abortion have made others feel can help us imagine our lives with each choice.

A final consideration is that there are three choices, although we often dismiss adoption. One 42 year old says, "I completely and absolutely support any woman's decision to have an abortion." At the same time, she says, "I know so many people who are desperately trying to get pregnant and desperately want to adopt a baby." Both her brother and sister were adopted. She comments, "I love them dearly. I can't imagine what it would have been like if they hadn't been in my life." Although she would not want to force adoption on anyone, and did not consider it herself when she ended a pregnancy at age 24, she wishes more women would think about giving children up for adoption.

Prepare for the Procedure

If we do choose abortion, it is important to select a facility carefully. One 27 year old had a bad experience with Planned Parenthood and tells women never to go there for an abortion. She notes that people assume Planned Parenthood is less expensive, when this may not be true. Many others have had fantastic experiences at Planned Parenthood and highly recommend it. One woman, age 47, points out that the clinic staff's philosophy matters most. She says, "Go to a good feminist-oriented clinic."

We may have a choice about the level of anesthetic we receive in the facility. People disagree about the advantages of being awake or asleep during an abortion. One 39 year old who has had five abortions reasons, "Have general [anesthesia]. Why have more pain than need be?" To make this choice, we may want to consider our threshold of pain, our need to be aware or unaware of the procedure, and the higher cost and risks of general anesthesia.

It can help to be prepared for the physical experience of abortion. For this reason, some women feel that the best advice they can give is a description of how it feels. One 25 year old laments, "I wish someone who'd had an abortion had given me insight into how it really feels, physically." She was surprised to find out what a "big deal" the physical experience is. Another woman, age 22, disagrees. She remarks, "It's not painful. It feels strange, like major cramps, but it's not horrible in any way." Unfortunately, while many women feel quite concerned about how much pain the procedure will cause, it can be difficult to tell someone else how much pain they will feel; the physical experience is quite subjective and varies from person to person. It may even differ for the same woman from abortion to abortion. Learning about the procedure might alleviate our anxieties, however. As one 47 year old says after six abortions, "Know as much about the procedure as possible before the abortion, so you're not afraid."

A good way to prepare for an abortion is investigating whether we can bring someone to the procedure. Many facilities allow a support person to be present during the operation. Some women regret that they did not know this beforehand. Having someone at the procedure can keep us from feeling that no one knows what we have experienced.

Find Support Throughout the Experience

It is important to have support, not just at the abortion facility, but during the whole experience. We may need to look for support from several people in order to obtain just what we need, and may have to tell them exactly what we want from them. Otherwise, we may feel let down that they have not read our minds. One woman, age 18, advises people to "find someone they could confide in and tell all their feelings." She says, "Get it out! But don't tell a lot of people." She cautions that because this is a volatile issue, we might want to limit the number of people who know. This is a good point. The number of listeners may not be as important, however, as the type of listener. We should share our feelings only with people who care about us and who can say helpful things.

We might turn to a counselor to listen and provide feedback in the way we need it. One 27 year old feels that this is the only way to limit gossip. She says, "Discuss it with a therapist, so that it is confidential! The first abortion, I wish I had kept it to myself. Too many found out about it." Counselors may also provide what friends cannot, in that they purport to be unbiased. They ought to be able to listen to any sort of feelings, not just ones that correspond to their ideology. Some women feel so positive about therapy that they say things like, "Even if you think you don't need it, seek counseling," and "All women going through this should be in some form of therapy."

We may find full support and understanding from our partners. But the tension of the pregnancy and abortion can dampen the relationship, at least temporarily. Some women offer advice to men, who may wonder what to do during this time. One 22 year old says, "She's not going to feel too good. Be really nice to her. Give her all the support she's going to want. Especially since you guys can't make love." Another woman, age 24, says that she often hears men "not knowing what to do or say," especially during an abortion experience. She comments, "I know for myself and others–love us. Be warm, tender. Hold us. Stay by our sides. We need you now more than you will ever know." Women, too, may need to try even harder for intimacy during this tense time. An 18 year old advises, "Don't push the man (boyfriend, husband, etcetera) away. Understand that he may also be affected, even if it doesn't show." We may not have a choice about pushing men away; they may leave on their own. If this is the case, the advice might be, "Don't give up on love. Not all men will disappoint you in the future."

Feel Your Feelings

Whether or not we have support as we go through an abortion, it is important that we support ourselves. One 22 year old says, "Go easy on yourself. Mourn. Be sad. Someday your pain will end. Things keep going on. This is making you wiser and stronger than you'll ever know." Another woman, age 31, concurs, "Being gentle with yourself is so important. It takes years sometimes to make sense of it." There are many ways to be kind to ourselves during this time. One 49 year old counsels, "Lavish yourself with gifts in whatever form. You are making a sacrifice; give yourself a break."

It is important to let all feelings come forward. Otherwise, they can fester and cause emotional or even physical problems. Twenty-three-year-old Toni addresses this matter when she says, "Whatever you're going to feel, allow yourself to feel it. My biggest problems come about when I try to stifle what I'm feeling." Another woman, also age 23, is on the same wavelength. She says, "The only way to feel is to feel honestly–if you're sad, you're sad. If you're relieved, you're relieved. Keeping yourself open to all emotions and not censoring them is the key." It is essential not to critique the feelings. Just go with them, as much as possible. A 34 year old has tried to do this with each abortion and says to other women, "Cry when you need to. Remember that you will get through it." A 25 year old elaborates on this, as she thinks of what she'd say to a woman going through what she did: "I would tell her to cut herself some slack. She might feel weird/crazy for a while. I would tell her lots of women have abortions and everybody is different, so whatever she feels or needs. I'd let her know that it might all be really intense right now, but it won't always be this intense, and she can move on with her life."

As she says, the feelings will fade in time. That is the biggest realization that 49-year-old Rhonda took away from her abortion more than twenty years ago. She states, "I want to tell people that it is possible to have an abortion, feel genuinely sorrowful about the act at the time, and get over it." Rhonda adds, "I think the fact that you might have some emotions about it does not mean it's the wrong thing to do–you'll have a lot more emotions about a kid, and if you didn't want one, they'll create much bigger problems than an abortion. Antichoice people manipulate women's emotions as if they're everything–but quality of life is more important than fleeting feelings." Rhonda blames both of the ideological camps for restricting her freedom to grieve for her abortion, and says, "I did feel feminists were and are minimizing the sad feelings of having an abortion. Even though mine did not last, they were intense and deserved to be respected–or given attention."

As Rhonda notes, many people have minimized the emotional experience of abortion, which only does a disservice to those who go through it. One 24 year old seeks to redress that through her advice to women having abortions. She comments that women should not "underestimate the possible emotional trauma," and notes, "I never expected it to be so difficult. I only saw it as a procedure. But it's a process." Similarly, one 27 year old regrets not knowing how much her abortion would affect her mentally. Two years after the abortion, she says, "I wish someone had told me that I would think about it, that I would wonder what that child would have looked like, been like."

For a variety of reasons, people may not be available to support us and we may find ourselves coping with our feelings alone. It is important to remember that even if we feel alone, millions of other women have had abortions and a sizable chunk of that group must have felt the way we do. One woman, age 23, mentions this when she advises, "So many women have had abortions; you are not an isolated incident."

Twenty-three-year-old Wanda has astute advice on the matter of feeling alone. She points out, "You have to walk into something like this and go, 'I am alone.' And accept that right off the bat." She says this is a statement of tolerance, not bitterness, and explains, "It's a choice you have to make alone. It's the ultimate taking responsibility for your actions. You're the one doing it. You're alone. Accept that and know that by yourself you can stand with this decision and deal with your feelings." Wanda adds, "Try to make sure there's somebody there. But realize there may not be." In her view, we should not expect others to help us with this experience.

Wanda is right. The reality is that many of us go through this without much support, or with some support, but with an overwhelming sense of loneliness, anyway. It is not too different from the way a cancer patient may feel with smiling and weeping family members by the bedside. She is surrounded and supported, and yet she's the one lying in that bed. When something happens in our body, there are some ways in which we simply cannot share the experience with others. For this reason, keeping a journal is helpful during an abortion experience. Thirty-two-year-old Oriana recommends this outlet to women. When she went through her most recent abortion, she found it helpful to reread her feelings about previous abortions. Oriana comments, "You don't have to be a writer. You've got feelings and thoughts and dreams. It really was helpful through all the pregnancies to write everything down. I'd go back and reread those sections and think, 'Wow, look how far I've come,' or in some cases, 'I've come full circle.' Instead of reading somebody else's experiences, you get to read your own thoughts and feelings and impressions. If you don't have access to a therapist or a support group, just put it down on paper." Not only is this cathartic, but Oriana says it provided her with her own support. She explains, "You start putting down whatever you feel without judging it. You get to go back and hold your own hand. You can say, 'Look where I am now. I have this career, traveling,' or whatever you've done, and see the positive aspects that have come from this period."

Accept Yourself

Women stress the importance of accepting oneself after an abortion. One 40 year old advises, "Forgive yourself if you need forgiveness, and treat yourself with love and respect, no matter what you choose." There is no reason for us to think less highly of ourselves after an abortion; the pregnancy and abortion in no way reflect an unworthy person. One young woman has insight into this issue. She notes, "I never thought I'd have an abortion. I looked down on people who got pregnant young. But here I am, twenty-three and two abortions in my life. Forgive yourself your snobbery.

Don't imagine yourself scarred or somehow marred–you will heal. Learn something about yourself in this experience–I found a strength I wasn't sure I possessed." Indeed, as she says, the pregnancy and abortion can highlight our assets, or give us more maturity and wisdom.

If we have self-doubts after the procedure, we may need to frame the abortion in a more positive light. Many of us look at abortion as something that has benefited our lives, saving us from having had a child when we felt unable to do so. One 49 year old feels that women who have abortions should "Know they're doing the right thing and be proud they're taking care of themselves." She views abortion as a form of self-protection. A 24 year old advises people to "find some purpose for the abortion, if they can. Turn it into a gift." There is a lot of wisdom in this recommendation. Once we can see how the pregnancy and abortion have enhanced our lives, not only can we stop regretting that we ever conceived in the first place, but we can readily accept that the whole thing happened. We may come to see it as an integral, indispensable part of our lives, one that helped make us who we are today. This may be especially true if the abortion causes us to engage in meaningful activities that we would not otherwise have undertaken. In this book, people have said that an abortion experience prompted them to run a support group for HIV-positive men; serve as a big sister to troubled youth; cease to take drugs; drop destructive friends or worthless boyfriends; donate eggs; use birth control regularly; begin therapy; plan on having a baby; feel clarified about not wanting children; investigate spirituality; volunteer at a clinic; become savvier about gender relations; speak to a large group about one's abortion; and make more female friends. There are countless ways in which unplanned pregnancy and abortion can motivate us to improve our lives.

CHANGING THE EXPERIENCE OF ABORTION

Clearly, many of us have ideas about how to make pregnancy and abortion experiences better on a personal level. It may also be possible for abortion facilities to improve the physical and psychological experiences of abortion for women.

Improving the Counseling

Currently, many abortion facilities are already stretched in several ways. They have lost patients to managed care, and therefore find themselves financially strapped. The political climate is so inhospitable that many abortion facilities must concern themselves with matters of security. It can be a major effort just to protect clients as they walk from the parking lot into the clinic. Clinicians may have no money or energy left over to improve the experiences their patients have once they enter the facility.

Still, it seems as if some changes should be made, particularly in counseling. Even some women who have worked as counselors at abortion clinics feel this way. For instance, Sally, who is 52 years old and who had an abortion twelve years ago, worked as a volunteer counselor for a short time after that. She says she was instructed to give "a fifteen- to twenty-minute counseling 'session' (which I thought was too brief). In reality it was ten minutes of paperwork, excuse yourself to do a urine test, present the results, and schedule an abortion. If there was an extreme reaction or inability to make a decision, a follow-up session with an intern psychologist could be scheduled in a week or so, but then you ran into the time limitations, since most women waited or could not get an appointment until they were pushing the time-limit boundaries." Twenty-five-year-old Cassie also volunteered in a clinic after her first abortion, but did not last long for several reasons. Cassie notes that the clinic, and the pro-choice camp in general, "doesn't want to admit that not everybody can go through this smiling the whole time." Because the clinic minimized the negative feelings that abortion can bring, it underemphasized counseling.

Although the counseling is good at many abortion facilities, there is much room for improvement. Financial realities aside, here are some suggestions–a wish list of sorts:

1. Counselors at abortion facilities are usually not licensed therapists, but people trained to ask certain questions. This set-up may not lend itself to an in-depth exploration of feelings. It is difficult for some women to trust that a counselor who is not a psychologist will know what to do if they express their true emotions. If abortion

facilities employed a therapist, the counseling sessions might be truly therapeutic.

2. The counseling that takes place right before the abortion procedure sometimes has little emphasis on feelings. Instead, the counselor discusses birth control, takes the patient's blood pressure, and fills out paperwork. The counselor, who must say and do certain things, ends up doing much of the talking. The clinic does need to communicate essential information to the patient. Perhaps clinicians could give this information on paper, requesting that the patient read the literature in the waiting room. This would help the patient pass time in the waiting room and allow the counseling session to be more of a free-form dialogue. The patient would have room to say whatever is on her mind and might feel heard and seen, not merely processed through the clinic. Plus, the counselor might connect better with the patient, which would be more rewarding for both.

3. Counselors should make sure that patients don't have any misinformation. Even if patients don't make misstatements, it would help if counselors discussed a list of myths and facts. For instance, many patients fear that abortion can lead to infertility or will cause them to have miscarriages later. Some women worry about being punished by having disabled children, or even interpret the bleeding that follows abortion as a punishment. Some have the wrong idea about how developed a fetus is or isn't at the time of their abortion. It would be a valuable service if counselors could address such topics and dispel fears. Again, they might do this on paper, which the patient could read in the waiting room and take home with her.

4. Many counseling sessions are limited in time, because it is important to keep patients flowing through the clinic. If the doctor is paid by the hour, it can be very expensive to have delays between operations. Consequently, both the counselors and the patients may sense pressure to move along, which might inhibit the patient from exploring her feelings during the counseling session. If clinics hired more counselors, and had a few rooms where counseling went on simultaneously, each woman could have enough time to vent her feelings. Whichever patient seemed most resolved about her feelings could have an abortion first. There would be no reason for a patient to have surgery before she felt ready.

5. Some patients feel that their counselors are biased. For instance, the counselor may insist that it is a fetus or tissue, not a baby. Telling a patient not to call it a baby is not the same as correcting misinformation. The patient may be well versed in fetal development and know quite well that a fetus is not the same as a full-term infant. In her mind and heart, however, it may be a baby. She has every right to choose the words she uses.

6. Abortion facilities sometimes deny abortions to women who seem too conflicted to go through with the procedure that day. While this is a laudable policy, and should certainly remain intact, it also has an unfortunate side effect. Some women refrain from mentioning certain feelings for fear that they will not be allowed to have an abortion. For this reason, counseling may achieve little. Instead, the patient may give all the "correct" answers. If the counselor senses that this is happening, it might help to encourage the patient to say whatever she feels. The counselor could explain that the clinic does have a certain policy about not allowing deeply conflicted women to have abortions that day, or whatever the policy may be, but might say that it is rare for the clinic to turn away patients. The counselor can also tell the patient that simply expressing ambivalence will not bar her from having the abortion that day, and could reassure her that it is all right to have some ambivalence or some negative feelings about an abortion both before and after the procedure. Hearing this point of view from the clinician would make it less confusing if some conflict does emerge later. The patient would no longer expect to have only positive feelings about the experience, and might accommodate negative feelings a little better.

On the flip side, there are some patients who want counselors to challenge their decisions, and who feel angry afterward if there has been no such opposition. To prevent patients from having such feelings of blame after the abortion, the counselor could emphasize that the decision ultimately remains in the patient's hands and that patients who feel fully responsible for their decision tend to cope with their abortions better.

7. Sometimes, the questions counselors ask about a patient's feelings only scratch the surface. "How do you feel about this decision?" and "Are you getting enough support?" are good starting points, but they may also elicit monosyllabic answers such as "fine"

and "yes." It may help the patient examine her feelings more deeply if the counselor asked, "What are your thoughts about being here today?" This question could help the counselor identify what is on the patient's mind, whether that involves feelings about the decision, anxiety about the procedure, or even the stigma that the patient might associate with an abortion facility. Plus, it would help counselors distinguish between patients who are truly resolved, because they frame the pregnancy or abortion in a certain way, versus those who are less certain of their choice. Patients who seem reticent as they answer this question may not benefit from further questioning; they might need to steel themselves for the surgery and might find further questioning intrusive. If a patient seems willing to explore her feelings, however, the counselor might ask, "What does the pregnancy mean to you? What positive or negative feelings do you have about the fetus and pregnancy? How do you view abortion?" This line of questioning might help the patient articulate what she is losing or gaining by ending the pregnancy. It might also gear the discussion toward her individual beliefs and values, rather than touching on issues generically.

In addition, a counselor might ask: "Do you feel a need to say goodbye to the fetus? If so, how would you do this?" The counselor could even ask these two questions at the patient's first visit, when they discuss the positive pregnancy test. If she is in shock about the test results, the question might be better suited to a handout that she could mull over at home. The literature might mention how other women have commemorated abortions.

8. Postabortion counseling is a must. Although nearly all abortion facilities require a two-week follow-up visit, they usually focus on the physical aftermath of an abortion, not a woman's emotional responses. Why not pay just as much attention to her feelings afterward as before? While she may not have had much to say in a preabortion counseling session, she may have a new perspective on her abortion two weeks later. It is essential to have counselors who can help women sort through their feelings at any time after an abortion. If any of the questions suggested in item 7 seem inappropriate on the day of the abortion (because some women are intent on getting through the procedure, not exploring their feelings), a counselor could ask those questions in a postabortion session.

9. Clinics could run ongoing postabortion support groups. People have so much trouble coming forward about their abortions that groups are hard to form and find in the outside world. But within an abortion facility, abortion is much more accepted and mentionable. It would be wonderful if clinics could further legitimize the experience and break through the taboo on abortion by providing forums for postabortion feelings. Then, women could meet other women who have been through the same thing.

10. After any of the patient's visits to the abortion facility, the counselor could give her written information. This might help her feel more supported and prepared if unsettling feelings arise when she is away from the clinic. These handouts could include the following:

- A brochure about possible emotional reactions to abortion. This would prepare the patient for the drop in hormones that she will experience when her pregnancy ends, and the emotional ramifications of that change. The brochure might also mention that some women feel sad, guilty, angry, or relieved after abortions.
- A list of local psychotherapists who specialize in postabortion work.
- Information about any postabortion support groups. The names of therapists who have run groups in the past might be helpful; if therapists receive several calls inquiring into a group, they might form another one.
- A list of women who want to be available to other women going through abortions in a big sister/little sister type of peer support network.
- Recommended reading about abortion, with a description of each text.

Such literature can mention many of the things a counselor might not have time to say.

Improving the Physical Experience of Abortion

The surgical method of abortion can feel invasive, and we may feel that we lose control as we lie on the table and let others work on us. Plus, the procedure can seem mechanical and cold. Several women have researched alternative methods to abortion.

Six women in this book tried using herbs or other natural ingredients to end their pregnancies. Twenty-five-year-old Nicola explains her thinking in taking this route: "I knew some women who had done herbal self-abortions, and their experiences were more positive than those of the women I knew who had been through clinical abortions. I drank cup after cup of bitter tea. I felt sick and drained. The whole thing was harder than I thought it would be." She took black and blue cohosh, tansy, rue, and pennyroyal, but figures that because she learned of the pregnancy too late, it did not work. In fact, five of the six women had no success with inducing abortion herbally. Another drawback was that after taking the herbs, one woman changed her mind about the pregnancy, but was told she had to have an abortion anyway, because the herbs could have harmed the fetus.

A sixth woman did have success with using natural ingredients. Forty-five-year-old Nadine ended a pregnancy after taking baths with mustard and red onions. The method failed her with two other pregnancies, but Nadine has used this method over the years when she has even suspected that she is pregnant. It may have worked for her ten times, for all she knows. It appeals to her because it works "with the spirit of the earth." Nadine believes that there should be networks of women exchanging information about herbal abortions. She says she finds the method empowering because, "I can take personal responsibility for my womb. I don't just depend on the medical establishment."

For more information on abortifacient herbs, see Joy Gardner's book, *A Difficult Decision*, in "Recommended Reading." Gardner gives instructions and warns about risks.

Gardner also supplies information about menstrual extraction, a do-it-yourself medical procedure that sucks out the uterine lining. One must insert a tube into the uterus, but this tube is much smaller than any used in a vacuum aspiration, so there is minimal pain. Menstrual extraction only works five to six weeks after the last period begins. One 26 year old says, "I recently had a friend at my house having a menstrual extraction as a means for abortion. It was very positive! She did not feel pain, just discomfort." She adds, "I advise looking for a woman's self-help group doing menstrual extractions."

It may not be ideal to end a pregnancy without supervision. What if problems arise with no practitioner present? Many women have died trying to obtain abortions outside medical facilities. That's why people have fought for legal abortion. The best bet may be to look to new advances as less invasive, more autonomous ways to end pregnancies.

Many of us have pinned our hopes on RU 486 combined with a prostaglandin as just such a panacea. With this method, women expel the fetus within four hours of receiving the prostaglandin, and need not always wait at a medical facility for this to occur. There have also been recent discoveries that combining an anticancer drug, Methotrexate, with a prostaglandin, Misoprostol, causes abortions. These newer methods have some drawbacks. RU 486 can fail, causing some women to need surgical abortions as well. It could be dangerous for clinicians not to witness or control the expulsion of the fetus. While there might be more privacy when the pregnancy ends, women may have to visit a medical setting up to four times, thus losing autonomy.

On the other hand, it certainly seems gentler and less invasive to swallow a pill, receive an injection, or use a vaginal suppository than to undergo suction abortion. Plus, it seems appealing not to lie on a table, feeling powerless. It is hard to know how the newer methods could affect the emotional experience of abortion. Perhaps we would feel more isolated if we were alone as the pregnancy ended. Maybe it would seem easier to deny the abortion to ourselves; for better or for worse, we might frame it more as a miscarriage. Alternatively, we might find it easier to mourn, both because we could perform some ritual in our own homes as the pregnancy ended, and because we would have seen the fetus and could visualize exactly what we had lost. We would not have misconceptions about the fetus's size or level of development and would be closer to the truth than we are when clinicians whisk away a jar filled with fetal tissue. If our bodies played more active roles in expelling the pregnancy, we might find it easier to take responsibility for our choice and might be less inclined to blame others for influencing us in certain ways. Those of us who felt that we lost control over our lives in having an accidental conception might feel that control return if we oversaw our own abortions. It is quite likely that we would feel less alienated from our bodies, as we would attend to their functions ourselves.

These newer methods might make abortions more accessible. According to the Fall 1995 *Feminist Majority Report*, a third of OB-GYNs who do not currently provide abortions would prescribe RU 486 when it became available in the United States. If it became easier to obtain abortions, not only would the stress of finding an abortion provider disappear, but we could go to more doctors' offices and not have to face picketers. Perhaps the political furor over the issue would die down and abortion would be less stigmatized. If so, then we might at last be able to speak of our abortion experiences freely and find more people to support us in our feelings and choices.

Recommended Reading

Help in Coping with Emotions

Buttenweiser, Sarah, and Reva Levine. Breaking silences: A post-abortion support model. In *From abortion to reproductive freedom: Transforming a movement*, Marlene Gerber Fried (ed.). Boston: South End Press, 1990.

- Article about a successful postabortion group, where counselors help women work through shame, guilt, and other emotions.

Lerner, Harriet Goldhor. *The dance of anger: A woman's guide to changing the patterns of intimate relationships*. New York: Harper Collins, 1985.

Panuthos, Claudia, and Catherine Romeo. *Ended beginnings: Healing childbearing losses*. South Hadley, MA: Bergin and Garvey Publishers, 1984.

Snow, Kimberley. *Keys to the open gate: A woman's spirituality sourcebook*. Berkeley: Conari, 1994.

- Includes ceremony for aborted fetuses.

Understanding Our Relationship with Our Bodies

Luker, Kristin. *Taking chances: Abortion and the decision not to contracept*. Berkeley: University of California Press, 1975.

- Proposes widely accepted theory of contraceptive risk taking.

Martin, Emily. *The woman in the body: A cultural analysis of reproduction*. Boston: Beacon Press, 1987.

- Feminist/Marxist analysis of how women experience their bodies and how the medical world views and treats women's bodies.

Emotional Issues Concerning Pregnancy and Motherhood

Colman, Libby Lee, and Arthur D. Colman. *Pregnancy: The psychological experience.* New York: Noonday Press, 1991.
- Shows how pregnancy affects emotions and body image, even in the early weeks.

Reti, Irene (ed.). *Childless by choice: A feminist anthology.* Santa Cruz, CA: HerBooks, 1992.

Rich, Adrienne. *Of woman born: Motherhood as experience and institution.* New York: Norton, 1976.

Information About Abortion Methods

Chalker, Rebecca, and Carol Downer. *A woman's book of choices: Abortion, menstrual extraction, RU-486.* New York: Four Walls, Eight Windows, 1992.

Gardner, Joy. *A difficult decision: A compassionate book about abortion.* Freedom, CA: Crossing Press, 1986; earlier edition was called *Abortion–A personal approach.*
- Both have information about abortant herbs, especially earlier edition.

Raymond, Janice, Renate Klein, and Lynette Dumble. *RU 486: Misconceptions, myths, and morals.* Cambridge, MA: Institute on Women and Technology, 1992.

Different Perspectives on Abortion

Baehr, Ninia. *Abortion without apology: A radical history for the 1990s.* Boston: South End Press, 1990.

Hardacre, Helen. *Marketing the menacing fetus in Japan.* Berkeley: University of California Press, 1997.

McDonnell, Kathleen. *Not an easy choice: A feminist re-examines abortion.* Boston: South End Press, 1984.

Paris, Ginette. *The sacrament of abortion.* Dallas: Spring Publications, 1992.
- Argument that abortion is a sacrifice to our futures.

Index